I0066502

Advanced Research in Pharmacology

Advanced Research in Pharmacology

Edited by Phoenix McWilliams

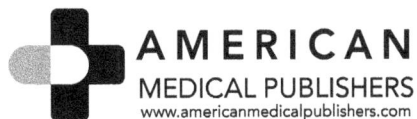

AMERICAN
MEDICAL PUBLISHERS
www.americanmedicalpublishers.com

American Medical Publishers,
41 Flatbush Avenue,
1st Floor, New York,
NY 11217, USA

Visit us on the World Wide Web at:
www.americanmedicalpublishers.com

© American Medical Publishers, 2022

This book contains information obtained from authentic and highly regarded sources. Copyright for all individual chapters remain with the respective authors as indicated. All chapters are published with permission under the Creative Commons Attribution License or equivalent. A wide variety of references are listed. Permission and sources are indicated; for detailed attributions, please refer to the permissions page and list of contributors. Reasonable efforts have been made to publish reliable data and information, but the authors, editors and publisher cannot assume any responsibility for the validity of all materials or the consequences of their use.

ISBN: 978-1-63927-553-3

Trademark Notice: Registered trademark of products or corporate names are used only for explanation and identification without intent to infringe.

Cataloging-in-Publication Data

Advanced research in pharmacology / edited by Phoenix McWilliams.
 p. cm.
Includes bibliographical references and index.
ISBN 978-1-63927-553-3
1. Pharmacology. 2. Drugs. 3. Pharmacy. 4. Chemicals--Physiological effect. I. McWilliams, Phoenix.
RM301 .A28 2022
615.1--dc23

Table of Contents

Preface

The purpose of the book is to provide a glimpse into the dynamics and to present opinions and studies of some of the scientists engaged in the development of new ideas in the field from very different standpoints. This book will prove useful to students and researchers owing to its high content quality.

Pharmacology is a biological discipline that is concerned with the study of a drug or medication action. A drug is a man-made, natural, or endogenous molecule that affects the cell, tissue, organ or organism, biochemically or physiologically. Pharmacology is the study of interactions between a living organism and chemicals that influence the normal and abnormal biochemical function. It blends the study of the drug composition and properties, synthesis and drug design, molecular and cellular mechanisms, molecular diagnostics, interactions, chemical biology and toxicology. Pharmacodynamics and pharmacokinetics are the two main branches of pharmacology that respectively study the effects of a drug on biological systems and the effects of biological systems on the drug. This book presents researches and studies performed by experts across the globe. Also included herein is a detailed explanation of the various concepts and applications of pharmacology. Those in search of information to further their knowledge will be greatly assisted by this book.

At the end, I would like to appreciate all the efforts made by the authors in completing their chapters professionally. I express my deepest gratitude to all of them for contributing to this book by sharing their valuable works. A special thanks to my family and friends for their constant support in this journey.

Editor

The Effects of Lyophilization on the Physico-Chemical Stability of Sirolimus Liposomes

Saeed Ghanbarzadeh[1,2], Hadi Valizadeh[3], Parvin Zakeri-Milani[4]*

[1] Drug Applied Research Center and Faculty of Pharmacy, Tabriz University of Medical Sciences, Tabriz, Iran.

[2] Student Research Committee, Tabriz University of Medical Sciences, Tabriz, Iran.

[3] Research Center for Pharmaceutical Nanotechnology and Faculty of Pharmacy, Tabriz University of Medical Sciences, Tabriz, Iran.

[4] Liver and Gastrointestinal Diseases Research Center and Faculty of Pharmacy, Tabriz University of Medical Sciences, Tabriz, Iran.

ARTICLE INFO

Keywords:
Liposome
Sirolimus
Lyophilization
Stability

ABSTRACT

Purpose: The major limitation in the widespread use of liposome drug delivery system is its instability. Lyophilization is a promising approach to ensure the long-term stability of liposomes. The aim of this study was to prepare sirolimus-loaded liposomes, study their stability and investigate the effect of lyophilization either in the presence or in the absence of lyoprotectant on liposome properties. *Methods:* Two types of multi-lamellar liposomes, conventional and fusogenic, containing sirolimus were prepared by modified thin film hydration method with different ratio of dipalmitoylphosphatidylcholine (DPPC), cholesterol and dioleoylphosphoethanolamine (DOPE), and were lyophilized with or without dextrose as lyoprotectant. Chemical stability investigation was performed at 4°C and 25°C until 6 months using a validated HPLC method. Physical stability was studied with determination of particle size (PS) and encapsulation efficiency (EE %) of formulations through 6 months. *Results:* Chemical stability test at 4°C and 25°C until 6 months showed that drug content of liposomes decreased 8.4% and 20.2% respectively. Initial mean EE % and PS were 72.8 % and 582 nm respectively. After 6 months mean EE % for suspended form, lyophilized without lyoprotectant and lyophilized with lyoprotectant were 54.8 %, 62.3% and 67.1 % at 4°C and 48.2%, 60.4 % and 66.8 % at 25°C respectively. Corresponding data for mean PS were 8229 nm, 2397 nm and 688nm at 4°C and 9362 nm, 1944 nm and 737 nm at 25°C respectively. *Conclusion:* It is concluded that lyophilization with and without dextrose could increase shelf life of liposome and dextrose has lyoprotectant effect that stabilized liposomes in the lyophilization process.

Introduction

Sirolimus (Rapamycin, SRL, Rapamune, $C_{51}H_{79}NO_{13}$, CAS No: 53123-88-9), a carbocyclic lactone-lactam macrolide antibiotic, is anatural fermentation product of the streptomyces hygroscopicus discovered in Rapa Nui (Easter Island). Although initially isolated as an antifungal agent with potent anticandida activity, subsequent studies revealed impressive antitumor and immunosuppressive activities. It binds to the immunophilin FKBP12 and interferes with the function of mTOR, thus blocking the progression from G1 to the S phase of the cell cycle and blockage of the response of T and B cells to cytokines and consequently cell proliferation. Although SRL and Tacrolimus are structural analogs, they have different mechanisms of action. Sirolimus is available in oral solution and tablet form. It is rapidly but poorly absorbed after oral administration with an estimated bioavailability of 15%.[1-8]

Liposomes are artificial vesicles, composed of lipidic amphiphiles, usually phospholipids, which organize themselves in water to form an aqueous core surrounded by a lipidic bilayer. This structure allows liposomes to transport both hydrophilic and lipophilic compounds and have led to their clinical use as drug carriers of several drug classes including antibiotics, antifungals and anticancer agents. Liposomes have a 50-year history of use with numerous applications. Their utility has included toxicity buffering of drugs, targeting to specific tissue sites, enhancement of drug efficacy or potency, dissolution of insoluble drugs and sustained release of drugs.[9-16]

However, its potential application as therapeutic agent is still challenged by its physical and chemical instabilities in aqueous dispersions (e.g., hydrolysis and oxidation of phospholipids, encapsulated solute leakage and liposome aggregation) for long-term storage.

Corresponding author: Parvin Zakeri-Milani, Department of Pharmaceutics, Faculty of Pharmacy, Tabriz University of Medical Sciences, Tabriz, Iran. 51664. E-mail: pzakeri@tbzmed.ac.ir

Liposome dispersions prepared from commercially available lipids do not meet the required standards for long-term stability of pharmaceutical preparations. If they are stored as aqueous dispersions the encapsulated drugs tend to leak out of the bilayer structureand the liposomes might aggregate or fuse on storage and it is generally necessary to use them within the first few months of preparation. Accordingly, many methods available for stabilization of liposome have been investigated, such as lyophilization, freezing, spray-drying and supercritical fluid technology. Among these, lyophilization is the main approach used toextend the shelf-life of liposomes, especially for liposome containing thermo-sensitive drugs. Some liposomal products in the market or in clinical trials are provided as a lyophilized powder.[17-21]

A variety of sugars, including sucrose, glucose, fructose, maltose, arabinose and trehalose have been shown to act as lyoprotectant during dehydration/rehydration of liposomes.[22-26]

In the present study, SRL-entrapped multilamellar liposomes were prepared using the thin film hydration method. Physical stability tests of liposomal formulations of SRL were performed at 4°C and 25°C. Moreover the prepared liposomes were lyophilized to study the effect of lyophilization with and without lyoprotectant and also to investigate the lyoprotectant effect to protect liposomes against fusion and leakage during storage at the same temperatures.

Materials and Methods

Materials

Sirolimus was obtained from Poli Company (Lazio, Italy). Dipalmitoylphosphatidylcholine (DPPC) and dioleoylphosphoethanolamine (DOPE) were purchased from Lipoid GMBH (Ludwigshafen, Germany). Cholesterol (Chol) was obtained from Merck Company (Darmstadt, Germany). All solvents were HPLC grade and all reagents were of analytical grade and were purchased from Merck Company (Darmstadt, Germany).

Liposome preparation

SRL multilamellar liposomal formulations with different molar ratios were prepared using the thin film hydration technique. The lipid components (DPPC and Chol) either alone or mixed with DOPE, in the case of fusogenic liposome, with different molar ratios were dissolved in chloroform:methanol mixture (3:1, % v/v) in a round-bottomed flask. The organic solvents were slowly removed under reduced pressure, using a rotary evaporator (Buchi, Zurich, Switzerland), at 45°C, above gel-liquid crystal transition temperature (Tc) of phospholipids, such that a very thin film of dry lipids was formed on the inner surface of the flask. The dry lipid film was slowly hydrated with 20 ml of phosphate buffered saline (PBS) (pH 7.4) containing SRL 500 μg/ml for 3 hrs in rotary leading to the formation of multi-lamellar liposomes. The resulting suspension was sonicated for 10 min to reduce liposome size.

Chemical stability of SRL

Samples of liposomal formulations in suspension and lyophilized form in 4°C and 25°C were investigated initially and monthly until 6 months using previously developed HPLC method.[27]

Lyophilization of liposomes and subsequent reconstitution

The lyoprotectant (dextrose) was dissolved in phosphate buffered saline at concentration of 10%. Liposomal suspensions in buffer with or without lyoprotectant were freeze-dried (ZIRBUS sublimator 400, ZIRBUS Technology, Bad Grund, Germany) where the liquid was frozen at-195°C. Dehydration step lasted for 2 days at temperature of -40°C until dried powder formed. The resulting lyophilized powderswere rehydrated to its original volume at room temperature with PBS, and following the addition of PBS the samples were equilibrated at room temperature for 30 min. Then the samples were subjected to the following tests.

Physical stability of liposomal formulations

Storage stability of all suspensions and lyophilized formulations was tested at 4°C and 25°C for six months.

Determination of drug content and encapsulation efficiency (EE %) of liposomes

Unentrapped drug was separated using dialysis method at temperature below gel-liquid-crystalline transition temperature (Tc) in sink condition after 24 hrs. Drug content in the liposome dispersion and unentrapped drug were analyzed with RP-HPLC system (Beckman, USA). The as follow: Knauer C18 column (4.6×150mm, 5μm) (Berlin, Germany) was used at 54°C, mobile phase consisting of acetonitril and ammonium acetate buffer (pH5.8)(70:30, % v/v) with flow rate of 1.5 ml/min, detection wavelength was set at 278 nm and injection volume was150μl. A linear response was observed over a concentration range of 125–2000 ng/ml (r^2> 0.991). For all quality control (QC) standards in intraday and interday assay, accuracy and precision ranges were 0.96 to 6.30 and 0.86 to 13.74 respectively, demonstrating the acceptable precision and accuracy over the analytical range.

EE %was calculated by the following equation:[28-32]

$$EE\ (\%) = [(C_{total} - C_{free})/C_{total}] \times 100$$

Where C_{total} is total drug concentration which was added and C_{free} is the concentration of unentrapped drug.

Measurement of particle size distribution of liposome

Mean vesicle size and size distribution profile of liposome was determined using particle size analyzer

(Shimadzu, Japan) which uses laser diffraction method. All sample measurements were conducted in triplicate.

Results and Discussion
Chemical stability of SRL
After six months storage at 4°C and 25°C, drug content of liposomes following disruption of liposome in methanol and after enough dilution was analyzed with RP-HPLC method. Results revealed that SRL content of liposomes after 6 months was 91.6 ± 2.3% at 4°C and 79.8 ±3.6% at 25°C for suspended form. Respective results for lyophilized form at the end of 6 months storage were 92.3 ±1.6% and 81.6±2.7% (Figure 1). Therefore it can be concluded that hydrolysis has small effect in SRL degradation.

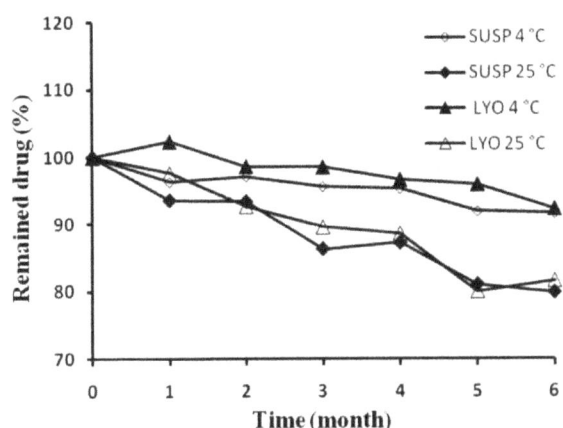

Figure 1. Chemical stability of SRL during 6 months in the suspension and lyophilized form

Physical stability studies
Physical stability study of SRL liposomes was conducted at refrigeration temperature (4°C) and at room temperature (25°C) for a period of 6 months. Drug entrapment of liposomes in suspension and reconstituted liposome was evaluated monthly. The results are demonstrated in Figure 2 in terms of percentage of SRL retained in the liposomes.

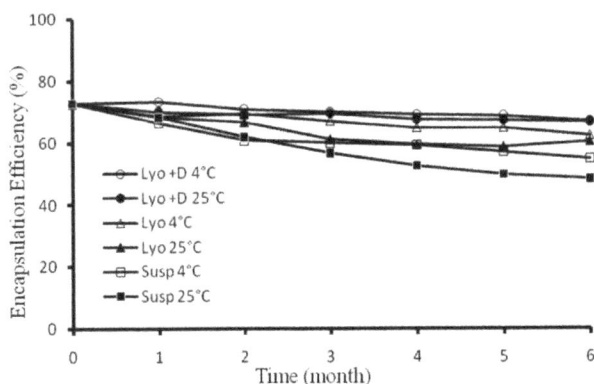

Figure 2. Mean EE % of different forms of multilamellar SRL liposomes stored at 4°C and 25°C

Mean initial EE % for liposomes was 72.8 % and average retained SRL percent in liposomal

formulations after 6 months were 54.8 %, 62.3 % and 67.1 % for suspended form, lyophilized without lyoprotectant and lyophilized with dextrose (Lyo + D) respectively. The retained drug in formulations after 6 months storage at 25°C was 48.2 %, 60.4 % and 66.8 % respectively (Figure 2).

Lyophilization increases the shelf-life of liposomal formulation and preserves it in dried form as a lyophilized cake to be reconstituted with water prior to administration. To maintain the same particle size distribution after lyophilization- rehydration cycle, a lyoprotectant needs to be added. Since the process of lyophilization is harmful for the liposome integrity, an obvious decrease in the encapsulation efficiency is seen for lyophilized formulations. In fact freeze-drying leads to destroy the membrane function of the phospholipid bilayer. In the present study we have used dextrose as protecting agent. It is well-known that sugars can be applied to prevent aggregation of nanoparticles during drying and storage. A literature review reveals that in previous studies various sugars were investigated for their ability to protect liposomes against fusion and leakage during lyophilization process. Glavas-Dodov et al, showed that particle size, EE % and release profile did not differ significantly after lyophilization with saccharose.[33] However, in this study dextrose showed protective effect for SRL liposomes. This protective ability can extend both prevention of vesicle fusion and retention of encapsulated drug within the liposome. The protective effect during liposome lyophilization is mainly determined by the formulation factors, such as the nature of the drug, the lipid bilayer composition, and the choice of lyoprotectants. The stabilization property of sugars has been explained by the particle isolation theory, water replacement hypothesis and vitrification theory.[34-38] Liposomes with lyoprotectant showed better stability, as indicated by higher drug retention. Suspended form liposomes had the less stability. Initial mean particle size of liposomes was 582 nm, which after 6 months storage at 4°C were increased up to 8229 nm, 2397 nm and 688 nm for suspended form, lyophilized without lyoprotectant and lyophilized with dextrose respectively. However in storage at 25°C particle sizes were increased more significantly up to 9362 nm, 1944 nm and 737 nm respectively (Figure 3). Considering 0.01 as significance level, only difference in particle size for formulation lyophilized with dextrose and stored at 4°C wasn't significant (P=0.026) and in all other formulations differences were significant (P<0.005).

As mentioned before more SRL retained in liposomes in lyophilized formulations compared to suspension form, but with using dextrose for lyophilization of multi-lamellar liposomes, EE % was higher. The leakage of entrapped SRL could be explained by the fact that in the suspension form, lyophilization and rehydration of a liposomal suspension can result in leakage of internal aqueous contents. Whereas, with using dextrose as a lyoprotectant and in the absence of protective agent, the amount of entrapped SRL didn't decrease significantly (P> 0.15).

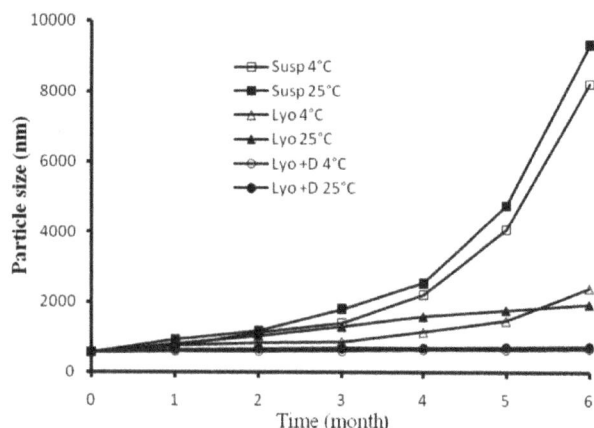

Figure 3. Mean particle size of different forms of multilamellar SRL liposomes stored at 4°C and 25°C.

Conclusion

Instabilities of liposomes during storage are a serious limiting factor for their applicability as drug delivery systems. Lyophilization is a commonly used drying technique for thermolabile pharmaceuticals and also various studies have demonstrated that lyophilization is an effective way to overcome the instability problems of liposomes in the aqueous state. The present work focuses on physicochemical characterization of lyophilized SRL loaded multi-lamellar liposomes and short-term storage stability studies of formulation. The process of lyophilization is often used to prepare pharmaceutical formulations to achieve commercially practicable shelf life and easy handling (shipping and storage). It is important to have a product of a desirable quality and maintain physicochemical characteristics of formulation during storage. It was observed that there was no significant change in drug content at 4°C and 25°C storage conditions for 6 months in lyophilized liposomes with and without dextrose as lyoprotectant (P>015) but decreasing drug content in suspension forms was significant at both 4°C and 25°C (P=0.009 and P=0.005 respectively). Whereas significant increase (P<0.005) in size were observed at the same temperatures over 6 months of storage in all formulations except lyophilized form with lyoprotectant (P=0.026). Taken together, studies showed superior stability of the lyophilized product after reconstitution in comparison with those of the suspension product, and physico-chemical stability of products which have dextrose was most superior. Then we could conclude that lyophilization with and without dextrose could increase shelf life of liposome and glucose has lyoprotectant effect that stabilized liposomes in the lyophilization process. Overall, studies on the optimization of formulation and technological parameters to improve the lyoprotective effect are still required for improving liposome lyophilization.

Acknowledgements

The authors would like to thank the authorities of Research Center for Pharmaceutical Nanotechnology, Tabriz University of Medical Sciences, for financial support. This article is based on a thesis submitted for PhD degree (No. 54) in Faculty of Pharmacy, Tabriz University of Medical Sciences, Tabriz, Iran.

Conflict of interest

The authors report no conflicts of interest.

References

1. Bargnoux AS, Bonardet A, Chong G, Garrigue V, Deleuze S, Dupuy AM, et al. Evaluation of an immunoassay (abbott-imx analyzer) allowing routine determination of sirolimus: Comparison with lc-ms method. *Transplant Proc* 2006;38(7):2352-3.

2. Campanero M, Cardenas E, Sadaba B, Garca Quetglas E, Muaoz-Juarez M, Gil-Aldea I, et al. Therapeutic drug monitoring for sirolimus in whole blood of organ transplants by high-performance liquid chromatography with ultraviolet detection. *J Chromatogr* 2004;1031(1-2):265-73.

3. Holt DW, Lee T, Johnston A. Measurement of sirolimus in whole blood using high-performance liquid chromatography with ultraviolet detection. *Clin Ther* 2000; 22 Suppl B:B38-48.

3. Holt DW, Lee T, Johnston A. Measurement of sirolimus in whole blood using high-performance liquid chromatography with ultraviolet detection. *Clin Ther* 2000;22 Suppl B:B38-48.

4. Ong ATL, van Domburg RT, Aoki J, Sonnenschein K, Lemos PA, Serruys PW. Sirolimus-eluting stents remain superior to bare-metal stents at two years: Medium-term results from the rapamycin-eluting stent evaluated at rotterdam cardiology hospital (research) registry. *J Am Coll Cardiol* 2006;47(7):1356-60.

5. Park D, Kim Y, Yun S, Kang S, Lee S, Lee C, et al. Comparison of zotarolimus-eluting stents with sirolimus- and paclitaxel-eluting stents for coronary revascularization: The zest (comparison of the efficacy and safety of zotarolimus-eluting stent with sirolimus-eluting and paclitaxel-eluting stent for coronary lesions) randomized trial. *J Am Coll Cardiol* 2010;56(15):1187-95.

6. Song Y, Hahn J, Choi S, Choi J, Lee S, Jeong M, et al. Sirolimus- versus paclitaxel-eluting stents for the treatment of coronary bifurcations: Results from the cobis (coronary bifurcation stenting) registry. *J Am Coll Cardiol* 2011;55(16):1743-50.

7. Sakurai R, Inajima T, Kaneda H, Nagai R, Hashimoto H. Sirolimus-eluting stents reduce long-term mortality compared with bare metal stents in st-segment elevation myocardial infarction: A meta-analysis of randomized controlled trials. *Int J Cardiol* 2012:In Press, doi: 10.1016/j.ijcard.2011.12.054.

8. Moeller S, Kegler R, Sternberg K, Mundkowski RG. Influence of sirolimus-loaded nanoparticles on physiological functions of native human polymorphonuclear neutrophils. *Nanomed Nanotechnol Biol Med* 2012;8(8):1293-300.

9. Agashe H, Lagisetty P, Awasthi S, Awasthi V. Improved formulation of liposome-encapsulated hemoglobin with an anionic non-phospholipid. *Colloids Surf B Biointerfaces* 2011;75(2):573-83.

10. Chang C, Liu D, Lin S, Liang H, Hou W, Huang W, et al. Liposome encapsulation reduces cantharidin toxicity. *Food Chem Toxicol* 2008;46(9):3116-21.

11. da Silva Malheiros P, Daroit DJ, da Silveira N, Brandelli A. Effect of nanovesicle-encapsulated nisin on growth of listeria monocytogenes in milk. *Food Microbiol* 2011;27(1):175-8.

12. Fallon MS, Chauhan A. Sequestration of amitriptyline by liposomes. *J Colloid Interface Sci* 2006;300(1):7-19.

13. Fillion P, Desjardins A, Sayasith K. Encapsulation of DNA in negatively charged liposomes and inhibition of bacterial gene expression with fluid liposome-encapsulated antisense oligonucleotides. *Biochim Biophys Acta* 2001;1515(1):44-54.

14. Franz-Montan M, Silva ALR, Fraceto LF, Volpato MC, Paula Ed, Ranali J, et al. Liposomal encapsulation improves the duration of soft tissue anesthesia but does not induce pulpal anesthesia. *J Clin Anesth* 2011;22(5):313-7.

15. Fresta M, Villari A, Puglisi G, Cavallaro G. 5-fluorouracil: Various kinds of loaded liposomes: Encapsulation efficiency, storage stability and fusogenic properties. *Int J Pharm* 1993;99(2-3):145-56.

16. Gabizon A, Shmeeda H, Horowitz AT, Zalipsky S. Tumor cell targeting of liposome-entrapped drugs with phospholipid-anchored folic acid-peg conjugates. *Adv Drug Del Rev* 2004;56(8):1177-92.

17. Arnold K, Okhi S, Krumbiegel M. Interaction of dextran sulfate with phospholipid surfaces and liposome aggregation and fusion. *Chem Phys Lipids* 1990;55(3):301-7.

18. Comiskey SJ, Heath TD. Leakage and delivery of liposome-encapsulated methotrexate-aspartate in a chemically defined medium. *Biochim Biophys Acta* 1990;1024(2):307-17.

19. SanAnna V, Malheiros P, Brandelli A. Liposome encapsulation protects bacteriocin-like substance p34 against inhibition by maillard reaction products. *Food Res Int* 2011;44(1):326-30.

20. Chen C, Han D, Cai C, Tang X. An overview of liposome lyophilization and its future potential. *J Controlled Release* 2010;142(3):299-311.

21. Suakowski WW, Pentak D, Nowak K, Sua KA. The influence of temperature, cholesterol content and pH on liposome stability. *J Mol Struct* 2005;744:737-47.

22. Sundaramurthi P, Suryanarayanan R. Calorimetry and complementary techniques to characterize frozen and freeze-dried systems. *Adv Drug Del Rev* 2012;64(5):384-95.

23. Abdelwahed W, Degobert G, Stainmesse S, Fessi H. Freeze-drying of nanoparticles: Formulation, process and storage considerations. *Adv Drug Del Rev* 2006;58(15):1688-713.

24. Wang W. Lyophilization and development of solid protein pharmaceuticals. *Int J Pharm* 2000;203(1-2):1-60.

25. Konan YN, Gurny R, Allamann E. Preparation and characterization of sterile and freeze-dried sub-200 nm nanoparticles. *Int J Pharm* 2002;233(1-2):239-52.

26. Wolf M, Wirth M, Pittner F, Gabor F. Stabilisation and determination of the biological activity of l-asparaginase in poly(d,l-lactide-co-glycolide) nanospheres. *Int J Pharm* 2003;256(1-2):141-52.

27. Islambulchilar Z, Ghanbarzadeh S, Emami S, Valizadeh H, Zakeri-Milani P. Development and validation of an hplc method for the analysis of sirolimus in drug products. *Adv Pharm Bull* 2012;2(2):135-9.

28. Nii T, Ishii F. Encapsulation efficiency of water-soluble and insoluble drugs in liposomes prepared by the microencapsulation vesicle method. *Int J Pharm* 2005;298(1):198-205.

29. Piel G, Piette M, Barillaro V, Castagne D, Evrard B, Delattre L. Betamethasone-in-cyclodextrin-in-liposome: The effect of cyclodextrins on encapsulation efficiency and release kinetics. *Int J Pharm* 2006;312(1-2):75-82.

30. Sanchez-Lapez V, Fernandez-Romero JM, Gamez-Hens A. Evaluation of liposome populations using a sucrose density gradient centrifugation approach coupled to a continuous flow system. *Anal Chim Acta* 2009;645(1-2):79-85.

31. Yuba E, Kojima C, Harada A, Tana G, Watarai S, Kono K. Ph-sensitive fusogenic polymer-modified liposomes as a carrier of antigenic proteins for activation of cellular immunity. *Biomaterials* 2010;31(5):943-51.

32. Modi S, Xiang T, Anderson BD. Enhanced active liposomal loading of a poorly soluble ionizable drug using supersaturated drug solutions. *J Controlled Release* 2012;162(2):330-9.

33. Glavas-Dodov M, Fredro-Kumbaradzi E, Goracinova K, Simonoska M, Calis S, Trajkovic-Jolevska S, et al. The effects of lyophilization on the stability of liposomes containing 5-fu. *Int J Pharm* 2005;291(1-2):79-86.

34. Kuo JHS, Hwang R. Preparation of DNA dry powder for non-viral gene delivery by spray-freeze drying: Effect of protective agents (polyethyleneimine and sugars) on the stability of DNA. *J Pharm Pharmacol* 2004;56(1):27-33.

35. Hinrichs WLJ, Sanders NN, De Smedt SC, Demeester J, Frijlink HW. Inulin is a promising cryo- and lyoprotectant for pegylated lipoplexes. *J Controlled Release* 2005;103(2):465-79.

36. Sun WQ, Leopold AC, Crowe LM, Crowe JH. Stability of dry liposomes in sugar glasses. *Biophys J* 1996;70(4):1769-76.

37. Van Winden ECA, Crommelin DJA. Long term stability of freeze-dried, lyoprotected doxorubicin liposomes. *Eur J Pharm Biopharm* 1997;43(3):295-307.

38. Komatsu H, Saito H, Okada S, Tanaka M, Egashira M, Handa T. Effects of the acyl chain composition of phosphatidylcholines on the stability of freeze-dried small liposomes in the presence of maltose. *Chem Phys Lipids* 2001;113(1-2):29-39.

Cytoprotective Effects of Organosulfur Compounds against Methimazole-Induced Toxicity in Isolated Rat Hepatocytes

Reza Heidari[1,2,3], Hossein Babaei[1,2], Mohammad Ali Eghbal[1,2]*

[1] Drug Applied Research Center, Tabriz University of Medical Sciences, Tabriz, Iran.

[2] Pharmacology and toxicology department, School of pharmacy, Tabriz University of Medical Sciences, Tabriz, Iran.

[3] Students' Research Committee, Tabriz University of Medical Sciences, Tabriz, Iran.

ARTICLE INFO

Keywords:
Isolated hepatocytes
Methimazole
Mitochondria
N-methylthiourea
Organosulfurs
Protein carbonylation

ABSTRACT

Purpose: Methimazole is a drug widely used in hyperthyroidism. However, life-threatening hepatotoxicity has been associated with its clinical use. No protective agent has been found to be effective against methimazole-induced hepatotoxicity yet. Hence, the capacity of organosulfur compounds to protect rat hepatocytes against cytotoxic effects of methimazole and its proposed toxic metabolite, N-methylthiourea was evaluated. *Methods:* Hepatocytes were prepared by the method of collagenase enzyme perfusion via portal vein. Cells were treated with different concentrations of methimazole, N-methylthiourea, and organosulfur chemicals. Cell death, protein carbonylation, reactive oxygen species formation, lipid peroxidation, and mitochondrial depolarization were assessed as toxicity markers and the role of organosulfurs administration on them was investigated. *Results:* Methimazole caused a decrease in cellular glutathione content, mitochondrial membrane potential ($\Delta\Psi$m) collapse, and protein carbonylation. In addition, an increase in reactive oxygen species (ROS) formation and lipid peroxidation was observed. Treating hepatocytes with N-methylthiourea caused a reduction in hepatocytes glutathione reservoirs and an elevation in carbonylated proteins, but no significant ROS formation, lipid peroxidation, or mitochondrial depolarization was observed. N-acetyl cysteine, allylmercaptan, and diallyldisulfide attenuated cell death and prevented ROS formation and lipid peroxidation caused by methimazole. Furthermore, organosulfur compounds diminished methimazole-induced mitochondrial damage and reduced the carbonylated proteins. In addition, these chemicals showed protective effects against cell death and protein carbonylation induced by methimazole metabolite. *Conclusion:* Organosulfur chemicals extend their protective effects against methimazole-induced toxicity by attenuating oxidative stress caused by this drug and preventing the adverse effects of methimazole and/or its metabolite (s) on subcellular components such as mitochondria.

Introduction

Methimazole is one of the most effective drugs in managing hyperthyroidism in humans.[1] However, serious adverse effects such as hepatotoxicity and agranulocytosis accompany its clinical use.[2,3] The mechanism(s) by which methimazole induces hepatotoxicity is not clearly understood yet and no protective agent has been found to be effective against its toxicity. In some investigations, it has been shown that reactive metabolites formed during methimazole metabolism could be the cause of cellular damage and toxicity. It was found that a kind of cytochrome P450 enzyme might be responsible for biotransformation of methimazole to its reactive metabolite that could be involved in cellular damage caused by this drug in olfactory mucosa.[4,5] N-methylthiourea is one of the methimazole metabolites which is generated by

cytochrome P450 enzymes and is suspected to be responsible for methimazole-induced hepatotoxicity.[6] N-methylthiourea is further metabolized to some reactive nucleophilic metabolites,[6] which are capable of binding to different cellular targets,[7] and causing cell dysfunction and toxicity. In another study, we have shown that methimazole cytotoxicity towards hepatocytes could be attributed to its reactive intermediates.[8]

Reactive metabolites interact with many cellular targets, especially proteins, and affect cell function. These events could result in toxicity and finally cell death. Glutathione is a thiol containing molecule that conjugate with electrophilic reactive intermediates of xenobiotics and prevent cellular damage.[9] In some experiments, it has been shown that glutathione had a

*Corresponding author: Mohammad Ali Eghbal, Faculty of pharmacy, Pharmacology and toxicology department, Tabriz University of Medical Sciences, Tabriz, Iran. E-mail: m.a.eghbal@hotmail.com

pivotal role in preventing methimazole-induced toxicity and this drug caused a severe hepatic injury in mice depleted of glutathione.[10] Depleting glutathione reservoirs had the same effects on the toxicity induced by methimazole in mice olfactory mucosa.[5] In another study, it was shown that methimazole inhibited some forms of CYP450 enzymes in the absence of glutathione, probably by its reactive metabolites.[11] 2-propen-1-thiol (Allyl mercaptan), and Diallyl disulfide, are small sulfur containing molecules derived from *Allium sativum* (garlic).[12] These compounds in contribution with other molecules are responsible for garlic odor and have been formed in breath after garlic ingestion.[12,13] It has been shown that organosulfurs had protective properties against xenobiotics-promoted cellular damage and oxidative stress in many cases such as carbon tetrachloride (CCl_4),[14] acetaminophen,[15,16] doxorubicin,[17,18] cyclophosphamide,[19] and aflatoxin B_1.[20] Another organosulfur chemical, N-acetylcysteine (NAC) has found its role in clinic and is used as a standard treatment in drugs-induced hepatotoxicity such as acetaminophen intoxication in humans.[21]

Because of their protective roles observed in previous investigations and their capability in scavenging reactive species,[22,23] this study attempted to evaluate the beneficial effects of organosulfur chemicals against methimazole-induced cellular injury in an *in vitro* model of isolated rat hepatocytes. Cell death, reactive oxygen species (ROS) formation, lipid peroxidation, protein carbonylation, and mitochondrial damage were considered as toxicity markers and the effects of organosulfur compounds on them were studied. Furthermore, the levels of cellular reduced and oxidized glutathione were measured to evaluate the ability of organosulfur compounds in preventing methimazole-induced hepatotoxicity.

Materials and Methods
Chemicals
Methimazole was purchased from Medisca pharmaceutique incorporation (Montreal, Canada). N-acetyl cysteine (NAC), 2-vinyl pyridine, Triethanolamine, Tris (hydroxymethyl) aminomethane, Oxidized glutathione (GSSG), and (4-(2-hydroxyethyl) 1-piperazine-ethanessulfonic acid (HEPES) were obtained from Acros (New Jersey, USA). Albumine bovine type was purchased from Roche diagnostic corporation (Indianapolis USA). 2-propen-1thiol (Allyl mercaptan), Diallyl disulfide (DADS), Rhodamine 123, 5,5'-dithio-bis(2-nitro-benzoicacid)(DTNB), 2,4-Dinitrophenyl hydrazine (DNPH), Guanidine, 2',7'Dichlorofluorescin diacetate, Glutathione reductase from baker's yeast, β-Nicotinamide adenine dinucleotide (NADPH), and Collagenase from clostridium histolyticum, were obtained from Sigma Aldrich (St. Louis, USA). Reduced glutathione (GSH), N-methylthiourea, Trichloro acetic acid (TCA), Ethyleneglycol-bis (ρ-aminoethylether)-N,N,N',N'-tetra

acetic acid (EGTA), and Trypan blue were obtained from Merck (Darmstadt, Germany). Thiobarbituric acid (TBA) was obtained from SERVA (Heidenberg, New York). All salts used for preparing buffer solutions were of analytical grade and obtained from Merck (Darmstadt, Germany).

Hepatocyte preparation
Male Sprague–Dawley rats weighing 250–300 g were cared in plastic cages in an ambient temperature of 25 ± 3 °C. Animals were fed a normal diet and water *ad libitum*. Collagenase perfusion method was used to isolate rat hepatocytes.[24] This technique is based on liver perfusion with collagenase after removal of calcium ion (Ca^{2+}) with a chelator (EGTA 0.5 mM). Liver was perfused with different buffer solutions through the portal vein. Collagenase containing buffer solution destructs liver interstitial tissue and cause hepatocyte to be easily isolated in next steps. Isolated hepatocytes (10 mL, 10^6 cells/mL) were incubated in Krebs-Henseleit buffer (pH 7.4) under an atmosphere of 95% O_2 and 5% CO_2, in 50 ml round bottom flasks which continuously rotating into a 37 °C water bath. Any of chemicals used for evaluating their protective effects, caused no significant toxicity toward hepatocytes as compared to the control cells when administered alone in given concentrations. The animals were handled and used, according the ethical guidelines of Tabriz University of Medical Sciences, Tabriz, Iran.

Cell viability
Trypan blue dye exclusion staining was used to assess the percentage of death cells.[25] Hepatocytes viability was determined at different time intervals to evaluate the effect of methimazole and N-methylthiourea on cell viability, determining LC_{50} (lethal concentration 50%) dose of the drugs and testing the protective effects of organosulfur compounds against cell death induced by methimazole or N-methylthiourea. Hepatocytes were at least 85% viable before their use.

Reactive oxygen species (ROS) formation
To control the extent of ROS formed during methimazole metabolism, 2, 7-dichlorofluorescein diacetate (1.6 µM) was added to the hepatocyte incubate. DCFH-DA became hydrolyzed to non-fluorescent dichlorofluorescein (DCFH) in hepatocytes. Dichlorofluorescin then reacted with reactive oxygen species to form the highly fluorescent dichlorofluorescein. 1mL (10^6 cells) of hepatocytes was taken and the fluorescence intensity was measured using a Jasco® FP-750 spectrofluorometer with excitation and emission wavelengths of 500 and 520 nm, respectively.[26]

Lipid peroxidation Measurement
Hepatocyte lipid peroxidation was determined by measuring the amount of thiobarbituric acid reactive

substances (TBARS) formed during the decomposition of lipid hydroperoxides. After treating 1mL aliquots of hepatocyte suspension (10^6 cells/mL) with trichloroacetic acid (70%w/v), the supernatant was boiled with thiobarbituric acid (0.8% w/v) for 20 minutes. The absorbance of appeared color was determined using an Ultrospec® 2000 UV spectrophotometer at 532 nm.[27]

Protein carbonylation assay

Total protein-bound carbonyl content was measured by derivatizing the carbonyl adducts with DNPH at 30, 90, and 180 minutes. Briefly an aliquot of the suspension of cells (0.5 mL, 0.5×10^6 cells) was added to 0.5 mL of 0.1% DNPH (w/v) in 2.0 N HCl and allowed to incubate for 1 hour at room temperature. This reaction was stopped and total cellular protein precipitated by adding 1.0 mL of 20% TCA (w/v). Cellular protein was rapidly pelleted by centrifugation at 10,000 rpm, and the supernatant was discarded. Excess unincorporated DNPH was extracted three times using 0.5 mL of ethanol: ethyl acetate (1:1) solution each time. Following the extraction, the recovered cellular protein was solubilized in 1 mL of Tris-buffered 8.0 M guanidine–HCl, pH 7.2. The resulting solubilized hydrazones were measured at 366–370 nm. The concentration of 2,4-DNPH derivatized protein carbonyls was determined using the extinction coefficient of 22,000 M^{-1} cm^{-1}.[28]

Mitochondrial membrane potential

Mitochondrial membrane potential was assessed as an indicator of toxicity induced by methimazole or N-methylthiourea. The fluorescent dye, rhodamine 123 was used as a probe to evaluate the mitochondrial membrane potential in rat hepatocytes. Samples (1 mL) were taken from the cell suspension at scheduled time points, and centrifuged at 1000 rpm for 1 minute. The cell pellet was then resuspended in 2 mL of fresh incubation medium containing 1.5 µM rhodamine 123 and gently shaked in a 37 °C thermostatic water bath for 10 minutes. Hepatocytes were separated by centrifugation (3000 rpm for one minute) and the amount of rhodamine 123 appearing in the incubation medium was measured fluorimeterically at 490 nm excitation and 520 nm emission wavelengths using a Jasco® FP-750 spectrofluorometer.[29]

Determination of Hepatocytes GSH/GSSG content

Hepatocytes reduced and oxidized glutathione (GSH and GSSG) content was determined using enzymatic recycling method.[30] For determination of GSH, a 1 ml aliquot of the cell suspension (10^6 cells) was taken and 2 ml of 5% TCA was added and centrifuged. Then 0.5 ml of Ellman's reagent (0.0198% DTNB in 1% sodium citrate) and 3 ml of phosphate buffer (pH 8.0) were added. The absorbance of developed color was determined at 412 nm using an Ultrospec® 2000 spectrophotometer. To assess the hepatocytes GSSG

level, cellular GSH content was covalently bonded to 2-vinylpyridine at first. Then the excess of 2-vinylpyridine was neutralized with thriethanolamine and GSSG was reduced to GSH using glutathione reductase enzyme and NADPH. The amount of GSH formed was measured as described for GSH using Ellman reagent (0.0198% DTNB in 1% sodium citrate).[30]

Statistical analysis

Results are given as the Means±SE for at least three independent experiments. Statistical analysis was performed by a one-way analysis of variance (ANOVA) followed by a Tukey's *post hoc* test (SPSS software; version 16.0). A P< 0.05 was considered as significant difference.

Results

Trypan blue exclusion test was used to determine the ability of hepatocytes to maintain their viability with different concentrations of methimazole or N-methylthiourea, alone or in combination with organosulfur compounds. It was previously found that methimazole caused cell death in a concentration dependent manner.[8] The concentration in which the drug caused 50 % loss in hepatocytes viability (LC_{50}) was found to be 10 mM (Table 1).[8] The LC_{50} for the methimazole metabolite, N-methylthiourea was 1 mM (Table 1).[8] To determine the effects of organosulfur compounds on cell death induced by methimazole and/or N-methylthiourea, Diallyl disulfide (DADS), Allyl mercaptan, and N-acetyl cysteine were added to incubation medium. For this purpose, the LC_{50} of methimazole (10 mM) and N-methylthiourea (1 mM) were selected.

It was found that NAC and the other two organosulfur agents, Allyl mercaptan, and/or DADS decreased cell death induced by methimazole or N-methylthiourea (Table 1) (P<0.05). In another study on methimazole cytotoxicity, we found that depleting glutathione reservoirs by using 1-bromoheptane[31] had a deleterious effect on methimazole and/or N-methylthiourea-induced cytotoxicity.[8] Only 5 µM methimazole was needed to cause 50% cell death in glutathione depleted cells (data not shown) and all glutathione depleted hepatocytes were dead when 1 mM of N-methylthiourea was added to the cellular media (data not given).[8] These findings suggest the pivotal role of glutathione in preventing methimazole-induced cytotoxicity. N-acetyl cysteine effectively prevented cell death in glutathione-depleted hepatocytes (data not shown).[8]

Since glutathione depletion had a dramatic effect on cell death induced by methimazole and its metabolite, cellular glutathione content was measured to further investigate if methimazole or N-methylhiourea toxicity is related to GSH reduction in hepatocytes. The results showed that hepatocytes glutathione reservoirs were decreased significantly (P<0.01) when cells were treated with methimazole and/or N-methylthiourea (Figure 1).[8] As previously showed in another study on methimazole,[8] this might indicate the importance of this thiol containing molecule to detoxify methimazole metabolites and preventing cellular damage induced by this drug. The presence of DADS in cellular media prevented glutathione (GSH) depletion induced by methimazole or its metabolite ($P<0.05$) (Figure 1). The amount of oxidized glutathione (GSSG) was elevated in hepatocytes treated with methimazole ($P<0.01$) (Figure 2), but there was no significant difference in

GSSG content between N-methylthiourea-treated cells and control group (Figure 2). Addition of 100 µM of DADS to cellular medium reduced ($P<0.0.05$) the amount of GSSG formed during methimazole administration (Figure 2). Elevation in oxidized glutathione in cells during chemical exposure is an indicator of the reactive oxygen species formation and occurrence of oxidative stress during toxic insult. Hence, the amount of ROS formation was evaluated to assess if methimazole or N-methylthiourea caused oxidative stress in isolated rat hepatocytes.[8]

Table 1. Methimazole and N-methylthiourea cytotoxicity in freshly-isolated rat hepatocytes.

	Cytotoxicity (% Trypan blue uptake)		
Incubation time (min):	60	120	180
Incubate			
Control (only hepatocytes)	20±2	25±2	29±2
+ Methimazole 10 mM	43±2 [a]	55±3 [a]	68±4 [a]
+ N-acetyl cysteine 200 µM	23±3 [b]	32±2 [b]	35±3 [b]
+ Diallyldisulfide 100 µM	28±2 [b]	39±3 [b]	46±2 [b]
+ Allylmercaptan 200 µM	24±1 [b]	33±2 [b]	43±2 [b]
+ N-methyl thiourea 500 µM	29±4	38±5	54±3 [a]
+ N-methyl thiourea 1 mM	39±2 [a]	54±1 [a]	65±3 [a]
+ N-acetyl cysteine 200 µM	24±1 [c]	28±2 [c]	33±2 [c]
+ Diallyldisulfide 100 µM	28±2 [c]	39±3 [c]	58±1
+ Allylmercaptan 200 µM	23±1 [c]	40±2 [c]	44±3 [c]
+ N-methyl thiourea 2 mM	48±3 [a]	59±4 [a]	75±7 [a]

Isolated rat hepatocytes (10^6 cells/mL) were incubated at 37 °C in rotating round bottom flasks with 95 % O_2 and 5 % CO_2 in Krebs-Henseleit buffer (pH 7.4).
The results shown represent the Mean± SE for three independent experiments.
[a] Significantly different from control group ($P < 0.05$).
[b] Significant as compared to methimazole-treated group ($P<0.05$).
[c] Significantly different from N-methylthiourea treated group ($P<0.05$).

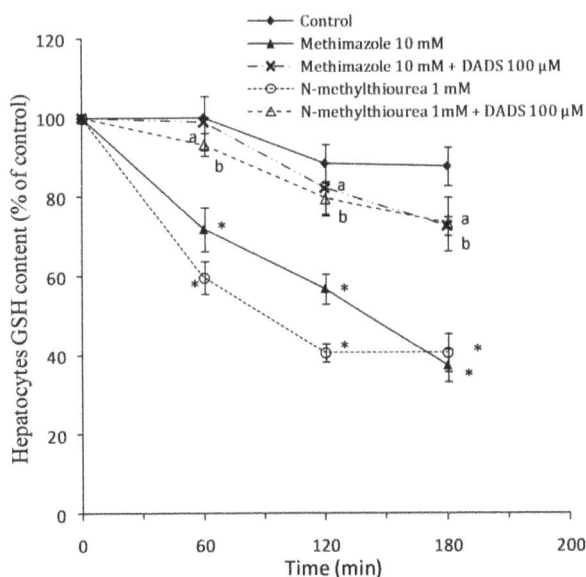

Figure 1. The effect of methimazole on hepatocytes GSH content. DADS: Diallyldisulfide.
Given data represent Means±SE for at least three separate experiments.
* Significantly different from control group ($P<0.01$).
[a] Significantly different from methimazole-treated group ($P<0.05$).

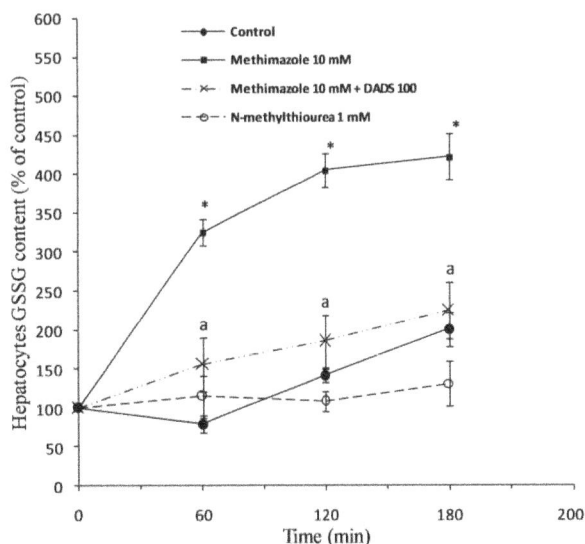

Figure 2. The level of oxidized glutathione (GSSG) formed after methimazole and N-methylthiourea. DADS: diallyldisulfide.
* Significantly different from control group ($P<0.01$).
[a] Significantly different from methimazole-treated group ($P<0.05$).

Treating rat hepatocytes with methimazole caused a significant elevation in reactive oxygen species formation (P<0.001) (Figure 3).[8] N-methylthiourea-treated hepatocytes showed no difference in ROS formation as compared to the control group (Figure 3).[8] Administration of organosulfur chemicals decreased ROS formation (P<0.05) induced by methimazole (Figure 3).

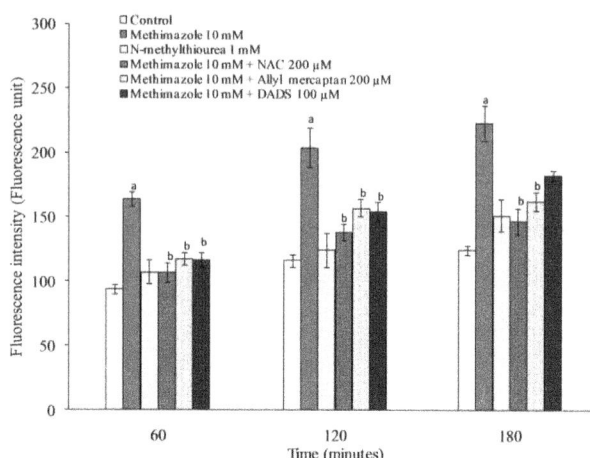

Figure 3. Methimazole-induced ROS formation in rat hepatocytes and the role of organosulfur compounds. DADS: Diallyl disulfide. NAC: N-acetylcysteine.
Data represent Mean±SE for three experiments.
[a] Significantly different from control group (P<0.001).
[b] Significantly different from methimazole-treated group (P<0.05).

Lipid peroxidation is a consequence of ROS formation and oxidative stress in biological systems.[32] It was found that a remarkable amount of thiobarbituric acid reactive substances (TBARS) was formed in methimazole-treated rat hepatocytes (P<0.001) as compared to the control group (Figure 4). This indicated the lipid peroxidation induced by cytotoxic concentrations of the drug. N-methylthiourea did not cause lipid peroxidation in rat hepatocytes.[8] Co-administration of NAC,[8] and/or other organosulfur chemicals considerably prevented (P<0.01) lipid peroxidation caused by methimazole (Figure 4).

The formation of carbonyl compounds is the most general and widely used marker of protein oxidation both *in vitro* and *in vivo*.[33] It was found that; protein carbonylation induced by methimazole was significantly higher (P<0.001) than the control level (Figure 5). Co-administration of organosulfur compounds reduced the level of protein carbonylation in methimazole-treated cells. The methimazole metabolite, N-methylthiourea caused an increase in carbonylated proteins (P<0.001) (Figure 5), which was significantly diminished (P<0.01) when organosulfur chemicals were added to hepatocytes incubation medium (Figure 5).

The changes in mitochondrial membrane potential (ΔΨ) as an important parameter of mitochondrial function were assessed previously to investigate if

cellular mitochondria are a target for methimazole and/or its metabolite.[8] The LC$_{50}$ dose of methimazole (10 mM) caused mitochondrial depolarization (P<0.05) as measured with rhodamine 123 test (Figure 6).[8] This indicates that mitochondria could be a target for methimazole or its reactive metabolite(s) to cause hepatocyte damage and consequently cell death. However, N-methylthiourea did not cause any significant reduction in mitochondrial membrane potential (Figure 6).[8] This finding suggested that other methimazole metabolite(s) rather than N-methylthiourea might be responsible for the adverse effect of methimazole on mitochondria.[8] Organosulfur compounds were administered with methimazole to investigate if they could alleviate mitochondrial injury induced by this drug. It was found that NAC, Allyl mercaptan, and DADS effectively prevented mitochondrial depolarization (P<0.05) caused by methimazole (Figure 6).

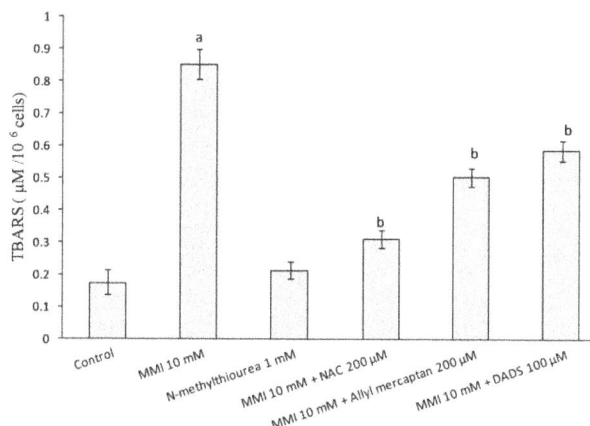

Figure 4. Methimazole-induced lipid peroxidation and the effect of organosulfur compounds. MMI: Methimazole (Methyl Mercapto Imidazole)
Data are shown as Mean±SE for three experiments as measured after 120 minutes.
[a] Significant as compared to control (P<0.001).
[b] Significant as compared to methimazole-treated group (P<0.01).

Discussion
Methimazole alone caused cell death in a concentration dependent manner. Methimazole-induced cytotoxicity was accompanied with ROS formation, lipid peroxidation, mitochondrial depolarization, and protein carbonylation. Furthermore, reduction in cellular glutathione (GSH) reservoirs, and increased hepatocytes' oxidized glutathione (GSSG) content was observed when hepatocytes were treated with methimazole. The suspected methimazole toxic metabolite, N-methylthiourea caused cell death concentration-dependently and reduced cellular glutathione content. In addition, a significant amount of carbonylated proteins was formed in N-methylthiourea treated hepatocytes, but no ROS formation, lipid peroxidation or changes in mitochondrial membrane potential were observed. Co-administration of organosulfur compounds diminished cell death induced

by methimazole or N-methylthiourea and reduced the consequences of methimazole induced toxicity such as ROS formation, lipid peroxidation, and mitochondrial damage.

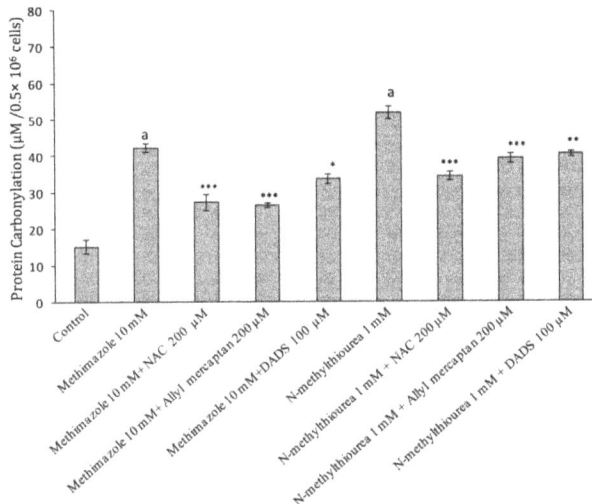

Figure 5. Protein carbonylation caused by methimazole and N-methylthiourea and the role of organosulfur compounds. DADS: Diallyl disulfide; NAC: N-acetyl cysteine.
Data are given as Mean±SE for three independent experiments as measured after 30 minutes of incubation.
[a] Significantly different from control (P<0.001).
[*] Asterisks indicate significant differences as compared to drug-treated groups (*P<0.05, **P<0.01 and ***P<0.001).

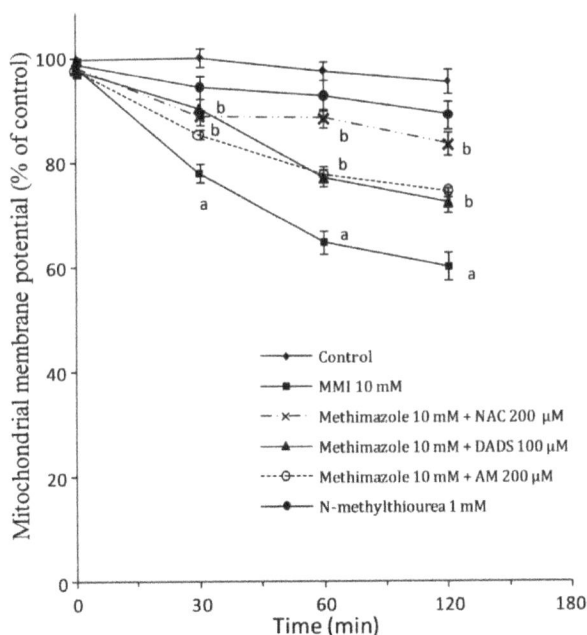

Figure 6. Methimazole-induced mitochondrial depolarization and the effects of organosulfur agents.
Data represent Mean±SE for three separate experiments.
[a] Different from control group (P<0.05).
[b] Significantly different from methimazole-treated group (P<0.05).

Reduction in glutathione reservoirs in hepatocytes treated with methimazole or N-methylthiourea,[8] indicates that GSH has a critical role in detoxifying methimazole metabolites and preventing cellular

damage. In previous studies it has been shown that glutathione depletion has deleterious effects on methimazole-induced toxicity in olfactory mucosa,[5] or mice liver.[10] Our results in isolated rat hepatocytes are in accordance with previous studies in this field.[8] Furthermore, our findings showed that methimazole caused an increase in ROS formation, lipid peroxidation, and reduction in hepatocytes mitochondrial membrane potential.[8] We found that the amount of oxidized glutathione (GSSG) was significantly raised in methimazole-treated cells, which indicates the occurrence of oxidative stress. Organosulfur chemicals such as diallyl disulfide significantly prevented glutathione reduction caused by methimazole or N-methylthiourea and reduced the GSSG formation during methimazole toxicity (Figure 2). This might indicate the importance of organosulfur chemicals in alleviating oxidative stress and scavenging reactive specie to prevent the consumption of glutathione as one of the main cellular defense mechanisms against toxic insults.

N-methylthiourea as the suspected toxic metabolite for methimazole[6] did not caused ROS formation, lipid peroxidation, or mitochondrial depolarization.[8] These finding suggest that other methimazole metabolite(s) rather than N-methylthiourea are responsible for observed adverse effects of methimazole in hepatocytes.[8] However, it has been shown that N-methylthiourea is further metabolized through flavin containing monooxygenase (FMO) enzyme to produce sulfenic acids.[6] Sulfenic acid species are reactive chemicals that covalently bind to nucleophilic sites.[7] Conjugating of sulfenic acids with glutathione could be a pathways for detoxifying them since N-methylthiourea caused reduction in cellular glutathione content and showed a sever toxicity profile in glutathione depleted cells. Binding of those reactive species to different targets such as proteins may cause cellular damage and toxicity. We found that N-methylthiourea caused an elevation in cellular carbonylated proteins level, which could be attributed to the cytotoxicity induced by N-methyl thiourea, and it is after head toxic metabolites. Since organosulfur agents significantly reduced protein carbonylation induced by N-methylthiourea (Figure 5), the protective effects of organosulfurs might be attributed to their effects on cellular protein damages caused by methimazole metabolite. In another investigation, we found that by administrating N,N-dimethylaniline as an FMO enzyme inhibitor,[34] the toxicity of N-methylthiourea in isolated hepatocytes was significantly reduced (Data not shown).[8]

The insignificant effect of N-methylthiourea on hepatocytes GSSG content supported the absence of oxidative stress during N-methylthiourea induced toxicity. This finding suggested that the reduction in hepatocytes glutathione (GSH) after treating cells with N-methylthiourea was due to conjugation of reactive metabolites with glutathione.[8]

The effect of methimazole and its metabolite on cell organelles such as mitochondria gives us an insight into the mechanisms by which this drug caused cytotoxicity toward isolated hepatocytes. Mitochondrial depolarization is accompanied by energy crisis and releasing of apoptotic signaling molecules, which could finally encounter cell death.[35] The insignificant effect of N-methylthiourea on mitochondrial membrane potential may indicate that the deleterious effect of methimazole on this organelle might be due to the other methimazole metabolite(s) rather than N-methylthiourea.[8] Administration of organosulfur chemicals might provide protection against methimazole-induced mitochondrial damage through their activity in attenuating oxidative stress and scavenging reactive species.

The use of glutathione-like thiol containing molecules such as allylmercaptan or other organosulfur compounds seems a reasonable choice to prevent methimazole-induced toxicity because of their non-enzymatic activities.[36] These compounds could scavenge reactive species[37,38] and chelating metal ions, which might have a role in preventing oxidative stress and lipid peroxidation.[39] The protective effects of organosulfur chemicals against methimazole and N-methylthiourea could be due to their capability in scavenging reactive metabolites. Furthermore, some organosulfur agents such as NAC might act as a glyoxal tarp and hence prevent methimazole-induced cytotoxicity.[8]

It seems that other methimazole metabolite(s) contributed with N-methylthiourea to induce cytotoxicity and the major part of organosulfurs protective effects in methimazole-induced toxicity might be due to their action against those metabolite(s). Further investigations including mass spectrometric analysis of conjugate formation is needed to elucidate subject.

The beneficial effect of organosulfur compounds against methimazole-induced toxicity proposes these agents as the subject of further studies for preventing different xenobiotics-induced liver damages, especially those accompanied with oxidative stress.

Conclusion
This study suggests that organosulfur chemicals extend their protective effects against methimazole-induced toxicity by attenuating oxidative stress caused by this drug. Furthermore, organosulfurs prevented the adverse effects of methimazole and its metabolite(s) on subcellular components such as mitochondria, which might has a role in attenuating the cytotoxicity induced by methimazole or its metabolite.

Acknowledgments
This study was funded (Grant number: 5/79/1436) by Drug Applied Research center of Tabriz University of Medical Sciences, Tabriz, Iran. The authors thanked Drug Applied Research Center of Tabriz University of Medical Sciences, Tabriz-Iran, for providing facilities and financial supports to carry out this study. This research was a part of Reza Heidari's PhD thesis that was supported by students' research committee. The authors are thankful to the students' research committee of Tabriz University of Medical Sciences, Tabriz-Iran, for providing supports to the study. The authors thank Dr. H. Hamzeiy and Dr. M.R. Satari for the proof reading of the manuscript.

Conflict of Interest
There is no conflict of interest in this study.

References
1. Franklyn JA. Thyroid gland: Antithyroid therapy--best choice of drug and dose. *Nat Rev Endocrinol* 2009;5(11):592-4.
2. Garcia D, Peon N, Torres F, Hip-Avagnina MI, Martinez A, di Crocce ME. Four cases of thiamazole-induced agranulocytosis. *Farm Hosp* 2008;32(3):183-5.
3. Livadas S, Xyrafis X, Economou F, Boutzios G, Christou M, Zerva A, et al. Liver failure due to antithyroid drugs: Report of a case and literature review. *Endocrine* 2010;38(1):24-8.
4. Brittebo EB. Metabolism-dependent toxicity of methimazole in the olfactory nasal mucosa. *Pharmacol Toxicol* 1995;76(1):76-9.
5. Bergström U, Giovanetti A, Piras E, Brittebo EB. Methimazole-induced damage in the olfactory mucosa: effects on ultrastructure and glutathione levels. *Toxicol Pathol* 2003;31(4):379-87.
6. Mizutani T, Yoshida K, Murakami M, Shirai M, Kawazoe S. Evidence for the involvement of N-methylthiourea, a ring cleavage metabolite, in the hepatotoxicity of methimazole in glutathione-depleted mice: structure-toxicity and metabolic studies. *Chem Res Toxicol* 2000;13(3):170-6.
7. Mansuy D, Dansette PM. Sulfenic acids as reactive intermediates in xenobiotic metabolism. *Arch Biochem Biophys* 2011;507(1):174-85.
8. Heidari R, Babaei H, Eghbal MA. Mechanisms of methimazole cytotoxicity in isolated rat hepatocytes. *Drug Chem Txicol* 2012: doi: 10.3109/01480545.2012.749272
9. Forman HJ, Zhang H, Rinna A. Glutathione: Overview of its protective roles, measurement, and biosynthesis. *Mol Aspects Med* 2009;30(1-2):1-12.
10. Mizutani T, Murakami M, Shirai M, Tanaka M, Nakanishi K. Metabolism-dependent hepatotoxicity of methimazole in mice depleted of glutathione. *J Appl Toxicol* 1999;19(3):193-8.
11. Kedderis GL, Rickert DE. Loss of rat liver microsomal cytochrome P-450 during methimazole metabolism. Role of flavin-containing monooxygenase. *Drug Metab Dispos* 1985;13(1):58-61.
12. Block E. The chemistry of garlic and onions. *Sci Am* 1985;252(3):114-9.
13. Rosen RT, Hiserodt RD, Fukuda EK, Ruiz RJ, Zhou Z, Lech J, et al. Determination of allicin, S-allylcysteine and volatile metabolites of garlic in breath, plasma or

simulated gastric fluids. *J Nutr* 2001;131(3s):968S-71S.

14. Fanelli SL, Castro GD, de Toranzo EG, Castro JA. Mechanisms of the preventive properties of some garlic components in the carbon tetrachloride-promoted oxidative stress. Diallyl sulfide; diallyl disulfide; allyl mercaptan and allyl methyl sulfide. *Res Commun Mol Pathol Pharmacol* 1998;102(2):163-74.

15. Sumioka I, Matsura T, Yamada K. Therapeutic effect of S-allylmercaptocysteine on acetaminophen-induced liver injury in mice. *Eur J Pharmacol* 2001;433(2-3):177-85.

16. Anoush M, Eghbal MA, Fathiazad F, Hamzeiy H, Kouzehkonani NS. The Protective Effect of Garlic Extract against Acetaminophen-Induced Loss of Mitochondrial Membrane Potential in Freshly Isolated Rat Hepatocytes. *Iran J Pharm Sci* 2009;5(3):141-50.

17. Mostafa MG, Mima T, Ohnishi ST, Mori K. S-allylcysteine ameliorates doxorubicin toxicity in the heart and liver in mice. *Planta Med* 2000;66(2):148-51.

18. Dwivedi C, John LM, Schmidt DS, Engineer FN. Effects of oil-soluble organosulfur compounds from garlic on doxorubicin-induced lipid peroxidation. *Anticancer Drugs* 1998;9(3):291-4.

19. Manesh C, Kuttan G. Alleviation of cyclophosphamide-induced urotoxicity by naturally occurring sulphur compounds. *J Exp Clin Cancer Res* 2002;21(4):509-17.

20. Sheen LY, Wu CC, Lii CK, Tsai SJ. Effect of diallyl sulfide and diallyl disulfide, the active principles of garlic, on the aflatoxin B(1)-induced DNA damage in primary rat hepatocytes. *Toxicol Lett* 2001;122(1):45-52.

21. Heard KJ. Acetylcysteine for Acetaminophen Poisoning. *N Engl J Med* 2008;359(3):285-92.

22. Zafarullah M, Li WQ, Sylvester J, Ahmad M. Molecular mechanisms of N-acetylcysteine actions. *Cell Mol Life Sci* 2003;60(1):6-20.

23. Kim JM, Chang HJ, Kim WK, Chang N, Chun HS. Structure-activity relationship of neuroprotective and reactive oxygen species scavenging activities for allium organosulfur compounds. *J Agric Food Chem* 2006;54(18):6547-53.

24. Heidari R, Babaei H, Eghbal MA. Ameliorative Effects of Taurine Against Methimazole-Induced Cytotoxicity in Isolated Rat Hepatocytes. *Sci Pharm* 2012;80:987-99.

25. Truong DH, Eghbal MA, Hindmarsh W, Roth SH, O'Brien PJ. Molecular Mechanisms of Hydrogen Sulfide Toxicity. *Drug Metab Rev* 2006;38(4):733-44.

26. Pourahmad J, Mortada Y, Eskandari MR, Shahraki J. Involvement of Lysosomal Labilisation and Lysosomal/mitochondrial Cross-Talk in Diclofenac Induced Hepatotoxicity. *Iran J Pharm Res* 2011;10(4):877-87.

27. Niknahad H, O'Brien PJ. Mechanism of sulfite cytotoxicity in isolated rat hepatocytes. *Chem Biol Interact* 2008;174(3):147-54.

28. Tafazoli S, O'Brien PJ. Amodiaquine-induced oxidative stress in a hepatocyte inflammation model. *Toxicology* 2009;256(1-2):101-9.

29. Eghbal MA, Pennefather PS, O'Brien PJ. H2S cytotoxicity mechanism involves reactive oxygen species formation and mitochondrial depolarisation. *Toxicology* 2004;203(1-3):69-76.

30. Rahman I, Kode A, Biswas SK. Assay for quantitative determination of glutathione and glutathione disulfide levels using enzymatic recycling method. *Nat Protoc* 2006;1(6):3159-65.

31. Khan S, O'Brien PJ. 1-bromoalkanes as new potent nontoxic glutathione depletors in isolated rat hepatocytes. *Biochem Biophys Res Commun* 1991;179(1):436-41.

32. Blokhina O, Virolainen E, Fagerstedt KV. Antioxidants, oxidative damage and oxygen deprivation stress: A review. *Ann Bot* 2003;91 Spec No:179-94.

33. Dalle-Donne I, Carini M, Orioli M, Vistoli G, Regazzoni L, Colombo G, et al. Protein carbonylation: 2,4-dinitrophenylhydrazine reacts with both aldehydes/ketones and sulfenic acids. *Free Radic Biol Med* 2009;46(10):1411-9.

34. Damani LA, Nnane IP. The assessment of flavin-containing monooxygenase activity in intact animals. *Drug Metabol Drug Interact* 1996;13(1):1-28.

35. Kroemer G, Galluzzi L, Brenner C. Mitochondrial membrane permeabilization in cell death. *Physiol Rev* 2007;87(1):99-163.

36. Yin MC, Hwang SW, Chan KC. Nonenzymatic antioxidant activity of four organosulfur compounds derived from garlic. *J Agric Food Chem* 2002;50(21):6143-7.

37. Pedraza-Chaverri J, Medina-Campos ON, Avila-Lombardo R, Berenice Zuniga-Bustos A, Orozco-Ibarra M. Reactive oxygen species scavenging capacity of different cooked garlic preparations. *Life Sci* 2006;78(7):761-70.

38. Garcia A, Haza AI, Arranz N, Delgado ME, Rafter J, Morales P. Organosulfur compounds alone or in combination with vitamin C protect towards N-nitrosopiperidine- and N-nitrosodibutylamine-induced oxidative DNA damage in HepG2 cells. *Chem Biol Interact* 2008;173(1):9-18.

39. Flora SJ. Structural, chemical and biological aspects of antioxidants for strategies against metal and metalloid exposure. *Oxid Med Cell Longev* 2009;2(4):191-206.

3

Dose-Dependent Effect of Flouxetine on 6-OHDA-Induced Catalepsy in Male Rats: A Possible Involvement of 5-HT$_{1A}$ Receptors

Hamdolah Sharifi[1], Alireza Mohajjel Nayebi[2]*, Safar Farajnia[2]

[1] Department of Pharmacology and Toxicology, Faculty of Pharmacy, Tabriz University of Medical Sciences.Tabriz, Iran.

[2] Drug Applied Research Center, Tabriz University of Medical Science, Tabriz, Iran.

ARTICLE INFO

Keywords:
Fluoxetine
6-Hydroxydopamine
Catalepsy
Rat

ABSTRACT

Purpose: Progressive loss of dopaminergic neurons of the substantia nigra pars compacta (SNc) in Parkinson's disease (PD) leads to impairment of motor skills. Several evidences show that the role of serotonergic system in regulation of normal movement is pivotal and mediates via 5-HT$_{1A}$ receptors. Our previous study has shown that fluoxetine in acute injections able to attenuate catalepsy in 6-hydroxydopamine (6-OHDA)-lesioned rats. Since drugs are used chronically in clinic, in this study we attempted to evaluate effect of chronic administration of fluoxetine on 6-OHDA-induced catalepsy. *Methods:* Catalepsy was induced by unilateral infusion of 6-OHDA (8 μg/2 μl/rat) into the central region of SNc and assayed by using bar-test. Fluoxetine (1, 2.5, 5 and 10 mg/kg) was injected intraperitonealy (ip) for 10 days and its anti-cataleptic effect was assessed at the 10th day. *Results:* Fluoxetine in high doses (5 and 10 mg/kg) worsened 6-OHDA-induced catalepsy while it had anti-cataleptic effect at the dose of 1mg/kg. The anti-cataleptic effect of fluoxetine (1mg/kg) was reversed by co-administration with NAN-190 (0.5 mg/kg, ip), as a 5-HT$_{1A}$ receptor antagonist. *Conclusion:* According to the results it can be concluded that fluoxetine has anti-cataleptic effect in parkinsonian rats only at low doses, whereas at higher doses it worsens catalepsy. It's anti-cataleptic effect is exerted through affecting on 5-HT$_{1A}$ receptors. However, at high doses other mechanisms may be involved. Further clinical studies are needed to prove it's possible clinical application as an adjuvant therapy in reducing catalepsy of PD.

Introduction

Parkinson's Disease (PD) is the second most common neurodegenerative disorder that is characterized by a marked loss of dopaminergic neurons of mainly the substantia nigra pars compacta (SNc) leading to a reduction of dopamine (DA) in the striatum. Dopamine deficiency results in motor disabilities, such as muscle rigidity, akinesia, tremor and postural abnormalities as well as cognitive disturbances.[1-3] Investigation of PD in animals is based on modeling of the disease by injection of some neurotoxins such as 6-OHDA that selectively destroys catecholaminergic neurons. Intracerebral injection of 6-OHDA into the rat nigrostriatal pathway degenerate virtually all dopaminergic neurons in the SNc and leading to stable motor deficits.[3,4]

In 6-OHDA-treated rats hyperinnervation of serotonergic (5-HT) fibers within the affected area takes place which compensate some activities of lost dopaminergic neurons.[5-7] All components of basal ganglia receive serotonergic neurons from dorsal raphe nucleus.[8] It seems that serotonergic system has a pivotal role in regulation of voluntary movements and disturbances in serotonine transmission might contribute to the neural mechanisms underlying disorders of basal ganglia such as PD, Tourette's syndrome and obsessive compulsive disorder.[5,9] Thus 5-HT transmission may be critical in treating the symptoms of PD and other motor disorders.[8] Several studies have shown anti-cataleptic effect of 5HT$_{1A}$ agonists in rodent model of PD but the effect of selective serotonin reuptake inhibitors (SSRIs) in improving of catalepsy is controversial.[9-11] Our previous study indicated that single-dose administration of flouxetine could abolish catalepsy in 6-OHDA lesioned rats.[5] Sinces the long-term effect of drugs can vary with their acute administration, therefore in this study we attempted to investigate the chronic effect of flouxetine in catalepsy induced by 6-OHDA.

Materials and Methods
Chemicals
All chemicals were purchased from Sigma Chemical Co. (USA). Solutions were prepared freshly on the days of experimentation. Fluoxetine and 1-(2-

*Corresponding author: Alireza Mohajjel Nayebi, Drug Applied Research Center, Tabriz University of Medical Sciences, Tabriz, Iran. E-mail: nayebia@tbzmed.ac.ir

methoxyphenyl)-4-[4-(2-phthalimido)buthyl]piperazine hydrobromide (NAN-190) were dissolved in 0.9% saline and 6-OHDA was dissolved in 0.9% saline containing 0.2% (w/v) ascorbic acid. The drugs were injected intraperitoneally (ip) except for 6-hydroxydopamine (6-OHDA) which was injected into right subestentia nigra pars compacta (SNc) in a total volum of 8 μl /rat with a constant injection rate of 0.2 μl/min.

Animals

The experiments were carried out on male Wistar rats weighing between 270-300 g. Before and during of study these animals were kept in polypropylene cages, four per cage, under standard conditions (12:12h) light/dark cycle at an ambient temperature about $25\pm2°C$ and had access to standard pellet and water ad labium. Animals were acclimated to the testing conditions 2 days before the behavioral assessments were done. All of the procedures were carried out under the ethical guidelines of Tabriz University of Medical Sciences.

Surgical procedures

The animals were anesthetized intrapitoenally by ketamine (50 mg/kg) and xylazine (5 mg/kg). After deep anaesthetization, rats were fixed in a stereotaxic frame in the flat skin positions. Scalp hairs of the rats were completely shaved with a standard electric shaving machine, swabbed with povidone iodine and a central incision made to reveal skull. A 0.7 millimeter bar hole was drilled and 23 gauge sterile stainless steel cannula, as a guide cannula inserted for subsequent injection of 6-OHDA in to the SNc. The coordinates for this site were based on the rat brain atlas[12]: anteroposterior (AP): -5.0 mm from the bregma; mediolateral (ML): ±2.1 mm from the midline and dorsoventral (DV):-7.7 from the skull. Desipramine (25 mg/kg) was injected intraperitoneally 30 min before intra-nigral injection of 6-OHDA to avoid degeneration of noradrenergic neurons. Then 6-OHDA (8 μg/ per rat in 2 μl saline with 0.02 % ascorbic acid) was infused by infusion pump at the flow rate of 0.2 μl/min into the right subestentia nigra pars compacta. At the end of injection, guide cannula was kept for an additional 2 min and then slowly was withdrawed. All of these procedures were repeated in Sham-operated animals but they were received only 2 μl vehicle of 6-OHDA (0.9% saline containing 0.2% (w/v) ascorbic acid). For approving the accuracy of the site of injection, we provided a histological slice of striatum region that showed the site of inserted guide cannula in accordance with rat brain atlas. After three weeks as a recovery period, only the rats that showed marked immobilization in bare test were subjected to further experimentation. Then parkinsonian rats were divided randomly into equal groups and received once daily (9 a.m.) injections of fluoxetine (1, 2.5, 5 and 10 mg/kg, ip) for 10 days. NAN-190 (0.5 mg/kg, ip), as a $5-HT_{1A}$

receptor antagonist, was injected concomitantly with the effective dose of fluoxetine.

Catalepsy test

Catalepsy was assessed by using of standard wooden bar test mean. Anterior limbs of rat gently extended on 9 cm high bar (0.9 cm in diameter). Elapsed time for each rat in this imposed posture was considered as a bar test time. The endpoint of catalepsy was designated to occur when both front pows were removed from the bar or if the animal moved its head in an exploratoty manner. The cut-off time of the test was 720 seconds. This test was carried out 5, 60, 120 and 180 minutes after drugs administration in the 10th day. All observations were made between 9 AM and 4 PM.

Statistical analysis

Statistical analysis of each data set was calculated by use of SPSS software (version 16.0). Data were expressed as the mean+SEM, and were analyzed by one-way ANOVA in each experiment. In the case of significant variation ($p<0.05$), the values were compared by Tukey test.

Results

Effect of Flouxetine on 6-OHDA induced catalepsy

Three groups of rats were shedoulded as normal (control), sham-operated (receiving 2 μl vehicle) and 6-OHDA (8 μg/2μl/rat, intra-SNc)-lesioned rats. As it has been shown in Figure 1, 6-OHDA could induce significant ($p<0.001$) catalepsy when compared with normal (control) and sham-operated animals. In other experiment five groups of 6-OHDA-lesioned rats received saline or one of four different doses of fluoxetine (1, 2.5, 5 and 10 mg/kg, ip), respectively for 10 days. The results showed that flouxetine decreased the severity of 6-OHDA-induced catalepsy dose dependently ($p < 0.001$) (Figure 2).

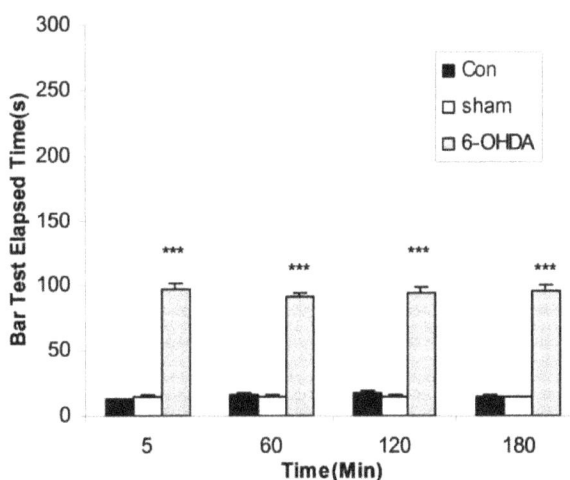

Figure 1. The results of bar test in control, Sham-operated and 6-OHDA (8μg/2μl/rat)-lesioned rats. Each bar represents the mean±SEM of elapsed time (s), n = 8 rats for each group; *** p<0.001 when compared with normal (Con) and sham operated groups.

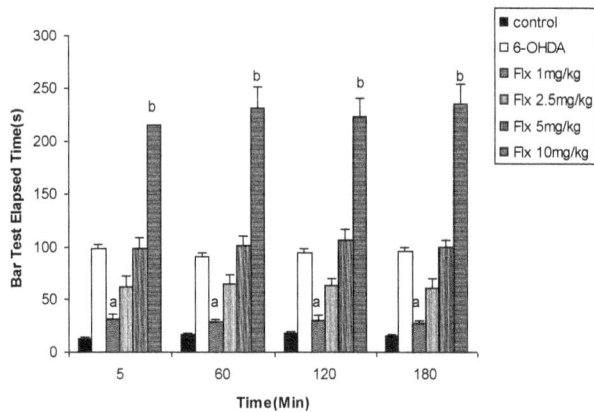

Figure 2. The bar test results of 6-OHDA (8 µg/2 µl/rat)-lesioned rats treated with Flouxetine (1, 2.5, 5 and 10 mg/kg, ip for 10 days). Each bar represents the mean ± SEM of elapsed time (s); n = 8 rats for each group; a p< 0.001 when compared with 6-OHDA-lesioned rats and b p< 0.001 when compared with control group.(Flx=Flouxetine)

Effect of NAN-190 co-treatment with flouxetine on 6-OHDA-induced catalepsy

Three groups of 6-OHDA-lesioned animals received saline, flouxetine (1 mg/kg, ip) or flouxetine (1mg/kg ip) with NAN-190 (1mg/kg ip) respectively. The results showed that catalepsy-ameliorating effect of flouxetine was reversed (p <0.001) by NAN-190 (Figure 3).

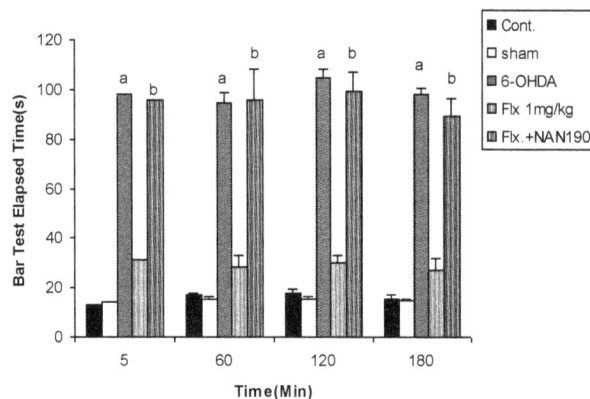

Figure 3. The bar test results from the co-administration of NAN-190 (0.5 mg/kg,ip) with flouxetine (1mg/kg, ip for 10 days) in 6-OHDA-lesioned rats. Each bar represents the mean ± SEM of elapsed time (s); n = 8 rats for each group; a p<0.001 when compared with 6-OHDA-lesioned rats; b p< 0.001 when compared with 6-OHDA-lesioned rats co-treated with NAN-190 and flouxetine.

Discussion

Striatal DA deficiency or direct striatal damage for any reason may lead to PD which is characterized by tremor at rest, muscle rigidity and slowness of voluntary movement.[4] 6-OHDA is a neurotoxin which is used generally to produce experimental model of PD.[5] In this study intra-SNc injection of 6-OHDA caused noticeable catalepsy when was assessed by bar test. This is standard test frequently used for evaluating catalepsy induced by 6-OHDA and neuroleptic drugs in rodents.[13] Our results showed that chronic injections of flouxetine for ten days attenuated 6-OHDA-induced

catalepsy only at low doses. The most anticatleptic effect was observed at the dose of 1mg/kg, whereas flouxetine at the high doses (5 and 10 mg/kg) trebeled catalepsy. This may be due to increase of flouextine dose and involvement of some other neuronal effects.

5-HT$_{1A}$ receptors are widely distributed through the basal ganglia. They are located on dorsal raphe neurons with efferents to the striatum, and are also localized on cortical neurons sending glutamatergic projections to the basal ganglia.[14,15] Release of dopamine following stimulation of 5-HT$_{1A}$ receptors in these regions is via the inhibition of adenyl cyclase and the opening of potassium channels. These findings show that modulation of 5-HT transmission by 5-HT$_{1A}$ receptor agonists can be a potential therapeutic approach in PD.[16,17] On the other hand it is supposed that the striatum is a central neuroanatomical site for both antidyskinetic and anti-parkinsonian actions of 5-HT$_{1A}$ receptor agonists.[18] In particular, the striatum and the output regions of the basal ganglia, the substantia nigra pars reticulata (SNr), and medial globus pallidus (GPm) receive a dense serotonergic input, thus suggesting a potential role for serotonin in PD.[19] Specific serotonin reuptake inhibitors (SSRIs) which increase serotonin levels in synaptic cleft may have similar effect through affecting on 5-HT$_{1A}$ receptors. In this study, NAN-190 (5-HT$_{1A}$ receptor antagonist) reversed the catalepsy-improving effect of fluoxetine in 6-OHDA lesioned rats. Thus, it seems that low doses of fluoxetine improves anti-cataleptic effect of 6-OHDA by affecting on 5-HT$_{1A}$ receptors. While high dose of fluoxetine worsened catalepsy. It has been shown that serotonin modulates dopamine in basal ganglia by inhibiting its production and release.[8] Furthermore, SSRIs may worsen the symptoms of pre-existing PD or depressive symptoms of anhedonia and social isolation.[11] Worsening of PD by SSRIs can be explained by two mechanisms:.First, over activation of serotonergic projections of dorsal raphe which project directly to the substantia nigra and subsequent inhibition of the dopaminergic neurons;[20] second, extrapyramidal side effects of SSRI.[19,21-23]

According to the results, we conclude that flouxetine improves catalepsy of parkinsonian rats in a dose-dependent manner. This effect is mediated by the stimulation of 5-HT$_{1A}$ receptors. We suggest a possible clinical application for fluoxetine in attenuating catalepsy of PD. To prove this hypothesis further clinical investigations should be carried out.

Acknowledgments
We wish to thank the Director of Drug Applied Research Center of the Tabriz University of Medical Sciences for supporting this study.

Conflict of interest
The authors report no conflicts of interest.

References

1. Singh N, Pillay V, Choonara YE. Advances in the treatment of Parkinson's disease . *Prog Neurobiol* 2007;81:29-44.
2. Di Filippoa M, Chiasserini D, Tozzi A, Picconi B, Calabresi P. Mitochondria and the link between neuroinflammation and neurodegeneration. *J Alzheimers Dis* 2010;20 (Suppl 2):S369-79.
3. Iancu R, Mohapel P, Brundin P, Paul G. Behavioral characterization of a unilateral 6-OHDA-lesion model of Parkinson's disease in mice. *Behav Brain Res* 2005;162(1):1-10.
4. Dauer W, Przedborski S. Parkinson's Disease: Mechanisms and Models. *Neuron* 2003;39(6):889-909.
5. Mahmoudi J, Nayebi AM, Reyhani-Rad S, Samini M. Fluoxetine improves the Effect of levodopa on 6-hydroxy dopamine-induced motor impairments in rats. *Adv Pharm Bull* 2012;2(2):149-55.
6. Maeda T, Kannari K, Huo SH, Arai A, Tomiyama M, Matsunaga M, et al. Increase of the striatal serotonergic fibers after nigrostriatal dopaminergic denervation in adult rats. *Int Congr Ser* 2003; 1251:211-5.
7. Brown P. Gerfen CR. Plasticity within striatal direct pathway neurons after neonatal dopamine depletion is mediated through a novel functional coupling of serotonin 5-HT2 receptors to the ERK 1/2 Map Kinase pathway. *J Comp Neurol* 2006;498(3):415-30.
8. Di Matteo V, Pierucci M, Esposito E, Crescimanno G, Benigno A, Di Giovanni G. Serotonin modulation of the basal ganglia circuitry: Therapeutic implication for parkinson's disease and other motor disorders. *Prog in Brain Res* 2008;172:423-63.
9. Caley CF, Friedman JH. Does fluoxetine exacerbate Parkinson's disease? *J Clin. Psychiatry* 1992;53:278-82.
10. Steur EN. Increase of Parkinson disability after fluoxetine medication. *Neurology* 1993;43(1):211-3.
11. Gönül AS, Aksu M. SSRI-induced Parkinsonism may be an early sign of future Parkinson's Disease. *J Clin Psychiatry* 1999;60(6):410.
12. Paxinos G, Watson C. The rat brain in stereotaxic coordinates. Sydney: Academic Press; 1982.
13. Pires JG, Bonikovski V, Futuro-Neto HA. Acute effects of selective serotonin reuptake inhibitors on neuroleptic-induced catalepsy in mice. *Braz J Med Biol Res* 2005;38(12):1867-72.
14. Mohajjel Nayebi AA, Sheidaei H. Buspirone improves haloperidol-induced Parkinson disease in mice through 5-HT(1A) recaptors. *Daru* 2010;18(1):41-5.
15. Navailles S, De Deurwaerdere P. Imbalanced dopaminergic transmission mediated by serotonergic Neurons in L-DOPA-induced dyskinesia. *Parkinsons Dis* 2012;2012:323686.
16. Nayebi AM, Rad SR, Saberian M, Azimzadeh S, Samini M. Buspirone improves 6-hydroxydopamine-induced catalepsy through stimulation of nigral 5-HT(1A) receptors in rats. *Pharmacol Rep* 2010;62(2):258-64.
17. Alex KD, Pehek EA. Pharmacologic mechanisms of serotonergic regulation of dopamine neurotransmission. *Pharmacol Ther* 2007;113(2):296-320.
18. Dupre KB, Eskow KL, Barnum CJ, Bishop C. Striatal 5-HT$_{1A}$ receptor stimulation reduces D1 receptor-induced dyskinesia and improves movement in the hemiparkinsonian rat. *Neuropharmacology* 2008;55(8):1321-8.
19. Fox SH, Chuang R, Brotchie JM. Serotonin and parkinson's disease: On movement, mood, and madness. *Mov Disord* 2009;24(9):1255-66.
20. Eltayb A, Svensson TH, Ahlenius S. Catalepsy induced by the 5-HT(1A) receptor antagonist WAY 100635 in rats pretreated with the selective serotonin reuptake inhibitor citalopram. *Eur J Pharmacol* 2001;411(3):275-7.
21. van de Vijver DA, Roos RA, Jansen PA, Porsius AJ, de Boer A. Start of a selective serotonin reuptake inhibitor (SSRI) and increase of antiparkinsonian drug treatment in patients on levodopa. *Br J Clin Pharmacol* 2002;54(2):168-70.
22. Schapira AH. Present and future drug treatment for parkinson's disease. *J Neurol Neurosurg Psychiatry* 2005;76(11):1472-8.
23. Arya DK. Extrapyramidal symptoms with selective serotonin reuptake inhibitors. *Br J Psychiatry* 1994;165(6):728-33.

4

Effect of Vitamin B6 on Clinical Symptoms and Electrodiagnostic Results of Patients with Carpal Tunnel Syndrome

Mahnaz Talebi[1]*, Sasan Andalib[1]*, Shohreh Bakhti[2], Hormoz Ayromlou[1], Alireza Aghili[2], Ashraf Talebi[3]

[1] Neurosciences Research Center, Tabriz University of Medical Sciences, Tabriz, Iran.

[2] School of Medicine, Tabriz University of Medical Sciences, Tabriz, Iran.

[3] School of Pharmacy, Tabriz University of Medical Sciences, Tabriz, Iran.

ARTICLE INFO

Keywords:
Carpal Tunnel Syndrome
Electrodiagnosis
NCV-EMG
Vitamin B6 treatment

ABSTRACT

Purpose: Carpal tunnel syndrome (CTS) refers to a cluster of signs and symptoms that stems from compression of the median nerve traveling through carpal tunnel. Surgery is a definite treatment for CTS; however, many conservative therapies have been proposed. The present study set out to assess the effect of vitamin B6 in patients with CTS. *Methods:* Forty patients (67 hands) with mild-moderate CTS were initially selected and randomly assigned into two groups as follows: 1) Case group with 20 subjects (32 affected hands) receiving vitamin B6 (120 mg/day for 3 months) and splinting. 2) Control group with 19 subjects (35 affected hands) only received splinting. One subject from the control group dispensed with continuing participation in the research. Daily symptoms and electrodiagnostic (NCV-EMG) results were assessed at baseline and after 3 months. *Results:* Nocturnal awakening frequency due to pain, daily pain, daily pain frequency, daily pain persistence, hand numbness, hand weakness, hand tingling, severity of nocturnal numbness and tingling, nocturnal awakening frequency owing to hand numbness and tingling, and clumsiness in handling objects improved significantly in the vitamin B6-treated patients; even so, only problem with opening a jam bottle and handling phone significantly reduced in the control group. The median nerve sensory latency mean decreased following the treatment; and the median nerve sensory amplitude mean and sensory conduction velocity mean increased. *Conclusion:* The present study suggests that vitamin B6 treatment improves clinical symptoms and sensory electrodiagnostic results in CTS patients, and thus is recommended for CTS treatment.

Introduction

Carpal tunnel syndrome (CTS) refers to a constellation of signs and symptoms that stems from compression of the median nerve traveling through the carpal tunnel.[1] It accounts for approximately 90% of entrapment neuropathies[2] and is more prevalent amongst females.[3] Paget first described the clinical manifestation of CTS.[4] CTS is classified into acute and chronic forms. Acute CTS is not prevalent and results from radius fractures, burns, coagulopathies, infections and local injections; however, chronic CTS is rather prevalent and patients present with its symptoms for several months or years.[2] CTS is also divided into primary and secondary forms. Secondary CTS can result from pregnancy,[5,6] rheumatoid arthritis,[7] acromegaly[8] and type 2 diabetes mellitus.[9] Furthermore, career is said to be involved in CTS. For instance, dentistry was suggested to be associated with CTS.[10] CTS is clinically diagnosed by Phalen's,[11] Hoffmann-Tinel's,[11] and Durkan[12] tests. In spite of the fact that conservative therapies are

proposed,[13] surgery is a definite treatment for CTS.[14] Initial therapies for CTS incorporate oral or local injection of corticosteroids,[15] splinting[16] and activity modification.[17] Moreover, vitamin B6 has been demonstrated to be effective in CTS treatment.[18,19] Vitamin B6 contributes to multiple metabolic pathways of neuronal function for instance, production of neurotransmitters, amino acid metabolism, synthesis and destruction of sphingolipids. Administration of vitamin B6 as add-on therapy for CTS has been introduced into western communities since 1980.[20] CTS is a common cause of patients' referral to neurology clinics and electrodiagnostic wards and patients with mild to moderate CTS do not necessitate surgery but to require treatment. Hence, it is difficult to ignore CTS conservative therapies such as vitamin B6 treatment. On the other hand, a literature search has offered contradictory results pertaining to impact of vitamin B6 upon CTS. Moreover, the preceding

Corresponding author: Mahnaz Talebi and Sasan Andalib. Neurosciences Research Center, Tabriz University of Medical Sciences, Tabriz, Iran. Emails: talebi511@yahoo.com and andalibsa@tbzmed.ac.ir

published research suffered major pitfalls, that is to say, limitation in sample size and methodology, uncontrolled CTS severity and difference in dose and duration of treatment. The present study attempted to iron out all aforesaid drawbacks of the preceding research and have a novel approach in order to achieve reliable results. Therefore, our aim was to assess the effect of vitamin B6 upon CTS. More to the point, the present study was designed in order to specifically identify the effect of vitamin B6 treatment upon clinical symptoms and electrodiagnostic results in CTS patients presenting with mild to moderate clinical symptoms. It was hypothesized that vitamin B6 treatment can improve CTS and specifically patients' electrodiagnostic results.

Materials and Methods
The whole study lasted for 18 months from 2009, Mar 21 to 2010, Jun 23. Forty patients with idiopathic CTS were initially recruited from Neurosciences Research Center, Tabriz University of Medical Sciences. Patients were randomly assigned into 2 groups as follows: 1) Case group including 20 patients with 32 affected hands 2) Control group involving 20 patients with 35 affected hands. Case group received splinting and was orally treated by vitamin B6 at a dose of 120 mg/day during 3 months; be that as it may, the control group received only splinting. Symptoms and electrodiagnostic results (Nerve Conduction Velocity [NCV] and Electromyography [EMG]) results were compared prior and subsequent to the treatment in both groups. All participants gave informed consent for the research. All the procedures were approved by ethical committee of Tabriz University of Medical Sciences. Of the study population, one subject from the control group dispensed with continuing participation in the research. Hence, we were ultimately studied a total number of 39 subjects with CTS. It is worth noting that we applied inclusion criteria of mild to moderate CTS for the study. Mild, moderate and severe CTSs were defined based upon electrodiagnostic results as follows: a) Mild: increased median nerve sensory latency of more than 3.1 ms or median-ulnar sensory latency difference of more than 0.5 ms b) Moderate: increased median nerve sensory latency and decreased median nerve sensory amplitude or increased median nerve motor latency c) Severe: decreased median nerve sensory amplitude or EMG results.[2,9] Moreover, patients with severe CTS, diabetes mellitus, acromegaly, wrist burns, wrist sesamoid fracture, pregnancy, hypothyroidism, cervical neuropathy and radiculopathy resulting in hand numbness and paresthesia were excluded from the study. It should also be noted that patients' hands, but not patients, were assessed in the present study. Therefore, at least 10 hands with mild or moderate CTS were assessed in each group. Electrodiagnostic tests including NCV and EMG tests, Phalen's and Tinel's tests and symptom assessments (standard Boston questionnaire) were

carried out prior to commencing the treatments. Aforesaid tests and assessments were repeated again 3 months later and changes were recorded. Splinting and activity modification were performed as usual. Patients' responses were scored from 1 to 5 in terms of severity of clinical symptoms. Ultimately, collected data incorporated age, gender, career, side of involvement, CTS severity, positive Phalen's and Tinel's tests, clinical symptoms and electrodiagnostic findings. Statistical analyses were performed using the SPSS statistical software package (Version 17.0). More precisely, statistical significance was analyzed for categorical variables using contingency tables, Chi-Square test, Fisher's exact test and McNemar test. In addition, comparisons were drawn for numerical variable using independent samples T-test, paired samples T-test and Wilcoxon test. The results were significant at P-value<0.05 level.

Results
In the present study, 40 participants including 20 cases and 20 controls were studied. Howbeit, one subject from the control group dispensed with continuing participation in the research. The recruitment was carried out for 3 months starting at 2009, June 20. Comparing the two results, no significant difference was found in the average age of the patients in the case and control groups which were 42.7±12.0 years (25 to 65 years) and 43.8±13.1 years (22 to 62 years), respectively(p=0.805). No significant difference was found in gender between the case and control groups (male cases [n=4; 20%], female cases [n=16; 80%], male controls [n=1; 5%] and female controls [n=19; 95%]) (p=0.342).The case group included 16 homemakers and 4 employed patients who constituted 80 % and 20%, respectively. To be more precise, the employed patients involved a carpet weaver and 2 self-employed individuals. However, the control group included 15 homemakers and 5 employed patients who made up 75% and 25%, respectively. More precisely, the employed patients involved a carpet weaver and 4 self-employed individuals. No significant difference was found in patients' career between these groups (p=0.647). In the case group, 19 subjects showed right hand involvement (59.4%), however, 13 subjects presented with left hand involvement (40.6%). In the control group, 24 subjects showed right hand involvement (68.6%); nonetheless, 11 subjects presented with left hand involvement (31.4%). In this regard, there was no significant difference between these groups (p=0.339). No significant difference was found between the case and control groups in the severity of CTS (22 [68.8%] and 10 [31.2%] controls with mild and moderate CTS, respectively, and 19 [54.3%] and 16 [54.7%] cases with mild and moderate CTS, respectively (p=0.177). In the case group, 14 hands with positive Phalen's and Tinel's tests were detected prior to treatment (43.8%) which were more than those observed subsequent to the treatment (11

[32.4%]). This difference was not statistically significant (p=0.727). In the control group, 12 hands with positive Phalen's and Tinel's tests were found prior to the treatment (43.3%) which were less than those detected following the treatment (16 [45.7%]). This difference was not statistically significant (p=0.359).

Table 1 provides a comparative breakdown pertaining to questionnaire responses of the patients in terms of clinical symptoms in the case and control groups. As can be decidedly noted, in the case group, nocturnal pain severity, nocturnal awakening frequency due to pain, daily pain, daily pain frequency, daily pain persistence, hand numbness, hand weakness, hand tingling, severity of nocturnal numbness and tingling, nocturnal awakening frequency owing to hand numbness and tingling, and clumsiness in handling objects decreased significantly following the treatment (amelioration). According to the table, problem with opening a jam bottle and handling phone significantly reduced in the control group (amelioration).

Table 1. A comparison of CTS patients' responses in the control and case groups in terms of distribution of clinical symptoms before and after treatment.

Variables	P value (Before and after treatment)	
	Case group	Control group
Nocturnal pain	0.040*	0.544
Nocturnal awakening frequency due to pain	0.027*	0.579
Daily pain	0.027*	0.865
Daily pain frequency	0.035*	0.725
Daily pain persistence	0.023*	0.185
Hand numbness	0.045*	0.936
Hand weakness	0.029*	0.675
Hand tingling	0.030*	0.865
Severity of nocturnal numbness and tingling	0.030*	0.253
Nocturnal awakening frequency owing to hand numbness and tingling	0.040*	0.166
Problem with handling objects	0.035*	0.558
Problem with writing	0.080	0.506
Problem with buttoning	0.287	0.344
Problem with holding book	0.306	0.075
Problem with holding phone	0.502	0.018*
Problem with opening bottle	0.223	0.029*
Problem with daily household chores	0.506	0.776
Problem with holding bag	0.306	0.258
Problem with bathing and dressing	0.333	0.644
* p<0.05		

Table 2 depicts a comparison of electrodiagnostic results in the case and control groups. It is apparent from the table that in the case group, median nerve sensory latency mean significantly diminished following the treatment; even so, median nerve sensory amplitude mean and median nerve sensory conduction velocity mean went up subsequent to the treatment (amelioration). It is apparent from the table that there was no significant difference amongst electrodiagnostic results in the control group.

Discussion

The present study was designed to assess the effect of administration of vitamin B6 with a dose of 120 mg/day for 3 months upon clinical symptoms and electrodiagnostic results in patients with mild to moderate CTS. Treatment with vitamin B6 in CTS patients in the case group alleviated several clinical symptoms such as nocturnal pain severity, nocturnal awakening frequency due to pain, daily pain, daily pain frequency, daily pain persistence, hand numbness, hand weakness, hand tingling, severity of nocturnal numbness and tingling, nocturnal awakening frequency owing to hand numbness and tingling, and clumsiness in handling objects. Moreover, there were improvements in sensory electrodiagnostic results incorporating increased median nerve sensory latency mean, increased median nerve sensory amplitude mean and increased sensory conduction velocity mean in this group. However, none of these results was observed in the control group. There were no significant differences in the results of Phalen's and Tinel's tests before and after treatment in both studied groups. To date, a large body of literature has investigated the effect of vitamin B6 upon symptoms and electrodiagnostic results in patients with CTS; nonetheless, the controversy about scientific evidence has raged unabated. Ellis et al. reviewed the literature concerning impact of vitamin B6 upon CTS and found that the influence of vitamin B6 upon CTS symptoms was demonstrated in 8 studies, although 6 studies did not corroborate these findings.[21] The authors also mentioned that the most important limitation for these studies lied in the relatively small sample size. Kasdan and Janes studied 1075 patients with CTS over 12 years symptoms were alleviated in 14.3 % of patients treated conservatively before 1980, with one or a combination of splinting anti-inflammatory drugs, job or activity modification, and steroid injections. Subsequent to vitamin B6 (pyridoxine) usage as a conservative treatment in 1980, Satisfactory improvement was achieved in 68 % of 494 patients treated with vitamin B6 at a dose of 100 mg.[20] Predicated upon this study, a course of treatment at aforementioned dose was recommended;[20] even so, two sources of uncertainty lied in this investigation. Firstly, it was a retrospective study. Secondly, it lacked a control group. These findings corroborated our results with respect to alleviation of CTS symptoms. On the other hand, Stransky et al. studied 15 patients with CTS receiving vitamin B6 and placebo for 10 weeks and reached different conclusions, finding no difference in symptoms and electrodiagnostic results before and after treatment in the cases and controls.[22] Spooner et al. reported that administration of vitamin B6 at a dose of 200 mg/day for 12 weeks did not exert any effect upon pain severity, nocturnal numbness and tingling in CTS patients.[19] Laso Guzman et al. traced the effect of vitamin B6 treatment with a dose of 150 mg/day for 3 months upon 12 CTS patients requiring surgery and observed that clinical symptoms and electrodiagnostic results improved in half of them.[23] The authors finally concluded that administration of vitamin B6 is beneficial for patients with CTS.[23] In contrast to these findings, the present study exhibited an improvement exclusively in sensory diagnostic results. Bernstein and Dinesen investigated the impact of vitamin B6 on and electrodiagnostic results and highlighted beneficial changes in pain severity and sensory latency results.[24] The authors also pointed to concurrent improvement of symptoms and electrodiagnostic results following vitamin B6 treatment.[24] Aufiero et al. reviewed the literature regarding administration of vitamin B6 for treatment of CTS and reported that in some studies the treatment produced positive effects upon symptoms and electrodiagnostic results; although they showed that some studies did not accord with the influence of vitamin B6 upon CTS.[25] The authors finally emphasized the administration of vitamin B6 to treat CTS.[25] They also recommended two mechanisms by which vitamin B6 treatment affects CTS as follows: 1) mitigation of vitamin B6 dependent-neurological problems 2) vitamin B6 effect as analgesic bringing about decreased pain threshold.[25] It is worth noting that there has been little agreement in the literature on the alleviation of vitamin B6 dependent-neurological problems. Lack of vitamin B6 in CTS patients has been demonstrated in a study;[21] howbeit, the association between lack of vitamin B6 and CTS was rejected elsewhere.[23] Results of the present study in terms of symptoms and electrodiagnostic assessments confirmed therapeutic effect of vitamin B6 upon CTS and were consistent with those of Bernstein and Dinesen.[24]

As mentioned above, preceding research findings into role of vitamin B6 has been inconsistent. There would be several plausible explanations for the disagreement in the following order: 1) Difference in sample size: some previous studies suffered from a serious drawback, that is, small sample size. This may result in erroneous or indefinite conclusions.[24] 2) Problems with methodology: a major weakness with the previous studies was old methods. Indeed, questions have raised about preciseness of preliminary studies. Moreover, it appears that conducting controlled and non-retrospective studies is essential in this regard. In fact, taking these issues into account was a strong point in the present study. 3) Difference in dose and duration of treatment with vitamin B6: in present study, CTS patients received a treatment at a dose of 120 mg/day for 3 months. Efficacy and safety of this dose of vitamin B6 have been demonstrated in the literature.[9] 4) Uncontrolled CTS severity: patients with mild to moderate CTS were exclusively assessed in the present study on the grounds of surgery indication for severe CTS. To clarify, Laso Guzman et al. investigated the impact of vitamin B6 upon CTS patients requiring surgery and observed that vitamin B6 treatment mitigated the symptoms, although it did not obviate the need for surgery.[23] Another study conducted by Folkers et al.[26] produced results which corroborated the findings of Laso Guzman et al..[23] Thereby, selection method is of crucial importance. Indeed, this was a benefit considered in the present study. 5) Method of investigation of symptoms: In order to assess the effect of vitamin B6 treatment upon CTS symptoms, a questionnaire was used that firstly covered all aspects of patients' life and secondly was simple and comprehensible and thirdly facilitated statistical comparison by quantifying answer choices (increasing the scores indicated symptom exacerbation).

Returning to the hypothesis posed at the beginning of this study, it is possible to state that administration of vitamin B6 in patients with mild to moderate CTS alleviates many clinical symptoms incorporating nocturnal pain severity, nocturnal awakening frequency due to pain, daily pain, daily pain frequency, daily pain persistence, hand numbness, hand weakness, hand tingling, severity of nocturnal numbness and tingling, nocturnal awakening frequency owing to hand numbness and tingling, and clumsiness in handling objects. The results of this study indicate that administration of vitamin B6 in patients with mild to moderate CTS ameliorates sensory diagnostic results. On another reading, it decreases median nerve sensory latency average, increases average of median nerve sensory amplitude and median nerve conduction velocity. Taken together, these results suggest that vitamin B6 treatment at a dose of 120 mg/day does not exert deleterious side effect and mitigates clinical symptoms. Thus, vitamin B6 at this dose is

recommended for CTS treatment. Additionally, a limitation of the current study was the relatively limited number of participants precluding us from studying the effect of different doses of vitamin B6 upon CTS. Hence, further investigation with various vitamin B6 doses, having more sample size and analysis of serum pyridoxine yields illuminating insight into treatment of CTS.

Table 2. A comparison of electrodiagnostic (NCV-EMG) results of CTS patients in the case and control groups before and after treatment.

Variables	P value (Before and after treatment)	
	Case group	Control group
Median nerve distal motor latency	0.178	0.879
Median nerve proximal motor latency	0.290	0.386
Median nerve distal motor amplitude	0.397	0.572
Median nerve proximal motor amplitude	0.506	0.518
Median nerve motor conduction velocity	0.498	0.514
Median nerve motor F	0.080	0.095
Median nerve sensory latency	0.001*	0.818
Median nerve sensory amplitude	0.008*	0.178
Median nerve sensory conduction velocity	0.034*	0.846
Ulnar nerve distal motor latency	0.592	0.732
Ulnar nerve proximal motor latency	0.427	0.921
Ulnar nerve distal motor amplitude	0.628	0.685
Ulnar nerve proximal motor amplitude	0.250	0.124
Ulnar nerve motor conduction velocity	0.948	0.278
Ulnar nerve motor F	0.159	0.299
Ulnar nerve sensory latency	0.642	0.737
Ulnar nerve sensory amplitude	0.072	0.752
Ulnar nerve sensory conduction velocity	0.892	0.579
Median nerve distal motor latency	0.178	0.879
* $p < 0.05$		

Conflict of interest
We declare that we do not have any conflict of interest.

References
1. Ashworth NL. Carpal tunnel syndrome. Clin Evid (Online) 2011;2011.
2. Lewis PJ. Pain in the hand and wrist. Pyridoxine supplements may help patients with carpal tunnel syndrome. *BMJ* 1995;310(6993):1534.
3. Balakrishnan C, Jarrahnejad P, Balakrishnan A, Huettner WC. Acute carpal tunnel syndrome as a result of spontaneous bleeding. *Can J Plast Surg* 2008;16(3):168-9.
4. Paget J. The first description of carpal tunnel syndrome. *J Hand Surg Eur Vol* 2007;32(2):195-7.
5. Ablove RH, Ablove TS. Prevalence of carpal tunnel syndrome in pregnant women. *WMJ* 2009;108(4):194-6.
6. Jurjevic A, Bralic M, Antoncic I, Dunatov S, Legac M. Early onset of carpal tunnel syndrome during pregnancy: case report. *Acta Clin Croat* 2010;49(1):77-80.
7. Ekim A, Armagan O, Tascioglu F, Oner C, Colak M. Effect of low level laser therapy in rheumatoid arthritis patients with carpal tunnel syndrome. *Swiss Med Wkly* 2007;137(23-24):347-52.
8. Iwasaki N, Masuko T, Ishikawa J, Minami A. Surgical efficacy of carpal tunnel release for carpal tunnel syndrome in acromegaly: report of four patients. *J Hand Surg Br* 2005;30(6):605-6.
9. Ryan-Harshman M, Aldoori W. Carpal tunnel syndrome and vitamin B6. *Can Fam Physician* 2007;53(7):1161-2.
10. Haghighat A, Khosrawi S, Kelishadi A, Sajadieh S, Badrian H. Prevalence of clinical findings of carpal

tunnel syndrome in Isfahanian dentists. *Adv biomed res* 2012;1:13.

11. Kachare M, Hahn E, Jr., Granick MS. Carpal tunnel syndrome. *Eplasty* 2013;13:ic8.

12. Wainner RS, Boninger ML, Balu G, Burdett R, Helkowski W. Durkan gauge and carpal compression test: accuracy and diagnostic test properties. *J Orthop Sports Phys Ther* 2000;30(11):676-82.

13. Gerritsen AA, De Krom MC, Struijs MA, Scholten RJ, De Vet HC, Bouter LM. Conservative treatment options for carpal tunnel syndrome: a systematic review of randomised controlled trials. *J Neurol* 2002;249(3):272-80.

14. Bickel KD. Carpal tunnel syndrome. *J Hand Surg Am* 2010;35(1):147-52.

15. Marshall S, Tardif G, Ashworth N. Local corticosteroid injection for carpal tunnel syndrome. *Cochrane Database Syst Rev* 2002(4):CD001554.

16. Viera AJ. Management of carpal tunnel syndrome. *Am Fam Physician* 2003;68(2):265-72.

17. De Pablo P, Katz JN. Pharmacotherapy of carpal tunnel syndrome. *Expert Opin Pharmacother* 2003;4(6):903-9.

18. Holm G, Moody LE. Carpal tunnel syndrome: current theory, treatment, and the use of B6. *J Am Acad Nurse Pract* 2003;15(1):18-22.

19. Spooner GR, Desai HB, Angel JF, Reeder BA, Donat JR. Using pyridoxine to treat carpal tunnel syndrome. Randomized control trial. *Can fam physician* 1993;39:2122-7.

20. Kasdan ML, Janes C. Carpal tunnel syndrome and vitamin B6. *Plast Reconstr Surg* 1987;79(3):456-62.

21. Ellis J, Folkers K, Levy M, Takemura K, Shizukuishi S, Ulrich R, et al. Therapy with vitamin B6 with and without surgery for treatment of patients having the idiopathic carpal tunnel syndrome. *Res Commun Chem Pathol Pharmacol* 1981;33(2):331-44.

22. Stransky M, Rubin A, Lava NS, Lazaro RP. Treatment of carpal tunnel syndrome with vitamin B6: a double-blind study. *South Med J* 1989;82(7):841-2.

23. Laso Guzman FJ, Gonzalez-Buitrago JM, De Arriba F, Mateos F, Moyano JC, Lopez-Alburquerque T. Carpal tunnel syndrome and vitamin B6. *Klin Wochenschr* 1989;67(1):38-41.

24. Bernstein AL, Dinesen JS. Brief communication: effect of pharmacologic doses of vitamin B6 on carpal tunnel syndrome, electroencephalographic results, and pain. *J Am Coll Nutr* 1993;12(1):73-6.

25. Aufiero E, Stitik TP, Foye PM, Chen B. Pyridoxine hydrochloride treatment of carpal tunnel syndrome: a review. *Nutr Rev* 2004;62(3):96-104.

26. Folkers K, Ellis J, Watanabe T, Saji S, Kaji M. Biochemical evidence for a deficiency of vitamin B6 in the carpal tunnel syndrome based on a crossover clinical study. *Proc Natl Acad Sci U S A* 1978;75(7):3410-2.

5

Diversity of *Helicobacter Pylori cag*A and *vac*A Genes and its Relationship with Clinical Outcomes in Azerbaijan, Iran

Reza Ghotaslou[1,2], Morteza Milani[1,2]*, Mohammad Taghi Akhi[2], Mohammad Reza Nahaei[2], Alka Hasani[2,3], Mohammad Saeid Hejazi[4], Mohammad Meshkini[2]

[1] *Liver and Gastroenterology Diseases Research Center, Tabriz University of Medical Sciences, Tabriz, Iran.*

[2] *Department of Microbiology, School of Medicine, Tabriz University of Medical Sciences, Tabriz, Iran.*

[3] *Infectious Diseases and Tropical Medicine Research Centre, Tabriz University of Medical Sciences, Tabriz, Iran.*

[4] *Department of Pharmaceutical Biotechnology, School of Pharmacy, Tabriz University of Medical Sciences, Tabriz, Iran.*

ARTICLE INFO

Keywords:
cagA gene
H. pylori
vacA gene

ABSTRACT

Purpose: The purpose of this research was to analyze *cag*A and *vac*A genotypes status in *H. pylori* isolates and relationship with clinical outcomes. *Methods:* Gastric biopsy specimens were cultured for *H. pylori* isolation and *cag*A and *vac*A genes were detected in these isolates. Data were collected and the results were analyzed using $\chi 2$ and Fishers exact tests by SPSS software version. 16. *Results:* Of the total 115 *H. pylori* isolates, 79 (68.7 %) were *cag*A positive and 82 (71.3%) of isolates contained the s1 allele which 33 (28.7%) were subtype s2. s1m2 was the most frequent *vac*A allelic combination in the *H. pylori* isolates examined (63 cases), followed by s2m2 (31 cases), s1m1 (19 cases) and s2m1 (2 case). Strains *cag*A positive were more frequent in peptic ulcer diseases patients than non ulcer diseases patients, as 47 (59.5%) and 32 (40.5%), while *cag*A negative were low, as 15 (41.7%) and 21 (58.3%), respectively. *Conclusion:* We found that the *cag*A and *vac*A status were not related to clinical outcomes in this area. Overall, in the present study, *vac*A s1/m2, *cag*A-positive strains were predominant irrespective of clinical outcome, but s2/m1 was rare.

Introduction

Helicobacter pylori (*H. pylori*), is a gram negative bacterial species that colonizes the human stomach and has been associated with human for at least tens of thousands of years.[1] This bacteria is permanently colonizes gastric epithelial cells in approximately 25% of the population in developed countries and 70–90% in developing countries, whereas most infected individuals are asymptomatic. Chronic *H. pylori* infection in susceptible individuals is associated with a variable degree of mucosal damage ranging from mild gastritis and ulcer disease to gastric carcinoma and mucosa-associated lymphoid tissue (MALT) lymphoma.[2] Colonization with these bacteria is usually without clinical consequences, but increases the risk of developing peptic ulcer disease, gastric adenocarcinoma and lymphoma.[3]

The clinical outcome of *H. pylori* infection has been associated with bacterial virulence factors, host gastric mucosal factors, and the environment.[4] It is estimated that 50% of the world's population is infected with *H. pylori*, but the factors associated with different outcomes, such as non-ulcer dyspepsia (NUD), peptic ulcer disease (PUD) or gastric carcinoma, are unknown.[5] This diverse clinical outcome may be associated with the expression of virulence factors. The cytotoxin-associated gene (*cag*A), which is not present in every *H. pylori* strain, is considered to be a marker for the cag pathogenicity island, and its expression is associated with severe infection.[6,7] In contrast, the vacuolating cytotoxin gene (*vac*A) is present in most *H. pylori* strains, although the VacA toxin may not be expressed in all cases.[8] The *vac*A gene contains a signal region and a middle region, both of which are divided into two allelic types: s1 or s2, and m1 or m2, respectively. These types are divided into the subtypes s1a, s1b or s1c, and m2a or m2b. Both s1/m1 and *cag*A-positive strains have been reported to be associated with PUD and gastric carcinoma.[9] The purpose of this research was to analyze *cag*A and *vac*A genotypes status in *H. pylori* isolates.

Materials and Methods
Patients

A total of 115 *H. pylori* isolates were obtained from gastric biopsies of patients with gastritis, peptic ulcer and gastroesophageal reflux diseases undergoing endoscopy. This study was approved by the ethical committee of regional Medical Research of Tabriz

*Corresponding author: Morteza Milani, PhD student of Bacteriology, Department of Microbiology, Faculty of Medicine, Tabriz University of Medical Sciences, Tabriz, Iran. Email: mohammadmilano@gmail.com

University of Medical Sciences and all patients provided written informed consent for this research.

H. pylori Culture and extraction of Genomic DNA

Briefly gastric biopsy samples were homogenized and cultured onto Brucella agar containing 5% sheep blood and antibiotics supplements. Culture plates were incubated at microaerophilic condition at 37 °C and high humidity for 5-7 days. Organisms were identified as H. pylori based on colony morphology, gram staining and positive oxidase, catalase and urease tests. Genomic DNA of total H. pylori strains was extracted by using CTAB[10] and stored at − 20 °C. Briefly, the loop full of bacteria was added to 1.5 ml sterile distilled water, vortexed well and was centrifuged in 1000 g for 10 min. The supernatant was discarded and 270 µl T/E buffer plus 30 µl SDS 10% plus 5 µl proteinase K was added to microtube and then incubated at 50 °C overnight. One hundred µl of 5 M NaCl solution was added to microtube and mixed well. Eighty µl of prewarmed CTAB/NaCl (65 °C) solution was added to microtube and vortexed well. Then the microtube was incubated at 65 °C for 10 minutes. Seven hundred µl of chloroform-isoamylalcohol (24:1) solution was added to the microtube and vortexed for 20 second. The suspension was centrifuged at 12000 g for 5-10 minute at 10 °C and aqueous phase was transferred into new microtube. Then, 200-300 µl isopropanol was added to each microtube and mixed gently, and incubated at -20 °C for 30 minute, finally centrifuged at 12000 g for 10 min. The supernatant was discarded and pellet was resuspended in 1 ml of 70% cold ethanol, and then centrifuged at 12000g for 5 min at 10 °C. The supernatant was discarded and after air drying, the DNA pellet was dissolved in 50 µl T/E (10:1) buffer and incubated at 37 °C for 30 min, then stored at 4 °C overnight.

Detection of cagA and vacA mosaicism distribution

In this study PCR was used to detect the H. pylori specific ureC gene for confirmation of H. pylori isolates, the virulence-associated vacA mosaic structure and the presence of cagA gene. All primer sets were selected from the published literatures (Table 1).[11,12] PCR reactions were performed in a volume of 50µL containing10mmol/L Tris-HCl, 1.5mmol/L MgCl$_2$, 0.2mmol/L of each deoxynucleotide, 25 pmol of each primer and 2.5 units of Taq polymerase (Geneone, Germany). PCR amplification conditions for cagA and glmM genes, involved 3 min of pre incubation at 94°C, followed by 35 cycles of 30 s at 94 °C, 30 s at 58 °C, and 30 s at 72 °C and 3min at 72°C for final extension. The vacA typing was performed with the following conditions: 3 min for pre incubation at 94 °C, followed by 35 cycles of 30 s at 94 °C, 30 s at 61 °C (for m1/m2), 50 °C (for s1/s2), 44 °C (for s1a), 52 °C (for s1b) for annealing, and 3 min at 72°C for final extension. PCR products were visualized by electrophoresis on 1.5% agarose gels with ethidium bromide. DNA from isolates with known genotypes was used as a positive control.

Table 1. Primers for amplification used in this study

DNA region amplified	Primer	Primer sequence	PCR products (bp)
ureC (glmM)	HP-F	GGATAAGCTTTTAGGGGTGTTAGGGG	294
	HP-R	GCTTACTTTCTAACACTAACGCGC	
cagA	cagA-Fm	AGG GAT AAC AGG CAA GCT TTT GA	352
	cagA-Rm	CTG CAA AAG ATT GTT TGG CAG A	
vacA-m1	ml -Fm	GGT CAA AAT GCG GTC ATG G	290
	ml -Rm	CCA TTG GTA CCT GTA GAA AC	
vacA-m2	m2-Fm	GGA GCC CCA GGA AAC ATT G	352
	m2-Rm	CAT AAC TAG CGC CTT GCA C	
vacA-s1 or s2	VA1-F	ATGGAAATACAACAAACACAC	259 or 286
	VA1-R	CTGCTTGAATGCGCCAAAC	
vacA-s1a	S1a-Fm	GTC AGC ATC ACA CCG CAA C	190
	S1a-Rm	CTG CTT GAA TGC GCC AAA C	
vacA-s1b	S1b-Fm	AGC GCC ATA CCG CAA GAG	187
	S1b-Rm	CTG CTT GAA TGC GCC AAA C	

Statistics analysis

Data were analyzed by SPSS version 16. The Pearson X^2 test was used to evaluate the relationship between individual genotypes and a variety of diseases. Logistic regression analysis was used to relate the different combinations of *vacA* and *cagA* genotypes of *H. pylori* to the presence of peptic ulcers.

Results

Fifty-three of our 115 patients were classified as non-ulcer diseases and, sixty-two patients had proven peptic ulcer disease based on observation during gastroscopy. There was no significant difference between the mean age of patients with and without ulcers. By using primers HP-F and HP-R to amplify the *ureC* gene, the expected PCR product of 294-bp was obtained in all strain isolates. Simultaneously using specific primers, *cagA* gene was detected in 79 (68.7 %) isolates.

In our study, strains carrying the *cagA* gene (*cagA*-positive) were more frequent in PUD patients than NUD patients, as 47 (59.5%) and 32 (40.5%), while

strains lacking *cagA* gene (*cagA*-negative) were low, as 15 (41.7%) and 21 (58.3%), respectively (Table 2 and 3).

In our study the presence of the *vacA* gene also was investigated in all of the isolates by PCR. Complete *vacA* s- and m-region genotypes were obtained in all samples. The majority of them (82 of 115; 71.3%) contained the s1 allele; most of them (80 of 82; 97.5%) were subtype s1a, and 2 of 82 (2.4%) were subtype s1b, However, 33 of 115 (28.7%) were subtype s2 (Figure 1). In this study, we did not find s1c. With regard to the middle region of 115 strains, 21(18%) samples were positive for the middle regions of the *vacA* genes (m1) and 94 (81.7%) were positive for the middle region (m2) by PCR. Meanwhile, PCR product size was 290 bp and 352 bp for m1 and m2, respectively.

Table 2. Distribution of *vacA* genotypes among 115 *cagA*-positive and *cagA*-negative *H. pylori* strains

Genotype	Number (%) of strains		Total (115)	Pv
	cagA-positive (n=79)	*cagA*-negative (n=36)		
s1/m1	19(100%)	0(0%)	19(16.5%)	0.005
s1/m2	53(84.1%)	10(15.9%)	63(54.8%)	0.001
s2/m1	0(0%)	2(100%)	2(1.7%)	0.005
s2/m2	7(22.6%)	24(77.4%)	31(26.9%)	0.001

Table 3. Relationship between clinical outcome and status of *cagA* and *vacA* genotypes by logistic regression analysis

Genotypes	Number (%) of isolates		Total (n=115)	Pv
	NUD (n=53)	PUD (n=62)		
*vac*As1	34(29.6%)	48 (41.7%)	82 (71.3%)	0.5
*vac*As1a	32 (27.8%)	47 (40.9%)	79 (68.7%)	1
*vac*As1b	1(0.9%)	1 (0.9%)	2 (1.8%)	1
*vac*As2	19 (16.5%)	14 (12.2%)	33 (28.7%)	0.1
vac*Am1	7 (6.1%)	14 (12.2%)	21 (18.3%)	0.3
vac*Am2	46 (40%)	48 (41.7%)	94 (81.7%)	0.1
*vac*As1m1	6 (5.2%)	13 (11.3%)	19 (16.5%)	0.1
*vac*As1m2	28 (24.3%)	35 (30.4%)	63 (54.8%)	0.1
*vac*As2m1	1 (0.9%)	1 (0.9%)	2 (1.8%)	0.1
*vac*As2m2	18 (15.7%)	13 (11.3%)	31 (27%)	0.1
*cag*A	32 (27.8%)	47 (40.9%)	79 (68.7%)	0.07

Discussion

The *cagA* gene is part of a 40 kb DNA insertion that is considered to have the typical features of a bacterial pathogenicity island (PAI) and may have originated from a non- helicobacter source. In the present study, 68.7% of the patients were infected with *cagA*-positive strains, similar to another Iranian study.[13] However,

this is different from studies from East to South Asian countries where more than 90% of the strains carry the *cagA* gene regardless of clinical outcomes.[14-16] Our result is consistent with studies reported from Europe and the USA where the prevalence of *cagA*-positive strains is between 60-70%.[9,17]

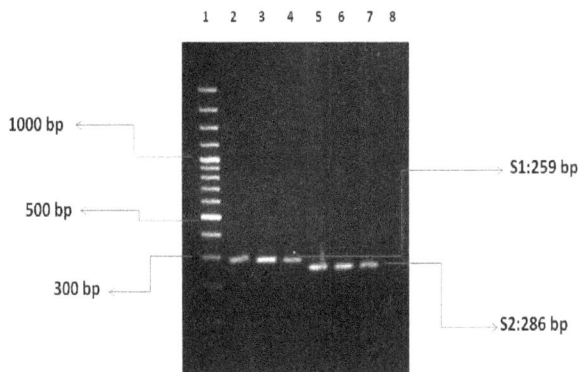

Figure 1. Amplified products of signal region alleles (S1 and S2) by PCR
Lane 1: 100-bp DNA ladder, Lane 2 and 3: S1 genotype *H. pylori*, Lane 4: S1 positive control of *H. pylori*, Lane 5 and 6: S2 genotype *H. pylori*, Lane 7: S2 positive control of *H. pylori*, Lane 8: negative control.

In this study, the relationship between *cag*A and clinical outcomes was assessed, and although we found that 59.5% of PUD and 40.5% of NUD patients were infected with *cag*A-positive strains, while this findings was not statistically significant (Pv > 0.05). This finding is in agreement with other reports from Iran,[18-20] but in contrast to many studies from Western countries where *cag*A positive strains are more often isolated from patients with PUD than with NUD.[21] For this difference in the *cag*A status, one possibility which exist is the large genomic variations in the *H. pylori* genomes (e.g., a PCR primer set) that amplifies the *cag*A gene of *H. pylori*.[22] There may be several distinct forms of the *cag*A gene with an uneven geographical distribution and these differences in *cag*A genotypes may provide a marker for differences in virulence among *cag*A-positive *H. pylori* strains and that only some forms of the *cag*A gene are associated with severe gastroduodenal diseases.[23]

All strains of *H. pylori* contain the *vac*A gene, but they vary in terms of their ability to produce cytotoxin.[24] Type s1 and m1 strains demonstrate more toxin activity than s2 and m2 strains.[11,25] The *vac*A genotypes are significantly different in each country. In Western studies, the presence of *vac*As1 and *cag*A has been shown to be significantly associated with peptic ulcers.[26] However, several studies in Asian populations have not confirmed this relationship, indicating that there are important geographic differences.[15] In this research, the frequency results of *vac*A alleles are in agreement with another study from Iran[27] which was reported frequency of s1, s2, m1 and m2 as 69%, 28%, 31% and 61%, respectively.

In our study, we evaluated the combination of *vac*A gene of different alleles in relation to clinical outcomes and no statistically significant correlation was found between these alleles and disease conditions (pv>0.05). In this study, predominance of s1 and s1m2 genotypes of *vac*A was observed in all clinical outcomes in patients which is in agreement with other studies from

Iran which showed s1 allele is associated with PUD, including DU and GU and also s1/m2 strain is dominant genotype among infected Iranian patients.[18,19,28-30] Similarly, s1/m2 genotype has been found to be predominant in Turkey and in Western countries.[31] However, the *vac*A s1/m1 genotype is more predominant from Afghanistan and India.[32,33]

In the present study, we examined the diversity of the *vac*A gene and the relationship between *vac*A genotypes and *cag*A status with clinical outcomes. The *vac*A s1/m1 genotype was the most virulent genotype, although the prevalence was even higher in PUD than in NUD patients (13 versus 6), but the differences were not statistically significant (Pv > 0.05). The prevalence of the s2/m2 genotype, which is reported to be less virulent, was even lower in PUD than in NUD patients (13 versus 18), but again the difference was not statistically significant (Pv > 0.05). We also analyzed the signal region and middle region separately, however, no significant relation was found between *vac*A s and m genotypes and clinical outcomes. There are many reports, that s1/m1 genotypes were associated with clinical outcomes such as PUD, whereas s2/m2 genotypes were associated with NUD.[34-36] However, we could not find any relationship between *vac*A genotypes and clinical outcomes. We found that s1/m2 was the most prevalent genotype irrespective of the clinical outcomes. Several studies have been published about the relationship between clinical outcomes and *vac*A and *cag*A status in Iranian populations,[29,30,37,38] where it has been concluded that the *vac*A genotypes are not a good marker for predicting clinical outcomes. In contrast, a study from Shiraz was reported that *vac*A genotypes were significantly different among gastritis, PUD and GC patients.[30] In addition, another study from Shiraz reported that *vac*A genotypes were more frequently found in PUD patients than in NUD patients;[37] since it is well known that almost all strains should possess the *vac*A gene, there finding are questionable.[37] The clinical relevance of the considered virulence- associated genes of *H. pylori* and geographical area is still a subject of controversy. The discrepancy between these reports may have several causes. First, patient selection is extremely important, and the study group should be sufficiently large and diverse with respect to genotypes and clinical symptoms. Second, the PCR assay and typing methods used should be adequate to determine the *vac*A and *cag*A genotypes.

Conclusion

In the present study relationship between *cag*A and *vac*A genotypes and clinical status was not found, which suggest that these genes are not helpful for the universal prediction of specific disease risk. Overall, we found that *vac*As1/m2, *cag*A-positive strains are predominant in our isolates irrespective of clinical outcome.

Acknowledgments
This project was financially supported by Liver and Gastrointestinal Diseases Research Center, Tabriz University of Medical sciences, Tabriz, Iran. This article was written based on a dataset of PhD thesis, registered in Tabriz University of Medical Sciences.

Conflict of interest
The authors report no conflicts of interest.

References
1. Ghose C, Perez-Perez GI, Dominguez-Bello MG, Pride DT, Bravi CM, Blaser MJ. East asian genotypes of helicobacter pylori strains in amerindians provide evidence for its ancient human carriage. *Proc Natl Acad Sci U S A* 2002;99(23):15107-11.
2. Milani M, Ghotaslou R, Akhi MT, Nahaei MR, Hasani A, Somi MH, et al. The status of antimicrobial resistance of Helicobacter pylori in Eastern Azerbaijan, Iran: comparative study according to demographics. *J Infect Chemother* 2012;18(6):848-52.
3. Suerbaum S, Michetti P. Helicobacter pylori infection. *N Engl J Med* 2002;347(15):1175-86.
4. McGee DJ, Mobley HL. Pathogenesis of helicobacter pylori infection. *Current opinion in gastroenterology* 2000;16(1):24-31.
5. Kim SY, Woo CW, Lee YM, Son BR, Kim JW, Chae HB, et al. Genotyping caga, vaca subtype, icea1, and baba of helicobacter pylori isolates from korean patients, and their association with gastroduodenal diseases. *J Korean Med Sci* 2001;16(5):579-84.
6. Catalano M, Matteo M, Barbolla R, Jimenez Vega D, Crespo O, Leanza A, et al. Helicobacter pylori vac a genotypes, cag a status and ure ab polymorphism in isolates recovered from an argentine population. *Diagn Microbiol Infect Dis* 2001;41(4):205-10.
7. Yamaoka Y, Kodama T, Kita M, Imanishi J, Kashima K, Graham DY. Relationship of vaca genotypes of helicobacter pylori to caga status, cytotoxin production, and clinical outcome. *Helicobacter* 1998;3(4):241-53.
8. Cover TL, Tummuru M, Cao P, Thompson SA, Blaser MJ. Divergence of genetic sequences for the vacuolating cytotoxin among helicobacter pylori strains. *J Biol Chem* 1994;269(14):10566-73.
9. Miehlke S, Kirsch C, Agha-Amiri K, Günther T, Lehn N, Malfertheiner P, et al. The helicobacter pylori vaca s1, m1 genotype and caga is associated with gastric carcinoma in germany. *Int J Cancer* 2000;87(3):322-7.
10. Sambrook J, Russell DW. Molecular cloning: A laboratory manual. 3rd ed New York: CSHL press; 2001.
11. Atherton JC, Cao P, Peek RM, Tummuru MKR, Blaser MJ, Cover TL. Mosaicism in vacuolating cytotoxin alleles of helicobacter pylori. *J Biol Chem* 1995;270(30):17771-7.
12. Van Doorn L, Figueiredo C, Rossau R, Jannes G, Van Asbroeck M, Sousa J, et al. Typing of helicobacter pylori vaca gene and detection of caga gene by pcr and reverse hybridization. *J Clin Microbiol* 1998;36(5):1271-6.
13. Jafarzadeh A, Rezayati MT, Nemati M. Specific serum immunoglobulin g to h pylori and caga in healthy children and adults (south-east of iran). *World J Gastroenterol* 2007;13(22):3117-21.
14. Tan HJ, Rizal AM, Rosmadi MY, Goh KL. Distribution of helicobacter pylori caga, cage and vaca in different ethnic groups in kuala lumpur, malaysia. *J Gastroenterol Hepatol* 2005;20(4):589-94.
15. Chomvarin C, Namwat W, Chaicumpar K, Mairiang P, Sangchan A, Sripa B, et al. Prevalence of helicobacter pylori vaca, caga, cage, icea and baba2 genotypes in thai dyspeptic patients. *Int J Infect Dis* 2008;12(1):30-6.
16. Datta S, Chattopadhyay S, Balakrish Nair G, Mukhopadhyay AK, Hembram J, Berg DE, et al. Virulence genes and neutral DNA markers of helicobacter pylori isolates from different ethnic communities of west bengal, india. *J Clin Microbiol* 2003;41(8):3737-43.
17. Van Doorn LJ, Figueiredo C, Megraud F, Pena S, Midolo P, Queiroz DM, et al. Geographic distribution of vaca allelic types of helicobacter pylori. *Gastroenterology* 1999;116(4):823-30.
18. Hussein NR, Mohammadi M, Talebkhan Y, Doraghi M, Letley DP, Muhammad MK, et al. Differences in virulence markers between helicobacter pylori strains from iraq and those from iran: Potential importance of regional differences in h. Pylori-associated disease. *J Clin Microbiol* 2008;46(5):1774-9.
19. Talebkhan Y, Mohammadi M, Mohagheghi MA, Vaziri HR, Eshagh Hosseini M, Mohajerani N, et al. Caga gene and protein status among iranian helicobacter pylori strains. *Dig Dis Sci* 2008;53(4):925-32.
20. Nahaei MR, Sharifi Y, Akhi MT, Asgharzadeh M, Nahaei M, Fatahi E. Heliobacter pylori caga and vaca genotypes and their relationships to peptic ulcer disease and non-ulcer dyspepsia. *Res J Microbiol* 2008;3(5):386-94.
21. Blaser MJ. Intrastrain differences in helicobacter pylori: A key question in mucosal damage? *Ann Med* 1995;27(5):559-63.
22. Miehlke S, Kibler K, Kim JG, Figura N, Small SM, Graham DY, et al. Allelic variation in the caga gene of helicobacter pylori obtained from korea compared to the united states. *Am J Gastroenterol* 1996;91(7):1322-5.
23. Zhou J, Zhang J, Xu C, He L. Caga genotype and variants in chinese helicobacter pylori strains and

relationship to gastroduodenal diseases. *J Med Microbiol* 2004;53(Pt 3):231-5.

24. Podzorski RP, Podzorski DS, Wuerth A, Tolia V. Analysis of the vaca, caga, cage, icea, and baba2 genes in helicobacter pylori from sixty-one pediatric patients from the midwestern united states. *Diagn Microbiol Infect Dis* 2003;46(2):83-8.

25. Ashour AA, Magalhaes PP, Mendes EN, Collares GB, de Gusmao VR, Queiroz DM, et al. Distribution of vaca genotypes in helicobacter pylori strains isolated from brazilian adult patients with gastritis, duodenal ulcer or gastric carcinoma. *FEMS Immunol Med Microbiol* 2002;33(3):173-8.

26. Atherton JC. The clinical relevance of strain types of helicobacter pylori. *Gut* 1997;40(6):701-3.

27. Jafari F, Shokrzadeh L, Dabiri H, Baghaei K, Yamaoka Y, Zojaji H, et al. Vaca genotypes of helicobacter pylori in relation to caga status and clinical outcomes in iranian populations. *Jpn J Infect Dis* 2008;61(4):290-3.

28. Dabiri H, Maleknejad P, Yamaoka Y, Feizabadi MM, Jafari F, Rezadehbashi M, et al. Distribution of helicobacter pylori caga, cage, oipa and vaca in different major ethnic groups in tehran, iran. *J Gastroenterol Hepatol* 2009;24(8):1380-6.

29. Siavoshi F, Malekzadeh R, Daneshmand M, Ashktorab H. Helicobacter pylori endemic and gastric disease. *Dig Dis Sci* 2005;50(11):2075-80.

30. Kamali-Sarvestani E, Bazargani A, Masoudian M, Lankarani K, Taghavi AR, Saberifiroozi M. Association of h pylori caga and vaca genotypes and il-8 gene polymorphisms with clinical outcome of infection in iranian patients with gastrointestinal diseases. *World J Gastroenterol* 2006;12(32):5205-10.

31. Saribasak H, Salih BA, Yamaoka Y, Sander E. Analysis of helicobacter pylori genotypes and correlation with clinical outcome in turkey. *J Clin Microbiol* 2004;42(4):1648-51.

32. Yamaoka Y, Kodama T, Gutierrez O, Kim JG, Kashima K, Graham DY. Relationship between helicobacter pylori icea, caga, and vaca status and clinical outcome: Studies in four different countries. *J Clin Microbiol* 1999;37(7):2274-9.

33. Chattopadhyay S, Datta S, Chowdhury A, Chowdhury S, Mukhopadhyay AK, Rajendran K, et al. Virulence genes in helicobacter pylori strains from west bengal residents with overt h. Pylori-associated disease and healthy volunteers. *J Clin Microbiol* 2002;40(7):2622-5.

34. Bolek BK, Salih BA, Sander E. Genotyping of helicobacter pylori strains from gastric biopsies by multiplex polymerase chain reaction. How advantageous is it? *Diagn Microbiol Infect Dis* 2007;58(1):67-70.

35. Kidd M, Lastovica A, Atherton J, Louw J. Heterogeneity in the helicobacter pylori vaca and caga genes: Association with gastroduodenal disease in south africa? *Gut* 1999;45(4):499-502.

36. Letley DP, Rhead JL, Twells RJ, Dove B, Atherton JC. Determinants of non-toxicity in the gastric pathogen helicobacter pylori. *J Biol Chem* 2003;278(29):26734-41.

37. Farshad S, Japoni A, Alborzi A, Hosseini M. Restriction fragment length polymorphism of virulence genes caga, vaca and ureab of helicobacter pylori strains isolated from iranian patients with gastric ulcer and nonulcer disease. *Saudi Med J* 2007;28(4):529-34.

38. Siavoshi F, Malekzadeh R, Daneshmand M, Smoot DT, Ashktorab H. Association between helicobacter pylori infection in gastric cancer, ulcers and gastritis in iranian patients. *Helicobacter* 2004;9(5):470.

6

Effect of *Phaleria macrocarpa* on Sperm Characteristics in Adult Rats

Saadat Parhizkar[1], Maryam Jamielah Yusoff[2], Mohammad Aziz Dollah[2]*

[1] *Medicinal Plants Research Centre, Yasuj University of Medical Sciences (YUMS), Yasuj, Iran.*

[2] *Biomedical Department, Faculty of Medicine and Health Sciences, University Putra Malaysia, Malaysia.*

ARTICLE INFO

Keywords:
Phaleria *macrocarpa*
Rats
Sperm Characteristics

ABSTRACT

Purpose: The purpose of this study was to determine the effects of *Phaleria macrocarpa* (PM) on male fertility by assessing its effect on the sperm characteristics which included the sperm count, motility, viability and morphology. *Methods:* Eighteen male rats were equally divided into three groups. Each group of rats was orally supplemented for 7 weeks either with PM aqueous extract (240 mg/kg), distilled water (0 mg/kg) or testosterone hormone, Andriol® Testocaps™ (4 mg/kg) respectively. On the last day of supplementation period, the rats were sacrificed and sperm was obtained from cauda epididymis via orchidectomy. The sperm count, motility, viability and morphology were determined. *Results:* PM aqueous extract significantly increased ($p<0.05$) the percentage of sperm viability. However, there was no significant effect of PM on the percentage of both sperm motility and morphology. The mean of body weight declined significantly in rats supplemented with PM aqueous extract compared to control groups ($p<0.05$). *Conclusion:* The results showed that PM significantly increased sperm viability without changing the sperm motility and morphology. Hence, this study suggests that PM offers an alternative way to improve male fertility by improving the sperm quality.

Introduction

Infertility is one of the most serious problems faced by some people around the world and the male counterpart contributes half of the infertility cases.[1] This problem is identifiable in about one out of thirteen couples who attempt to conceive.[2] According to United States Food and Drug Administration (FDA), infertility can be caused by androgen deficiency or low testosterone level. Testosterone deficit in men may exhibit symptoms such as decrease libido and erectile quality, low or zero sperm in semen, decrease body hair, decrease lean body mass and changes in mood.[3] The diagnostic testing can be done from the history, physical examination and of course, semen analysis.[2] The evaluation of infertility can aid in determining the underlying cause of infertility as well as giving treatment to allow conception to occur.[4] According to Schulte *et al.*,[5] sperm characteristics assessment has been increasingly important in reproductive studies. According to Concept Fertility Centre Kuala Lumpur,[6] approximately 13% of men have untreatable sterility, 11% have treatable conditions and 76% have disorders of sperm production or function which do not usually have clearly defined effective treatments. Medical practitioner initiates Testosterone Replacement Therapy (TRT) when clinical complaints are accompanied by testosterone decline. But, side effects may take place if TRT is used in excess amount. Some examples are nausea, acne, headache, fluid retention, liver toxicity, sleep apnea, tender breasts, polycytemia and prostate hyperplasia.[3,7] Over the past decades, herbal medicines have been accepted universally due to the various adverse reactions of hormone therapy. Traditional medicines continue to play an important role in healthcare system of a large number of world's population including Indian, Chinese, African, American and other people.[8-10] A National Centre for Complementary and Alternative Medicine has also been established in USA.[11]

Phaleria macrocarpa which is also known as mahkota dewa is an Indonesian herbal plant (Figure 1a, 1b) that was claimed to have various medicinal properties. Traditionally, Phaleria macrocarpa has been used to treat impotency, control cancer, haemorrhoids, diabetes mellitus, allergies, liver and heart disease, kidney disorder, blood diseases, acne, stroke, migraine and various skin diseases.[12] *Phaleria macrocarpa* has also been claimed to improve fertility in man, but its potential is still unknown. Besides that, there is still not enough scientific data to prove the claim to be true. Therefore the purpose of current study was to determine the effects of PM on male fertility by assessing its effect on the sperm characteristics.

*Corresponding author: Mohammad Aziz Dollah, Biomedical Department, Faculty of Medicine and Health Sciences, University Putra Malaysia, 43400 Serdang, Selangor, Darul Ehsan, Malaysia. Email: mohdaziz@medic.edu.my

Materials and Methods

Extraction of Phaleria macrocarpa

Phaleria macrocarpa (Voucher no. SK1929/11) fresh fruits were supplied by Associate Prof. Dr. Mohammad Aziz bin Dollah. 250 g of dried Phalera macrocarpa fruits slices were soaked in 4L of hot water boiled until the water become half. After that, the mixture solution was filtered and the filtrate was centrifuged at 3000rpm for 15minutes. The supernatant was freeze-dried to obtain crystal or powder form of the extract. The powder of the extract was weighted and kept in the freezer at -20 °C for later used. The extraction process was repeated till about 3kg of dried fruit slices was extracted.

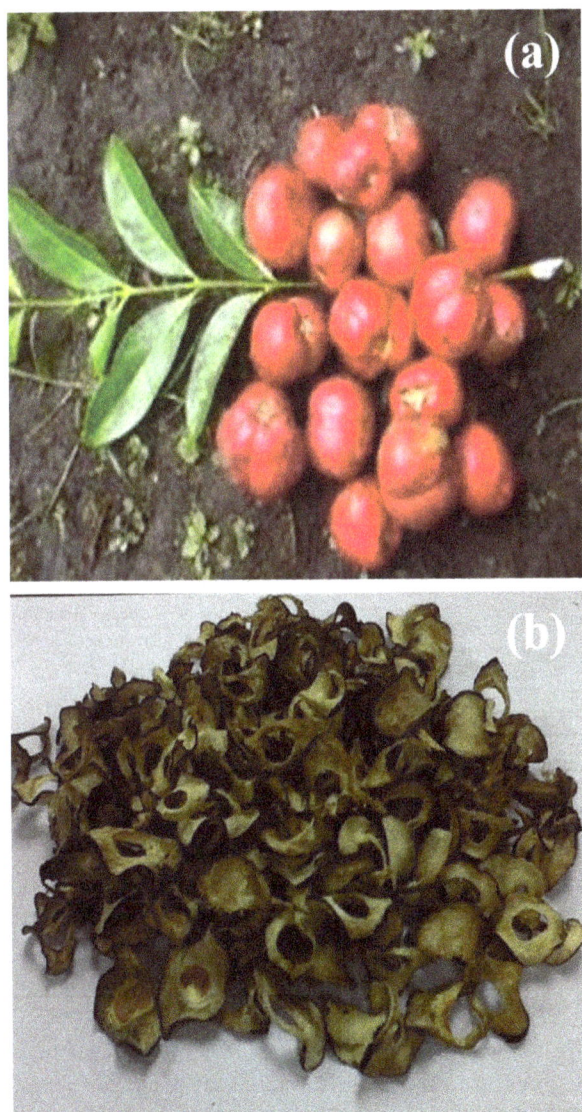

Figure 1. (a): *P. macrocarpa* fresh fruit. (b): *P. macrocarpa* dried fruit slices.

Working Solutions

There are three treatment groups in this study; negative control, positive control and supplemented with aqueous extract of *Phaleria macrocarpa*. In negative control, distilled water was used as supplement and in positive control; commercial testosterone drug (Andriol® Testocap™) was used as supplement. The *Phaleria macrocarpa* supplemented groups was given 240 mg/kg of aqueous extract of *Phaleria macrocarpa*. The *Phaleria macrocarpa* extract was weighted using electronic balance (AND GF3000) and reconstitute in distilled water. While the working solution for the commercial drug was used directly from the original product that was purchased from Schering-plough Sdn. Bhd. All of the working solutions were kept at -4 °C. The working solutions were prepared once a week to prevent any deactivation of the active compound in the extract and to maintain the quality of the working solution.

Experimental Animals

Eighteen Sprague Dawley male rats and ninety Sprague Dawley female rats with body weight 250-300 g, and two months old were used. They were kept in the animal house of Faculty Medicine and Health Sciences, University Putra Malaysia, under room temperature (29-32 °C), with 70-80% humidity, and automatic 12 hours light-dark cycle. The rats evaluated to be free from diseases and deformities. The rats were acclimatized for one week before starting treatments. They were group fed with pellet and drinking water was given *ad libitum*.

Experimental Design

Randomized experimental design with 3 supplementations was used for this study. Experiments were carried out according to the guidelines for the use of animals and approved by the Animal Care and Use Committee of the Faculty of Medicine and Health Sciences, University Putra Malaysia. The rats in each group were force fed with working solution according to their treatment groups (distilled water, 240 mg/kg Phaleria macrocarpa extract, Andriol® Testocap™) for seven weeks.

Parameters

Body Weight Measurement

The body weight of male rats were measured weekly by using electronic balance (Scaltec SBA5T) throughout the experiment period.

Cauda Epididymal Sperm Collection

Animals were killed after ether anaesthesia and the cauda epididymidis was quickly removed. The adherent fat, blood vessels and connective tissue were cut away and the organ from each animal was placed in a hollow plate that contained normal saline to wash out the blood. The cauda epididymidis were cut longitudinally with a pair of fine-pointed scissors and compressing with forceps. The sperm were released by mincing the cauda epididymis into pieces on the Petri dishes that contained phosphate buffer saline (PBS) for sperm characteristics analysis. Since epididymis came in pairs, one cauda epididymis was put in a Petri dish containing 10 ml of 0.1M PBS specifically for sperm count and sperm motility analysis while the other cauda epididymis was put in another Petri dish containing 1 ml 0.1M PBS for sperm viability and sperm morphology. The spermatozoa were allowed to flow out from cauda epididymis into the buffer. Then, the sperm suspensions were left at room temperature for 10 minutes for the suspension to allow sperm to swim out of the lumen of the cauda epididymidis for sperm characteristics analysis.

Sperm Characteristic Analysis
Sperm count analysis: Sperm count was determined using the haemocytometer under light microscope. A cover slip was placed on the haemocytometer before a drop with 10 µl of caudal epididymal sperm solution was loaded under the cover slip. The haemocytometer was placed under the light microscope and viewed under x400 magnification. Sperm count was done by counting 4×4 squares (horizontally or vertically) as shown in Figure 2. Sperm count was determined using the formula below as described previously by Rathje et al.[13]

Sperm count=total no. of sperm in 5 squares x 50,000 x 100 (cells/ml)

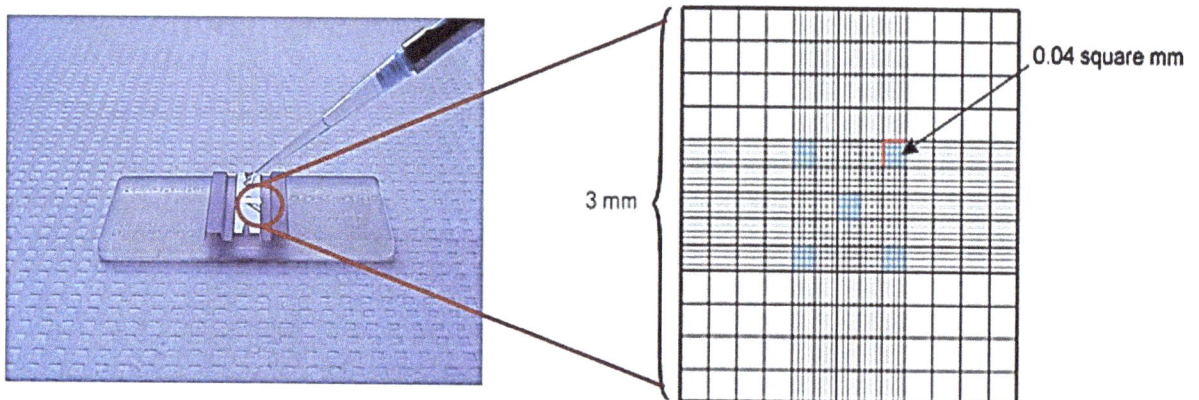

Figure 2. Haemocytometer showing the counting area (blue) for sperm count and motility.

Counting was only done for sperm heads that was found within the squares areas.
Sperm motility analysis: Haemocytometer was again used for sperm motility analysis. A cover slip was placed on the haemocytometer before a drop with 10 µL of caudal epididymal sperm solution was loaded under the cover slip. The haemocytometer was placed under the light microscope and viewed under x400. The light from the microscope was kept dim to reduce the

heat effect on the sperm which can reduce its motility and kill them. The sperm was counted when it entered the 4×4 squares (horizontally or vertically) according to its motility grade as shown in Table 1. Before statistically analysed, the raw data were tabulated in the form of percentage using the formula:

$$\text{Percentage of sperm for particular grade} = \frac{\text{no. of sperm for particular grade} \times 100\%}{\text{Total no of sperm from all grades}}$$

Table 1. Sperm Motility Characteristics.

Grade	characteristic
Grade 1	Sperm are immotile and fail to move.
Grade 2	Sperm known as non-progressive motility. They do not move forward despite the fact that they move their tail (vibrating-like movement).
Grade 3	Sperm known to have non-linear motility. They also move forward but tend to travel in a curved or crooked motion.
Grade 4	Sperm have progressive motility meaning that they are the strongest and swim fast in a straight line.

Sperm viability analysis: This analysis used the sperm from the other cauda epididymis that was put in a Petri dish with 1 ml 0.1M PBS. On a clean glass slide, 1 drop of sperm suspension was gently mixed with 3 drops of eosin using the sharp glass slide end. After 30 seconds, 1 drop of nigrosin was mixed together with the solution and a smear was made. The smear was then air-dried and observed under x200 magnification of imaging microscope. The sperm was counted based on the degree of membrane permeability. The dead sperm showed pink colouration of the head whereas the viable sperm showed whitish or colourless head. Before statistically analysed, the raw data were tabulated in the form of percentage using the following formula:

$$\text{Percentage of viable} = \frac{\text{No. of viable sperm} \times 100\%}{\text{Total no of dead and viable sperm} x}$$

Sperm morphology analysis: Sperm morphology analysis used the same sperm smear made for sperm viability analysis. This time, the sperm were observed under x400 magnification of imaging microscope to clearly evaluate the morphology of the sperm head, neck and tail. The sperm were generally classified as normal or abnormal without further characterized the types of abnormality found on the sperm. The normal sperm was given a score of 100 and the abnormal one will be given score of 0 to enable statistical analysis by using Statistical Analysis System (SAS) to be carried out easily.

Statistical Analysis

Data analysis was performed using Statistical Analysis System (SAS) version 9.2. Data of body weight, serum testosterone, mounting latency and mounting frequency were subjected to analysis of variance (ANOVA) to analyze the significant treatment effect and the mean between group was compared using Duncan Multiple Range Test if F value was significant at p<0.05.

Results
Body Weight

The means of rats' body weight supplemented with aqueous extract of *Phaleria macrocarpa* for 6 weeks period was shown in Table 2. The mean of body weights of the negative control, *Phaleria macrocarpa* and positive control groups before the study was 344, 317 and 310 g respectively, while at the end of the study, their mean body weights were 341, 321 and 342 g respectively. The ANOVA showed that the body weight was significantly affected (p<0.05) by the treatment. The mean of body weight for the rats supplemented with *P.macrocarpa* aqueous extract was significantly lower (p<0.05) than the control groups.

Table 2. Effects of distilled water, *P. macrocarpa* aqueous extract and Andriol® Testocaps™ supplementation on the body weight (mean ± SE) (g) of adult male rats.

Weeks	Treatment		
	Negative Control (Distilled water) (0 mg/kg)	Supplementation (*P.macrocarpa* aqueous extract) (240 mg/kg)	Positive Control (Andriol* Testocaps™) (4 mg/kg)
1	344.00 ± 7.61	317.00 ± 6.40	310.00 ± 9.68*
2	324.00 ± 7.68	287.00 ± 8.59**	359.00 ± 10.29*
3	305.00 ± 8.07*	342.00 ± 7.99	339.00 ± 8.92
4	368.00 ± 12.81	329.00 ± 5.68*	347.00 ± 8.49
5	343.00 ± 9.50	330.00 ± 6.56	323.00 ± 4.28
6	341.00 ± 10.00	321.00 ± 5.07*	342.00 ± 5.56
Total	337.00 ± 4.11	321.00 ± 3.88*	337.00 ± 4.87

Data are presented as Mean ±Standard Error of Mean
* indicate significant variation at p < 0.05
** indicate significant variation at p < 0.01

Sperm Count

The mean value of sperm count treated with distilled water (0 mg/kg), *P. Macrocarpa* aqueous extract (240 mg/kg) and Andriol® Testocaps™ (4 mg/kg) illustrated in Figure 3. The mean of sperm count is significantly highest in rats treated with 4 mg/kg Andriol® Testocaps™ (1112 million cells/ ml), followed by distilled water (712 million cells/ ml) and 240 mg/kg *P. macrocarpa* aqueous extract (707 million cells/ml). The results indicated that there was no significant difference between *P. macrocarpa* aqueous extract and negative control, while sperm count in positive control group was significantly different from those of *P. macrocarpa* aqueous extract and negative control.

Sperm Motility

Generally the percentage of motile sperm following treatment period did not change from baseline in all groups which illustrated graphically in Figure 4.

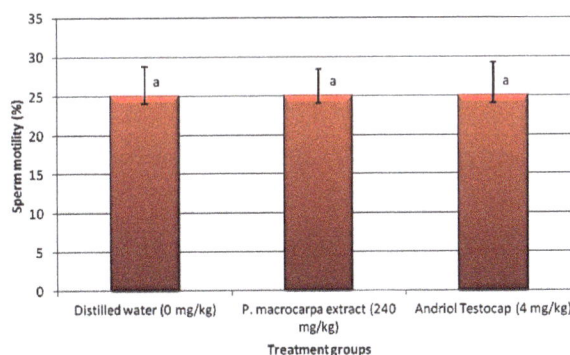

Figure 4. Means of motile sperm percentage in rats supplemented with *P.macrocarpa* aqueous extract and control groups for 6 weeks.
abc: different superscript indicated significance at p<0.05

However, grading of motility was done; the result showed that percentage of rats' motile sperm that treated with 240 mg/kg *P. macrocarpa* aqueous extract detected an increasing pattern from grade 1 to grade 3. Percentage of motile sperm with grade 3 from this group also was significantly higher than those control groups (p < 0.05). For grade 4 motility; there was no

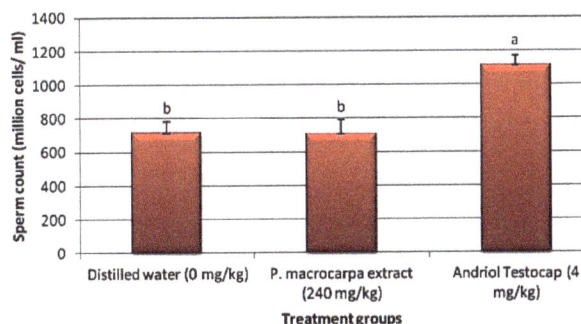

Figure 3. Means of sperm count in rats supplemented with *P.macrocarpa* aqueous extract and control groups for 6 weeks.
abc: different superscript indicated significance at p<0.05

significant difference between motile sperm percentage of *P. macrocarpa* aqueous extract and positive control group, but when compared with negative control group, the percentage of sperm treated with *P. macrocarpa* showed significant difference (p < 0.05).

Sperm Viability

The sperm viability in rats treated with *P. macrocarpa* aqueous extract (240 mg/kg) was significantly higher (p < 0.05) as compared to rats treated with distilled water (0 mg/kg). Whereas, there was no significant difference between rats treated with *P. macrocarpa* aqueous extract (240 mg/kg) and Andriol® Testocaps™ (4 mg/kg) (Figure 5). The percentage of sperm viability was significantly increased (p < 0.05) in response to 6 weeks treatment with *P. macrocarpa* aqueous extract and Andriol® Testocaps™ (65.26%, 37.22% and 70.46% for *P. macrocarpa*, distilled water and Andriol® Testocaps™ respectively) (Figure 6).

sperm morphology were 50% across all supplementation groups.

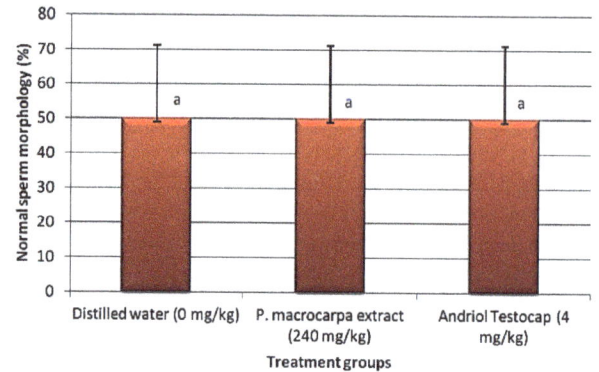

Figure 7. Percentage of normal sperm morphology in rats supplemented with *P.macrocarpa* aqueous extract and control groups for 6 weeks.
abc: different superscript indicated significance at p<0.05

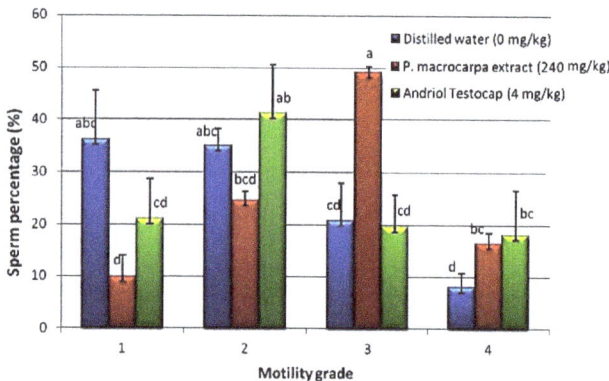

Figure 5. Means of sperm percentage in rats supplemented with *P.macrocarpa* aqueous extract and control groups according to motility grade.
abc: different superscript indicated significance at p<0.05

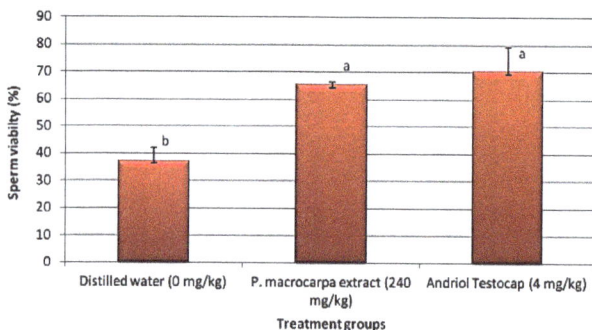

Figure 6. Means of viable sperm percentage in rats supplemented with *P.macrocarpa* aqueous extract and control groups for 6 weeks.
abc: different superscript indicated significance at p<0.05.

Sperm Morphology

The study showed that sperm morphology did not affect by treatment protocol and there was no difference in percentage of sperm morphology after 6 weeks supplementation by either *P. macrocarpa* or distilled water and Andriol® Testocaps™ (Figure 7 and Figure 8 a, b, c) and the percentage of normal

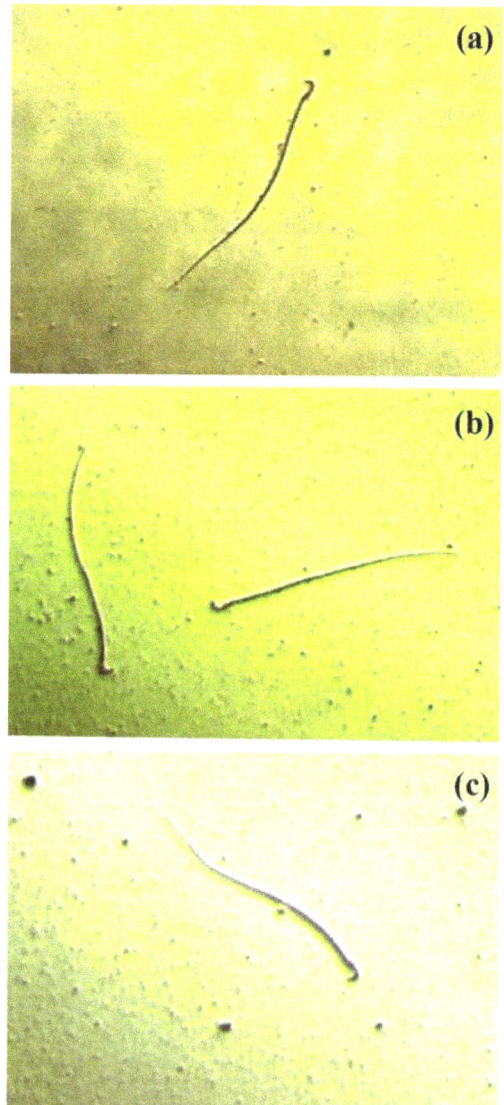

Figure 8. Normal sperm morphology observed (x 400) in male rats supplemented with **a)** distilled water **b)** *P. macrocarpa* (240 mg/kg) **c)** Andriol® Testocaps™ (4 mg/kg).

Discussion

This study aimed to evaluate the effect of *Phaleria macrocarpa* on sperm characteristics of adult rats during 7 weeks supplementation in comparison to either testosterone hormone as positive control or distilled water as negative control. In order to monitor the health condition of the rats, their body weight was measured every week. After 6 weeks of treatment, the mean of body weight for rats given 240 mg/kg *Phaleria macrocarpa* fruit aqueous extract was decline significantly as compared to both control groups. The reduction of body weight of rats supplemented with *Phaleria macrocarpa* might be due to its saponin content that has stimulatory effect on testosterone hormone. Gray *et al.*[14] reported that long-term treatment with high dose of testosterone reduce body weight gain and carcass fat content. Besides that, a study by Chong[15] showed that *Phaleria macrocarpa* significantly reduce body weight gain, total cholesterol, triglyceride, HDL and LDL and up regulated hepatic LDL receptor.

For the purpose of monitoring the fertility of rats, some andrological parameters f the Sprague Dawley rats were evaluated including sperm count, sperm motility, viability and morphology. The mean of sperm count of rats from *Phaleria macrocarpa* treated group showed no significant difference when compared with negative control group. The reduction seen in sperm count of rats treated with *Phaleria macrocarpa* can be due to the increase in mounting frequency in rats of the same group. This result is consistence with result found by Che Zairieha[16] who observed that the testosterone concentration level and mounting frequency was the highest in rats supplemented with *Phaleria macrocarpa*. Mounting frequency is a strong indicator of the occurrence of sexual performance. In addition, *Phaleria macrocarpa* contain saponin as one of its active compound. Saponin-rich extracts are able to improve the sexual performance as seen in rat model.[17]

In this study, sperm was collected from cauda epididymis, which is the primary sperm storage site prior to ejaculation. During the storage period, the cauda epididymis accumulates sperm to ensure that a sufficient number is available at the time of ejaculation.[18] During the seventh week of the treatment, the female rats were put in the cages of the male rats to enable the assessment of libido behavior. This assessment was carried out for five consecutive days. After 24 hours, the rats were sacrificed to obtain the sperm. This study design did not give the rats any sexual rest to allow the cauda epididymis to be sufficiently filled with mature sperm. Gloria *et al.*[19] also reported that sperm concentration in the cauda epididymis could depend on factors such as sexual rest and semen collection frequency. Besides that, there is a general agreement that semen volume and sperm concentration increase with prolonged sexual abstinence as reported by some scholars.[20-22] This

explained the lower sperm count retained in the cauda epididymis in *Phaleria macrocarpa* treated rats.

According to Oyeyemi *et al.*,[23] sperm motility is one of the most important indices determining the ability of a male to produce viable sperm. It is expressed in a percentage of all moving sperm in a sample. In this study, total mean percentage of motile sperm was not changed in all groups of treatments. The mean value of percentage of motile sperm was 25% across all treatment groups. This might be due to the sperm sampling which was collected from cauda epididymis. A study conducted by Gloria *et al.*,[19] reported that progressive motility for epididymal sperm was lower than ejaculated sperm. A correlation between mitochondrial activities and motile sperm has been shown using cytochemical techniques and flow cytometry. Hung *et al.*,[24] also showed rhesus macaques that ATP from mitochondria contributes to sperm motility. Besides that, the ejaculated sperm may have better progressive motility due to the presence of fructose in the fluid secreted by seminal vesicle. Fructose is the simple sugar that acts as the energy source for the sperm to keep swimming in its journey to fertilize an ovum. To compare, fluid from epididymis only allow sperm to survive for a few weeks instead of keeping them motile.

However, the increasing pattern of the percentage of motile sperm from grade 1 to grade 3 motility for rats supplemented with *Phaleria macrocarpa* indicated favorable effect of *Phaleria macrocarpa* in exerting motility of sperm compared to the negative and positive control groups. In order to fertilize an ovum, an ideal sperm should at least have graded as 3. For grade 4 motility, the percentage of sperm for rats treated with *Phaleria macrocarpa* was significantly higher than distilled water group. This result indicated that *Phaleria macrocarpa* supplementation increased the sperm motility by increasing the percentage of the sperm with higher motility grade.

Viable sperm can be defined as sperm that is alive and capable of fertilizing an ovum. In motility analysis, grade 1 sperm are immotile and fail to move. But, in certain cases, immotile sperm are still viable. Therefore, in cases of low motility as well as to further confirm the status of viability of the sperm, viability analysis was carried out. By using the eosin-nigrosin staining method, the viable and dead sperm was able to be differentiated. According to Björndahl *et al.*,[25] this classification was based on the degree of membrane permeability of dead spermatozoa which heads showed pink or red coloration due to the breakage of the membrane.

Phaleria macrocarpa showed significant increase in percentage of viable sperm as compared to negative control group. This may be due to *Phaleria macrocarpa* potential in increasing secretion of testosterone hormone through the presence of saponin. This result is in agreement with Koumanov *et al.*,[26] who found that saponin has the potency to increase testosterone hormone level which is the principal male reproductive hormone and this hormone play a huge role that affects sperm quality.

The increase in percentage of viable sperm in rats given *Phaleria macrocarpa* was also parallel with the result from Che Zairieha[16] that found significantly highest testosterone concentration in *Phaleria macrocarpa* treated rats as compared to rats given distilled water and Andriol® Testocaps™. In addition, a study conducted by Nakayama et al.,[27] found that sperm ATP concentration in testosterone-injected group is higher than control group. Generally, the function of mitochondria is the production of energy in the form of ATP. According to Gloria et al.,[19] viability and mitochondrial activity were higher in epididymal sperm as compared to ejaculated sperm. Therefore, measurement of sperm ATP concentration may become a possible biochemical method to measure actual fertilizing potential of sperm.[28]

Morphology can be defined as the structure and form of organisms to include the anatomy, histology and cytology at any stage of its life history.[29] Several studies in the literature have reported that percentage of normal sperm morphology is an essential characteristic for in vivo fecundity and in vitro fertilization.[30] Most of these studies indicate that morphology is the best predictor among all of the sperm characteristics. Based on the result obtained, the percentage of normal sperm morphology was not affected across all treatment groups including the rats given *Phaleria macrocarpa*. This indicate that *Phaleria macrocarpa* maintain sperm morphology and does not cause any defect to the morphology of the sperm produced.

Conclusion
The study showed an increment in sperm characteristics in response to *Phaleria macrocarpa* without causing any defect to the morphology of the sperm produced. This indicated that *Phaleria macrocarpa* was at the safe level and did not have toxic effects on the sperm. Thus, it can be concluded that *Phaleria macrocarpa* offers an alternative way to improve male fertility by improving the sperm quality.

Conflict of Interest
The authors report no conflicts of interest.

References
1. Miyamoto T, Tsujimura A, Miyagawa Y, Koh E, Namiki M, Sengoku K. Review Article: Male Infertility and Its Causes in Human. *Adv Urol 2012;* 33(3):483-7.
2. Stahl PJ, Stember DS, Goldstein M. Contemporary Management of Male Fertility. *Annu Rev Med* 2012;63:181-6.
3. Jose-miller AB, Boyden JB, Frey KA. Infertility. *Am Fam Physician* 2007;75(6):849-56.
4. Kolettis PN. Evaluation of the subfertile man. *Am Fam Physician* 2003;67(10):2165-72.
5. Schulte RT, Ohl DA, Sigman M, Smith GD. Sperm DNA damage in male infertility: etiologies, assays, and outcomes. *J Assist Reprod Genet* 2010;27(1):3-12.
6. Concept Fertility Centre. Malaysia 2006; Available from: http://www.conceptfertility.com.my/.
7. Werner MA. New York Andropause Centre. 2012; Available from: http://www.andropausespecialist.com.
8. Akarele O. Medicinal Plants and primary care: An agenda for action. *Fitoterapia* 1988;59:355-65.
9. Brandt HD, Osuch E, Mathibe L, Tsipa P. Plants associated with accidental poisoned patients presenting at Ga-Rankuwa Hospital, Pretoria. *S Afr J Marine* 1995;9:57-9.
10. Koduru S, Grierson DS, Afolayan AJ. Ethnobotanical information of medicinal plants used for the treatment of cancer in the Eastern Cape province, South Africa. *Curr Sci* 2007;92(7):906-8.
11. Pearson NJ, Chesney MA. The National Center for Complementary and Alternative Medicine. *Acad Med* 2007;82(10):967.
12. Zhang YB, Xu XJ, Liu HM. Chemical constituents from Mahkota dewa. *J Asian Nat Prod Res* 2006;8(1-2):119-23.
13. Rathje TA, Johnson RK, Lunstra DD. Sperm production in boars after nine generations of selection for increased weight of testis. *J Anim Sci* 1995;73(8):2177-85.
14. Gray JM, Nunez AA, Siegel LI, Wade GN. Effects of testosterone on body weight and adipose tissue: role of aromatization. *Physiol Behav* 1979;23(3):465-9.
15. Chong SC, Dollah MA, Chong PP, Maha A. Phaleria macrocarpa (Scheff.) Boerl fruit aqueous extract enhances LDL receptor and PCSK9 expression in vivo and in vitro. *J Ethnopharmacol* 2011;137(1):817-27.
16. Che Zairieha CZ. Effect of phaleria macrocarpa in serum testosterone level and libido behavior in rats. Malaysia: Universiti Putra Malaysia; Unpublished Thesis. 2012.
17. Arletti R, Benelli A, Cavazzuti E, Scarpetta G, Bertolini A. Stimulating property of Turnera diffusa and Pfaffia paniculata extracts on the sexual-behavior of male rats. *Psychopharmacology (Berl)* 1999;143(1):15-9.
18. Sostaric E, Aalberts M, Gadella BM, Stout TA. The roles of the epididymis and prostasomes in the attainment of fertilizing capacity by stallion sperm. *Anim Reprod Sci* 2008;107(3-4):237-48.
19. Gloria A, Contri A, Amicis ID, Robbe D, Carluccio A. Differences between epididymal and ejaculated sperm characteristics. *Anim Reprod Sci* 2011;128(1-4):117-22.
20. Le Lannou D, Colleu D, Boujard D, Le Couteux A, Lescoat D, Segalen J. Effect of duration of abstinence on maturity of human spermatozoa nucleus. *Arch Androl* 1986;17(1):35-8.

21. Blackwell JM, Zaneveld LJ. Effect of abstinence on sperm acrosin, hypoosmotic swelling, and other semen variables. *Fertil Steril* 1992;58(4):798-802.

22. Pellestor F, Girardet A, Andreo B. Effect of long abstinence periods on human sperm quality. *Int J Fertil Menopausal Stud* 1994;39(5):278-82.

23. Oyeyemi MO, Ola-Davies OE, Oke AO, Idehen CO. Morphological changes in sperm cells during epididymal transit in West African dwarf bucks. *Trop Vet* 2000;18(3-4):207-12.

24. Hung PH, Miller MG, Meyers SA, Vandevoort CA. Sperm mitochondrial integrity is not required for hyperactivated motility, zona binding, or acrosome reaction in the rhesus macaque. *Biol Reprod* 2008;79(2):367-75.

25. Bjorndahl L, Soderlund I, Kvist U. Evaluation of the one-step eosin-nigrosin staining technique for human sperm vitality assessment. *Hum Reprod* 2003;18(4):813-6.

26. Koumanov F, Bozadjieva E, Andreeva M, Platonova E, Ankova V. Clinical trial of Tribestan. *Exp Med* 1982;4: 211-5.

27. Nakayama H, Hidaka R, Ashizawa K. Effects of testosterone injection on semen quality in boars during high ambient temperature. *Anim Reprod Sci* 1991;25(1):73-82.

28. Comhaire F, Vermeulen L, Ghedira K, Mas J, Irvine S, Callipolitis G. Adenosine triphosphate in human semen: a quantitative estimate of fertilizing potential. *Fertil Steril* 1983;40(4):500-4.

29. Industrial Reproductive Toxicology Discussion Group (IRDG) Guideline Document: Rat Sperm Morphology Assessment. 1-15.2000.

30. Nallella KP, Sharma RK, Aziz N, Agarwal A. Significance of sperm characteristics in the evaluation of male infertility. *Fertil Steril* 2006;85(3):629-34.

7

Gene Therapy, Early Promises, Subsequent Problems, and Recent Breakthroughs

Saeideh Razi Soofiyani[1,2], Behzad Baradaran[1,2]*, Farzaneh Lotfipour[3], Tohid Kazemi[2], Leila Mohammadnejad[2]

[1] Drug Applied Research Center, Tabriz University of Medical Sciences, Tabriz, Iran.

[2] Immonuology Research Center, Tabriz University of Medical Sciences, Tabriz, Iran.

[3] Faculty of Pharmacy, Tabriz University of Medical Sciences, Tabriz, Iran.

ARTICLE INFO

Keywords:
Gene therapy
Recombinant DNA technology
Viral vectors
Non-viral vectors

ABSTRACT

Gene therapy is one of the most attractive fields in medicine. The concept of gene delivery to tissues for clinical applications has been discussed around half a century, but scientist's ability to manipulate genetic material via recombinant DNA technology made this purpose to reality. Various approaches, such as viral and non-viral vectors and physical methods, have been developed to make gene delivery safer and more efficient. While gene therapy initially conceived as a way to treat life-threatening disorders (inborn errors, cancers) refractory to conventional treatment, to date gene therapy is considered for many non–life-threatening conditions including those adversely influence on a patient's quality of life. Gene therapy has made significant progress, including tangible success, although much slower than was initially predicted. Although, gene therapies still at a fairly primitive stage, it is firmly science based. There is justifiable hope that with enhanced pathobiological understanding and biotechnological improvements, gene therapy will be a standard part of clinical practice within 20 years.

Introduction

Gene therapy is a form of molecular medicine based on the insertion of a functional gene into cells to correct a cellular dysfunction or to provide a new cellular function.

Gene therapy was originally developed as a strategy to treat inherited monogenic disease such as cystic fibrosis, but now gene therapy is considered for many non–life-threatening conditions including those adversely affecting a quality of life of patient.[1-5]

The idea of gene therapy was introduced by Joshua Lederberg in 1963; but on the whole, research on human genetics did not hasten until the 1980s.[6-8]

Afterwards, the first FDA approved clinical gene therapy was doen by Anderson et al in 1990. In that study, a 4 years old girl with adenosine deaminase (ADA)deficiency was treated by transfecting the ADA gene into her white blood cells, resulting in remarkable improvements in her immune system.[6,9-11]

In 1990, Rosenberg et al used a retroviral vector to introduce the neomycin resistance marker gene into tumor-infiltrating lymphocytes obtained from 5 patients with metastatic melanoma. Then these lymphocytes were expanded in-vitro and later reinfused into the respective patients.

That was the first practice showed that that retroviral gene delivery was safe and practical, it led to many other studies.[6,10,12] Since 1990, more than 1700 clinical trials have been conducted using different techniques for gene therapy.[13]

Development of recombinant DNA technology made gene therapy possible between 1963 and 1990.

In comparison to other traditional medicine, a strong theoretical advantage of gene therapy is the possibility to achieve a long-lasting therapeutic effect in the target tissue by a single administration of the gene without systemic side effects.[1]

Gene therapy classification
Gene therapy may be classified into the two types:

Germ line gene therapy
In germ line gene therapy, Germ cells, i.e., sperm or eggs, are modified by the introduction of functional genes, which are integrated into their genomes. This would let the therapy to be heritable and carried on to later generations. If this should, in theory, be highly effective in counteracting genetic disorders and hereditary diseases, many jurisdictions prohibit this for application in human beings, at least for the present, for different technical and ethical reasons.[14,15]

*Corresponding author: Behzad Baradaran, Faculty of Medicine, Immunology Research Center, Tabriz University of Medical Sciences, Tabriz, Iran., Email: behzad_im@yahoo.com

Somatic gene therapy

In somatic gene therapy, the therapeutic genes are introduced into the somatic cells, or body, of a patient. Any modifications and effects will be limited to the individual patient only, and will not be inherited by the patient's offspring or future generations. The purpose of somatic gene therapy is to alter the genetic material of living cells in order to achieve therapeutic benefit to the individual.

Somatic gene therapy shows the mainstream line of current basic and clinical research, where the therapeutic DNA transgene (either integrated in the genome or as an external episome or plasmid) is used to treat a disease in an individual.[14,16,17] Somatic gene therapy is also being evaluated specifically to cure various kinds of cancer. With time, it is optimism that the number of diseases subject to treat by this gene therapy will increase drastically. Numerous trials are being conducted under the supervision of medical experts in the laboratories to make the most of this gene therapy.

Some scientists believe that somatic gene therapy is better than germ line gene therapy. Somatic gene therapy is easier to use in comparison to the germ line gene therapy. Moreover, it does not harm the germ cells and thus the genetic alterations are not passed. It cures the symptoms of the problem and not the root cause.[18,19]

Strategies in gene therapy

The progression in the field of gene therapy have developed into two different strategies: ex vivo and in vivo gene therapy.[20] Ex vivo gene therapy includes the harvesting of cells from a patient followed subsequently by genetically modification ex vivo in a laboratory. The genetically modified cells are usually amplified in number, then the transduced cells are returned to the patient.[12,15,21]

Ex vivo gene therapy is a new therapeutic strategy especially well- suited to targeting a specific organ rather than for treating a whole organism .Therefore the eye and visual pathways make a suitable target for this approach. With blindness still so prevalent worldwide, new strategies to treatment would also be widely applicable and an important advance in improving quality of life. Despite being a relatively new approach, ex vivo gene therapy has already gained significant progresses in the treatment of blindness in pre-clinical trials. Particularly, advances are being taken in corneal disease, glaucoma, retinal degeneration, stroke and multiple sclerosis through genetic re-programming of cells to replace degenerate cells and through more refined neuroprotection.[22]

But ex vivo gene therapy is far less useful when the target organ is internal such as the lung, heart or brain. The lack of immune response is an apparent advantage of ex-vivo gene therapy.[23]

In vivo gene therapy

Ex vivo gene therapy was not successful to treat internal disorders, because of that the concept of in vivo gene therapy was established. In vivo gene therapy is a strategy in which genetic material usually in the form of DNA, is applied to modify the genetic repertoire of target cells for therapeutic goals.

This technology is now being developed in clinical trials as a treatment for hereditary disorders, and is also being considered as a potential treatment of acquired diseases, including atherosclerotic arterial disease, restenosis after vascular interventions, and cardiacallograft rejection.[24-29]

Vectors

There are two general approaches to deliver genes into a cell: viral and non-viral.

Gene delivery mediated by viral vectors is referred to as transduction and gene delivery mediated by non-viral vectors is referred to as transfection.

Viral vectors are highly efficient at introducing genes but can create some safety risks.

Non-viral vectors are remarked to be much safer than viral vectors, but at present, they are somehow inefficient at transferring genes.[30-33]

Viral systems

Viral vectors, which can deliver genetic materials into host cells, are biological systems derived from naturally developed viruses. Viruses used in gene therapy have been modified to enhance safety, increase specific uptake, and improve efficiency.[34-36]

Viral vectors are derived from viruses with either RNA or DNA genomes and are shown as both integrating and non-integrating vectors.

The former promises of lifelong expression of the deficient gene-product.

Efficient gene transduction can also be attained from vectors that are maintained as episomes, particularly in non-dividing cells.

The viral vectors include RNA virus such as retrovirus and DNA virus such as adenovirus, Herpes simplex virus and Adeno-associated virus (AAV), and poxvirus (vaccine virus).[37]

The most commonly used DNA viral vectors are based on adenoviruses and AAVs. Though, there are some drawback in the safety and toxicity of these vectors and the size of the transfected genetic material.

Therefore, great warning should be exercised when using viral vectors for the treatment of human diseases, and this topic should be investigated further.[34,36]

Adenoviral vectors

Adenoviral vectors are belonged to the family of adenoviride.

Adenoviral vectors are DNA viruses, can be produced in high titers, and efficiently transfer transgene into both dividing and non-dividing cells. Human cells are suitable candidate for adenoviral mediated gene delivery. They remain episomal and direct transient gene expression. Cell division causes fast loss of transgene. The infectivity and expression of adenoviral vector is dependent on the expression of adenovirus specific receptors on the desirable cells and immune response.

The adenovirus envelope fiber protein is important in first attachment and penton protein is mediated in virus internalization.

The adenoviral vectors are currently used are highly immunogenic, so the short term expression of transgene is observed. In addition to elict inflammatory and toxic reaction in the host, immune response may decrease gene delivery efficiency by omitting transduced cells and limiting the readministrations by generation of neutralizing antibodies. In some disease such as cancer, immunological reactions may be beneficial for the host.

Adenoviral vectors are employed, where the high level of transgene expression is required, such as pathological condition like cancer and angiogenesis.[36-41]

Adeno-associated virus

Adeno-associated viruses (AAVs) are human parvoviruses that normally require a helper virus, such as adenovirus, to mediate a productive infection. Most studies to date have focused on AAV-2. There is no known disease associated with AAV infection making it an ideal candidate for gene therapy. AAV vectors have been shown to transduce cells both through both episomal transgene expression and by random chromosomal integration.[42-45]

Retroviral and Lentiviral Vector

Retroviral and Lentiviral vectors are RNA-viruses and belong to the family of retroviride. Retroviral vectors are based on Molomy murine leukemia virus (MoML) and they have been used in many clinical trails for the treatment of cancer, inherited and acquired monogenic disorders, and AIDS.[46]

Lentiviral vectors are based on human immunodeficiency virus-1 (HIV-1), non-human immunodeficiency (SIV), or feline immunodeficiency viruses(FLV). Lentiviral Vectors are efficient and stable gene transfer tool to various cells like stem cells. Minimizing the possibility of recombination among various viral genetic elements has increased the safety of Lentiviral vectors .This has been gained by involving less than %5 of the viral genome into the vector and generating self-inactivating vectors.[47-49]

Retroviral and Lentiviral vectors could lead to a stable integration of the transfected gene into the host genome and a long lasting expression of the transgene. A restriction of the Retroviral vectors is their relatively low titer, which decrease in vivo gene transfer efficiency. Retroviral vectors need to cross the nuclear membrane for integration and can only infect dividing cells. This is a limitation, so the Retroviral vectors are not suitable for non-dividing cell.[1]

Non-viral system

The limitation related to viral vectors have Inspired researchers to emphasize on non-viral systems. Several methods have been developed for the Non-virus-mediated delivery of genetic materials including non-viral vectors.

Non-viral vectors are safe, can be constructed and modified by simple methods, and show high gene encapsulation ability.

The non-viral vectors consist of naked DNA delivered by injection, liposomes (cationic lipids mixed with nucleic acids), nanoparticles, and other ways.

Though non-viral vectors can be produced in relatively large scale and are likely to present minimum toxic or immunological problems, now they suffer from inefficient gene delivery. Furthermore, expression of the foreign gene tends to be transient, precluding their application to many diseased states in which sustained and high-level expression of the transgene is needed.[33,36]

It is likely that future gene therapy protocols will use new innovations to improve on the efficiency of non-viral vector systems, often building upon observations from viral vector transduction. Non-viral vectors are remarked to be much safer than viral vectors, but at present, they are somehow inefficient at transferring genes.

Enhancment in efficiency have made naked DNA gene delivery a viable method for gene therapy.[37,50]

Evolution in non-viral gene delivery include

- Injection of naked DNA in muscle causes in-vivo cell transfection available.
- Electroporation increases uptake of injected plasmid DNA into muscle and skin.
- Intravascular transfer of plasmid DNA results in a very effective gene Delivery to hepatocytes.
- Tail vein pDNA delivery is an easy and effective method to liver cells transfect in mice and rats.[1]

Physical methods for gene delivery

Over the last decade, physical methods of plasmid delivery have evaluated the efficiency of non-viral gene delivery, in some cases reaching the efficiencies of viral vectors.[50]

Electroporation and other physical methods

Electroporation (EP) is an efficient and easy method to DNA transfer.

This method is relied on the principle that applying electric pulses across the cell membrane creates a trans membrane potential difference, allowing transient membrane permeation and facilitating the insertion of DNA through the destabilized membrane.

EP is a safe and possible treatment approach and has been used to deliver genes into the cells of skeletal muscles, tumors, brain, liver, skin, and other tissues. Among these experiments, 38% are related to cancer treatment.

In addition, genes related to immune response are mostly used in EP mediated tumor treatment.[51,52]

Ultrasound

Ultrasound can generally be used to deliver ultrasound energy directly to an object and to enhance the delivery of therapeutic drugs and genes.

Ultrasound can enhance gene delivery by altering vascular permeability in a method called sonoporation. Sonoporation has been applied in many tissues, including tumors, and has been used to deliver oligonucleotides and small interfering RNA (siRNA) to tumors.

In the treatment of prostatic tumors, microbubble and ultrasound have been applied to target siRNA to the androgen receptor.[53-55]

Hydrodynamic based method

The hydrodynamic based method brought efficient gene delivery and expression by fast injection of a large volume of DNA solution through the tail vein of an animal. But this technique may be harmful for the experimental animal.[56]

Gene gun

Gene gun immunization through the skin is a trustful and reproducible method of DNA vaccine delivery. This method can induce immune response against both infectious diseases causing agent sand cancer in animal models.

DNA delivery using this approach requires 205-250 times less DNA than the standard method of intramuscular delivery.

Furthermore, the gene gun immunization is a highly efficient method of achieving antigen presentation.[57]

Clinical Trials

More than 600 clinical trials using gene therapy have been done or are underway, with the enrollment of thousands of patients in the world wide .A portion of these trials (over 70%) are for cancer and are often carried out using end-stage patients. Lots of the clinical trials are in Phase I or II, with less than 1%in Phase III, and so, now there are no commercially approved gene therapy treatments.

Gene delivery into multi potent hematopoietic stem cells has received much attention because of its relevance for a wide variety of human diseases, ranging from hematological disorders to cancer.[58]

Retroviral vectors based on MLV were the first viral vectors to be administered - in a gene therapy trial and continue to be the used more.

The first clinical trial tried to treat SCID patients suffering from adenosine deaminase (ADA) deficiency, using retroviral vectors to transduce T lymphocytes.[59]

A main drawback for the field happened in September 1999, when a broadly publicized death resulting from a gene-therapy trial was reported.[60]

Jesse Gelsinger (an 18-year-old man), died in a clinical trial at the University of Pennsylvania which used a modified Ad5 vector to deliver the gene for ornithine decarboxylase, a deficient hepatic enzyme.

Regarding to an investigation by the university, Gelsinger died from a massive immune response to the Ad5 vector.

Luckily for the gene therapy field, less than 1 year after Gelsinger died, the first report of a remarkable success in gene therapy trial was published. In 2000, Cavazzana-Calvo et al in Paris described results from a study involving two children suffering from a severe combined immune deficiency disorder (SCID-XI), which had restricted them to life in an isolated environment.[11] These studies used a MOMLV vector to deliver a curative gene (γc cytokine receptor subunit) into the patients lymphocytes ex vivo, and after proliferation of the cells, returned them to the patients both patients were able to leave the hospital and resume normal lives. After that, several other patients were treated and cured in these studies. However, there was a downside of around 11 early patients treated with the MoMLV vector, 3 developed leukemia directly as a result of the gene-transfer procedure.[61]

In another clinical study, patients suffering from hemophilia B, a bleeding disorder caused by a deficiency of coagulation factor IX, were treated with AAV vectors expressing human factor IX.

These patients attended in a Phase I trial and received intramuscular injections of AAV vectors. Though only very low levels of secreted factor IX could be detected in the plasma of one patient, the treated patients represented some clinical benefits and a reduced intake of factor.

One of the earliest hopes of gene therapy approaches was the possibility of using viral vectors to either introduce a lethal gene to cancer cells or to boost the immune system so as to recognize the tumor cell as foreign furthermore to using viruses to transfer.[62,63]

Tumor suppressors, apoptotic inducers, suicide genes, and cytokines, another interesting approach to cancer gene therapy is to harness the lytic action of replicating viruses for tumor-specific killing.[64]

Immune responses to gene therapy vectors

Circumventing the immune response to the vector is a principle challenge with all vector types likely to induce an immune response, particularly those, like adenovirus and AAV, which express immunogenic epitopes within the organism. The first immune response happening after vector delivery emerges from the innate immune system, consisting in a rapid, inflammatory cytokines and chemokines secretion around the administration site.

This reaction is high with adenoviral vectors and somehow null with AAV.[65,66] It is noteworthy that plasmid DNA vectors, because of CpG stimulatory islets, also stimulate the innate immunity via the stimulation of TLR receptors on leukocytes.[67-69]

Acquired immune response leading to antibodies production and T lymphocytes activation also occurs within a few days after vector introduction. Capsid antigens are mostly responsible for specific immunity toward adenoviruses, and are also involved in the response against AAV.

Even, viral gene-encoded proteins can also be immunogenic.[70-73]

The pre-existing humoral immunity coming from early infections with wild-type AAV or Adenovirus could avoid efficient gene delivery with the corresponding vectors.[73,74]

Some parameters like route of administration, dose, or promoter type have been described as critical factors influencing vector immunity.[75]

Conflict of Interest
The authors report no conflicts of interest.

References

1. Lehtolainen P, Laukkanen MO, Ylä-Herttuala S. Biotechnology. in: Gene therapy. Vol. XI, Encyclopedia of Life Support Systems (EOLSS), 2005. Available at: [http://www.eolss.net].

2. Ehmann WC, Rabkin CS, Eyster ME, Goedert JJ. Thrombocytopenia in HIV-infected and uninfected hemophiliacs. Multicenter Hemophilia Cohort Study. *Am J Hematol* 1994;54(4):296-300.

3. Kay MA, Manno CS, Ragni MV, Larson PJ, Couto LB, Mcclelland A, et al. Evidence for gene transfer and expression of factor IX in haemophilia B patients treated with an AAV vector. *Nat Genet* 2000;24(3):257-61.

4. Mannucci PM, Tuddenham EG. The hemophilias-- from royal genes to gene therapy. *N Engl J Med* 2001;344(23):1773-9.

5. Culver K. Gene Therapy-A Handbook for Physicians. New York: Mary Ann Liebert Inc; 1994.

6. Blaese RM, Culver KW, Miller AD, Carter CS, Fleisher T, Clerici M, et al. T lymphocyte-directed gene therapy for ADA- SCID: initial trial results after 4 years. *Science* 1995;270(5235):475-80.

7. Friedmann T. A brief history of gene therapy. *Nat Genet* 1992;2(2):93-8.

8. Friedmann T, Roblin R. Gene therapy for human genetic disease? *Science* 1972;175(4025):949-55.

9. Sheridan C. Gene therapy finds its niche. *Nat Biotechnol* 2011;29(2):121-8.

10. Edelstein ML, Abedi MR, Wixon J, Edelstein RM. Gene therapy clinical trials worldwide 1989-2004-an overview. *J Gene Med* 2004;6(6):597-602.

11. Cavazzana-Calvo M, Hacein-Bey S, Yates F, De Villartay JP, Le Deist F, Fischer A. Gene therapy of severe combined immunodeficiencies. *J Gene Med* 2001;3(3):201-6.

12. Rosenberg SA, Aebersold P, Cornetta K, Kasid A, Morgan RA, Moen R, et al. Gene transfer into humans--immunotherapy of patients with advanced melanoma, using tumor-infiltrating lymphocytes modified by retroviral gene transduction. *N Engl J Med* 1990;323(9):570-8.

13. J Gene Med. Gene Therapy Clinical Trials Database. Available from: http://www.wiley.com/legacy/wileychi/genmed/clinical.

14. Strachan T, Read AP. Human Molecular Genetics. 3rd ed. New york: Garland Publishing; 2004.

15. Akhtar N, Akram M, Asif HM, Usmanghani K, Ali Shah SM, Rao SA, et al. Gene therapy, a review article. *J Med Plant Res* 2011;5(10):1812-7.

16. Brenner MK. Human somatic gene therapy: progress and problems. *J Intern Med* 1995;237(3):229-39.

17. Berg P, Singer MF. The recombinant DNA controversy: twenty years later. *Proc Nat Acad Sci USA* 1995; 92:9011-3.

18. Gould DJ, Favorov P. Vectors for the treatment of autoimmune disease. *Gene Ther* 2003;10(10):912-27.

19. Mountain A. Gene therapy: the first decade. *Trends Biotechnol* 2000;18(3):119-28.

20. Canver MC. Evaluation of the Clinical Success of Ex Vivo and In Vivo Gene Therapy. *J Young Invest* 2009;19(7):1-10.

21. Templeton, NS. Gene and Cell Therapy: Therapeutic Mechanisms and Strategies. New York: CRC Press; 2008.

22. Gregory-Evans K, Bashar AM, Tan M. Ex vivo gene therapy and vision. *Curr Gene Ther* 2012;12(2):103-15.

23. Rejali D, Lee VA, Abrashkin KA, Humayun N, Swiderski DL, Raphael Y. Cochlear implants and ex vivo BDNF gene therapy protect spiral ganglion neurons. *Hear Res* 2007;228(1-2):180-7.

24. Lafont A, Guerot C, Lemarchand P. Prospects for gene therapy in cardiovascular disease. *Eur Heart J* 1996;17(9):1312-7.

25. Crystal RG. The gene as the drug. *Nat Med* 1995;1:15-7.

26. Nabel EG. Gene transfer for vascular diseases. *Atherosclerosis* 1995;118(26):51-6.

27. Muller DW. Gene therapy for cardiovascular disease. *Br Heart J* 1994;72(4):309-12.

28. Crystal RG. The Gordon Wilson Lecture. In vivo gene therapy: a strategy to use human genes as therapeutics. *Trans Am Clin Climatol Assoc* 1995;106:87-99.

29. Wilson JM. Gene therapy for cystic fibrosis: challenges and future directions. *J Clin Invest* 1995;96(6):2547-54.

30. Cotrim AP, Baum BJ. Gene Therapy: Some History, Applications, Problems, and Prospects. *Toxicol Pathol* 2008;36:97-103.

31. Friedmann T. The Development of Human Gene Therapy. New York: Cold Spring Harbor Laboratory Press; 1999.

32. Kay MA, Glorioso JC, Naldini L. Viral vectors for gene therapy: the art of turning infectious agents into vehicles of therapeutics. *Nat Med* 2001;7(1):33-40.

33. Zhang C, Wang QT, Liu H, Zhang ZZ, Huang WL. Advancement and prospect of tumor gene therapy. *Chinese J Cancer Res 2011;30(3):182-8.*

34. Miller N, Vile R. Targeted vectors for gene therapy. *FASEB J* 1995;9(2):190-9.

35. Verma IM, Weitzman MD. Gene therapy: twenty-first century medicine. *Annu Rev Biochem* 2005;74:711-38.

36. El-Aneed A. An overview of current delivery systems in cancer gene therapy. *J Control Release* 2004;94(1):1-14.

37. Kaneda Y, Tabata Y. Non-viral vectors for cancer therapy. *Cancer Sci* 2006;97(5):348-54.

38. Verma IM, Weitzman MD. Gene therapy: twenty-first century medicine. *Annu Rev Biochem* 2005;74:711-38.

39. Benihoud K, Yeh P, Perricaudet M. Adenovirus vectors for gene delivery. *Curr Opin Biotechnol* 1999;10(5):440-7.

40. Brody SL, Crystal RG. Adenovirus-mediated in vivo gene transfer. *Ann N Y Acad Sci* 1994;716:90-101; discussion -3.

41. Kovesdi I, Brough DE, Bruder JT, Wickham TJ. Adenoviral vectors for gene transfer. *Curr Opin Biotechnol* 1997;8(5):583-9.

42. Muzyczka, N. Use of adeno-associated virus as a general tranduction vector for mammalian cells. *Curr Top Microbiol Immunol* 1992;158:97-129.

43. Duan D, Sharma P, Yang J, Yue Y, Dudus L, Zhang Y, et al. Circular intermediates of recombinant adeno-associated virus have defined structural characteristics reponsible for long-term episomal persistence in muscle tissue. *J Virol* 1999;73(1):8568-77.

44. Nakai H, Iwaki Y, Kay MA, Couto LB. Isolation of recombinant adeno-associated virus vector-cellular DNA junctions from mouse liver. *J Virol* 1999;73(7):5438-47.

45. Miao CH, Snyder RO, Schowalter DB, Patijn GA, Donahue B, Winther B, et al. The kinetics of rAAV integration in the liver. *Nat Genet* 1998;19(1):13-5.

46. Coffin J, Hughes SH, Varmus HE. Retroviruses. New York: Cold Spring Harbor Laboratory Press; 2000.

47. Vigna E, Naldini L. Lentiviral vectors: excellent tools for experimental gene transfer and promising candidates for gene therapy. *J Gene Med* 2000;2(5):308-16.

48. Bukrinsky MI, Haffar OK. HIV-1 nuclear import: in search of a leader. *Front Biosci* 1999;4:D772-81.

49. Naldini L, Blomer U, Gallay P, Ory D, Mulligan R, Gage FH, et al. In vivo gene delivery and stable transduction of nondividing cells by a lentiviral vector. *Science* 1996;272(5259):263-7.

50. Nie S, Xing Y, Kim GJ, Simons JW. Nanotechnology applications in cancer. *Annu Rev Biomed Eng* 2007;9:257-88.

51. Heller LC, Heller R. In vivo electroporation for gene therapy. *Hum Gene Ther* 2006;17(9):890-7.

52. Andre F, Mir LM. DNA electro transfer: its principles and an updated review of its therapeutic applications. *Gene Ther* 2004;11(Suppl 1):S33-42.

53. Newman CM, Bettinger T. Gene therapy progress and prospects: ultrasound for gene transfer. *Gene Ther* 2007;14(6):465-75.

54. Frenkel V. Ultrasound mediated delivery of drugs and genes to solid tumors. *Adv Drug Deliv Rev* 2008;60(10):1193-208.

55. Haag P, Frauscher F, Gradl J, Seitz A, Schafer G, Lindner JR, et al. Microbubble-enhanced ultrasound to deliver an antisense oligodeoxynucleotide targeting the human androgen receptor into prostate tumours. *J Steroid Biochem Mol Biol* 2006;102(1-5):103-13.

56. Liu F, Song Y, Liu D. Hydrodynamics-based transfection in animals by systemic administration of plasmid DNA. *Gene Ther* 1999;6(7):1258-66.

57. Fynan EF, Webster RG, Fuller DH, Haynes JR, Santoro JC, Robinson HL. DNA vaccines: protective immunizations by parenteral, mucosal, and gene-gun inoculations. *Proc Natl Acad Sci U S A* 1993;90(24):11478-82.

58. Kohn DB, Sadelain M, Dunbar C, BodineD, Kiem HP, Candotti F, et al. American Society of Gene Therapy (ASGT) ad hoc subcommittee on retroviral-mediated gene transfer to hematopoietic stem cells. *Mol Ther 2003;*8(2):180-7.

59. Blaese RM, Culver KW, Miller AD, Carter CS, Fleisher T, Clerici M, et al. T lymphocyte-directed gene therapy for ADA- SCID: initial trial results after 4 years. *Science* 1995;270(5235):475–80.

60. Raper SE, Chirmule N, Lee FS, Wivel NA, Bagg A, Gao GP, et al. Fatal systemic inflammatory response syndrome in a ornithine transcarbamylase deficient patient following adenoviral gene transfer. *Mol Genet Metab* 2003;80(1-2):148-58.

61. Fischer A, Abina SH, Thrasher A, von Kalle C, Cavazzana-Calvo M. LM02 and gene therapy for severe combined immunodeficiency. *N Engl J Med* 2004;350(24):2526-7.

62. Nielsen LL, Maneval DC. P53 tumor suppressor gene therapy for cancer. *Cancer Gene Ther* 1998;5(1):52-63.

63. Gottesman MM. Cancer gene therapy: an awkward adolescence. *Cancer Gene Ther* 2003;10(7):501-8.

64. Nettelbeck DM. Virotherapeutics: conditionally replicative adenoviruses for viral oncolysis. *Anticancer Drugs* 2003;14(8):577-84.

65. Worgall S, Wolff G, Falck-Pedersen E, Crystal RG. Innate immune mechanisms dominate elimination of adenoviral vectors following in vivo administration. *Hum Gene Ther* 1997;8(1):37-44.

66. Zsengeller Z, Otake K, Hossain SA, Berclaz PY, Trapnell BC. Internalization of adenovirus by alveolar macrophages initiates early proinflammatory signaling during acute respiratory tract infection. *J Virol* 2000;74(20):9655-67.

67. Yasuda K, Ogawa Y, Kishimoto M, Takagi T, Hashida M, Takakura Y. Plasmid DNA activates murine macrophages to induce inflammatory cytokines in a CpG motif-independent manner by complex formation with cationic liposomes. *Biochem Biophys Res Commun* 2002;293(1):344-8.
68. Yi AK, Krieg AM. Rapid induction of mitogen-activated protein kinases by immune stimulatory CpG DNA. *J Immunol* 1998;161(9):4493-7.
69. Roman M, Martin-Orozco E, Goodman JS, Nguyen MD, Sato Y, Ronaghy A, et al. Immunostimulatory DNA sequences function as T helper-1-promoting adjuvants. *Nat Med* 1997;3(8):849-54.
70. Chirmule N, Hughes JV, Gao GP, Raper SE, Wilson JM. Role of E4 in eliciting CD4 T-cell and B-cell responses to adenovirus vectors delivered to murine and nonhuman primate lungs. *J Virol* 1998;72(7):6138-45.
71. Molinier-Frenkel V, Gahery-Segard H, Mehtali M, Le Boulaire C, Ribault S, Boulanger P, et al. Immune response to recombinant adenovirus in humans: capsid components from viral input are targets for vector-specific cytotoxic T lymphocytes. *J Virol* 2000;74(16):7678-82.
72. Kafri T, Morgan D, Krahl T, Sarvetnick N, Sherman L, Verma I. Cellular immune response to adenoviral vector infected cells does not require de novo viral gene expression: implications for gene therapy. *Proc Natl Acad Sci U S A* 1998;95(19):11377-82.
73. Chirmule N, Propert K, Magosin S, Qian Y, Qian R, Wilson J. Immune responses to adenovirus and adeno-associated virus in humans. *Gene Ther* 1999;6(9):1574-83.
74. Cichon G, Boeckh-Herwig S, Schmidt HH, Wehnes E, Muller T, Pring-Akerblom P, et al. Complement activation by recombinant adenoviruses. *Gene Ther* 2001;8(23):1794-800.
75. Bessis N, Garciacozar FJ, Boissier MC. Immune responses to gene therapy vectors: influence on vector function and effector mechanisms. *Gene Ther* 2004;11 Suppl 1:S10-7.

8

GABAB Receptor Blockade Prevents Antiepileptic Action of Ghrelin in the Rat Hippocampus

Zohreh Ataie[1], Shirin Babri[1,2], Mina Ghahramanian Golzar[1], Hadi Ebrahimi[1], Fariba Mirzaie[1], Gisou Mohaddes[1,2]*

[1] Neuroscience Research Centre (NSRC), Tabriz University of Medical Sciences, Tabriz, Iran.

[2] Neuroscience Research Centre, Shahid Beheshti Universiy of Medical Sciences, Tehran, Iran.

ARTICLE INFO

Keywords:
Ghrelin
Hippocampus
Epilepsy
PTZ
CGP35348

ABSTRACT

Purpose: Ghrelin has been shown to have antiepileptic function. However, the underlying mechanisms by which, ghrelin exerts its antiepileptic effects are still unclear. In the present study; we investigated antiepileptic mechanism of ghrelin through GABAB receptors using CGP35348 (selective GABAB receptor antagonist). *Methods:* Male Wistar rats' hippocampi were bilaterally microinjected with the single dose or 10-day ghrelin (0.3 nmol/µl/side). CGP35348, GABAB receptor antagonist, (12.5 µg/µl/side) or saline injected into the dorsal hippocampus 20 minutes before ghrelin administration. Thirty min after ghrelin microinjection, a single convulsive dose of pentylenetetrazole (PTZ) (50 mg/kg) was injected intraperitoneally (i.p). Afterwards, seizure duration and total seizure score (TSS) were assessed for 30 minutes in all animals. *Results:* Our results demonstrated that acute and chronic intrahippocampal (i.h.) injection of ghrelin could significantly ($p<0.001$) attenuate the severity of seizures. Ghrelin 0.3 nmol/µl/side decreased duration of seizure significantly both in acute ($p<0.001$) and chronic ($p<0.01$) injections. The ghrelin antiepileptic effect was completely antagonized by GABAB blockade. The suppression of both duration and TSS induced by ghrelin in hippocampus was significantly ($p<0.001$) blocked by CGP35348 in PTZ-induced seizures. *Conclusion:* In summary, our findings suggest that GABAB receptors may mediate the antiepileptic action of ghrelin in the hippocampus. Therefore, it is possible to speculate that ghrelin acts in the hippocampus to modulate seizures via GABA.

Introduction

Epilepsy is one of the oldest neurological conditions known to humankind and as a major public health problem worldwide, it afflicts 0.5–1% of the population in industrialized countries.[1,2] There are many therapeutic strategies for epilepsy such as pharmaceutical agents, administration of gonadal steroids, neurotrophic factors, dietary interventions and hormones. The effects of hormones either peripheral or endogenous on the nervous system have been well-established.[3] Ghrelin is a brain-gut hormone, which is mainly produced by stomach.[4,5] Other tissues that express ghrelin include different hypothalamic nuclei such as arcuate nucleus, ventromedial nucleus, dorsomedial nucleus, paraventricular nucleus; ependymal layer of third ventricle, pituitary, hippocampus, immune cells, lung, placenta, kidney, ovary and testis.[6] Ghrelin receptor is located in hypothalamus nuclei, hypophysis, and different brain regions such as CA1, CA2, CA3 and

dentate gyrus of hippocampal formation, substantia nigra, ventral tegmental region, raphe nucleus, nodose ganglion and cortex.[6,7] Therefore, hippocampus could be a target for the central effects of ghrelin.[8]

Ghrelin is a multifaceted peptide hormone.[5] Ghrelin stimulates GH secretion, increases food intake, and decreases fat utilization.[9] Concerning ghrelin's behavioral effects, it has been reported that intracerebroventricular administration in rats induced anxiety and improved memory retention.[10] Recently, Obay etal 2007, demonstrated that dose-dependent ghrelin administration significantly delay the onset time of the first myoclonic jerk, generalized clonic seizure and tonic generalized extension, diminish the duration of tonic generalized extension and suppress the onset time of PTZ-induced seizures.[11] Moreover, activation of the ghrelin receptor results in the attenuation of seizures in pilocarpine-induced limbic seizures in rats.[12] Ghrelin protects against cell death

*Corresponding author: Gisou Mohaddes, Department of Physiology, Faculty of Medicine, Tabriz University of Medical Sciences, Tabriz, Iran.
Emails: mohaddesg@tbzmed.ac.ir, gmohades@yahoo.com

of hippocampal neurons in pilocarpine-induced seizures in rats and promotes the formation of spine synapses in the stratum radiatum of the CA1 subfield of the hippocampal formation.[7,13]

Epilepsy is thought to be due to an imbalance between glutamate mediated excitatory and GABAergic inhibitory networks, changes in ionotropic receptor function and composition, altered calcium-mediated second messenger activity, or altered endogenous anticonvulsant and neuroprotective activities.[14]

GABA is the major inhibitory neurotransmitter in the central nervous system (CNS) and as such plays a key role in modulating neuronal activity.[15] GABA acts on two types of receptors, namely $GABA_A$, the ligand-operated ion channels, and $GABA_B$, the G protein coupled metabotropic receptors. $GABA_A$ receptors are responsible for fast inhibitory postsynaptic potential (IPSP), whereas $GABA_B$ receptors cause slower IPSP.[16] Postsynaptic $GABA_B$ receptors trigger the opening of K^+ channels through the G subunits. This results in a hyperpolarization of the postsynaptic neuron. Moreover, $GABA_B$ activates Ca^{2+} sensitive K^+ channels and small conductance K^+ channels in rat hippocampal neurons.[15]

Ghrelin may exert modulatory effects on neurotransmission.[9] The possible involvements of GABA in the ghrelin-mediated effects have been previously shown. Orexigenic action and appetite stimulation of ghrelin, directly or indirectly is mediated through GABA.[9,17-19]

The present study was designed to investigate ghrelin possible antiepileptic mechanism through $GABA_B$ receptor using CGP 35348 (a selective $GABA_B$ receptor antagonist).

Materials and Methods
Chemicals and Drugs
Rat ghrelin, CGP3534 and PTZ were purchased from Tocris Bioscience (Bristol, UK). Ghrelin was dissolved in saline (1mg/100µl), and stocked at -20°C. Immediately before i.h. microinjection, ghrelin was diluted with 0.9% saline to give a final concentration of 0.3nmol/µl. The control group received equal amount of saline (1µl). CGP35348 was dissolved in saline (1mg/100µl) and i.h. injection of 12.5 µg/µl/side performed.

Animals and Treatment
The Regional Ethics Committee of Tabriz University of Medical Sciences approved all experimental procedures. Every effort was made to minimize the number of used animals and their suffering. Animals were obtained from the colony of Tabriz university of Medical Sciences. The experiments were performed in adult male Wistar rats (n=50) weighing 220-250 g at the beginning of experiments. They were housed in a temperature (22±2 °C) and humidity-controlled room. The animals were maintained under a 12:12-h light/dark cycle, with lights off at 8:00 p.m. Food and water

provided *ad libitum* except for the periods of behavioral testing. The behavioral testing was done during the light phase.

Surgery
Rats were implanted with bilateral canula aimed at the dorsal hippocampus. Before surgery, animals were anesthetized with i.p. injection of ketamine (60 mg/kg) and xylazine (12 mg/kg). The animals were mounted into a stereotaxic frame used to position the 22-gauge stainless steel guide canula in the dorsal hippocampus. Coordinates obtained from Paxinos and Watson brain atlas (mm from bregma: AP= -3.8; ML = ± 2.2; DV = -2.7).[20] The guide canula was anchored to the skull using stainless steel screws and acrylic cement. The animals were allowed 7 days recovery after guide canula surgeries before the behavioral test.

Microinjection Procedure
All microinjections were done slowly (1 µl/2 min) using a 5µl Hamilton syringe connected by Pe-20 polyethylene tube. The stainless steel injection needle (30 G) was cut to protrude 0.5 mm beyond the tips of the guide cannulae and left in place for 1 min after injection to allow diffusion of the solution and to prevent back flow.

Saline or ghrelin 0.3 nmol/µl were injected bilaterally in dorsal hippocampus for 10 day. At the tenth day, ghrelin was injected 30 min before intraperitoneally (i.p.) injection of PTZ with a single convulsive dose of 50 mg/kg.

CGP 35348 was used to evaluate the role of $GABA_B$ receptors in antiepileptic effect of ghrelin. The conscious animals were gently restrained by hand, the injection needle was inserted through the guide cannulae, and saline or CGP 35348 and ghrelin (0.3 nmol/µl), were sequentially injected. A twenty min interval between i.h. injection of receptor antagonist or saline and ghrelin was considered. Thirty minutes after the last microinjection, a single convulsive dose of PTZ (50 mg/kg) was administered intraperitoneally. The doses and administration schedule of antagonist were established in accordance with some earlier studies. The dose of ghrelin was obtained according to the lowest effective dose to inhibit seizure.[21] Microinjections were done between 9:00 and 12:00 a.m. to prevent variations determined by circadian rhythms.

Seizure Assessment
The rats were housed in Plexiglas cages (50 cm × 50 cm × 40 cm) after PTZ injection and their behavior was observed and videotaped for 30 min. The latency to seizure onset, duration, and severity of seizures were monitored as parameters of seizure in all animals. Then videotapes were reviewed, and detected seizures were scored based on Racine's scale as following: (0) normal, nonepileptic activity; (1) mouth and facial movements, hyperactivity,

grooming, sniffing, scratching, wet dog shakes; (2) head nodding, staring, tremor; (3) forelimb clonus, forelimb extension; (4) rearing, salivating, tonic clonic activity; (5) falling, status epilepticus.[22] Rats were assigned a seizure score (SS) for each 5 min interval over the course of the 30 min session, after which a mean SS was calculated for the entire 30 min session for each rat and referred as total seizure score (TSS).[23]

Experimental Design

After 7 days of recovery rats were randomly divided into five groups (n = 10) as follows:

- Group (saline): 1 µl/side saline i.h.
- Group (acute ghrelin): a single dose of 0.3 nmol/µl/side ghrelin i.h.
- Group (chronic ghrelin): 0.3 nmol/µl/side ghrelin i.h. for 10 days
- Group (saline + ghrelin): 1µl/side saline 20 min before 0.3 nmol/µl/side ghrelin i.h.
- Group (CGP35348 + ghrelin): 12.5 µg/µl/side CGP35348, 20 min before 0.3 nmol/µl/side ghrelin i.h.

Then, PTZ (50 mg/kg) was injected intraperitoneally 30 min after the administration of ghrelin or saline in all groups.

On completion of each experiment, the rats were sacrificed, their brains were removed, fixed in formalin, and injection sides were verified in coronal sections. Only animals with the correct injection sides were taken for a further analysis.

Statistical Analysis

Data are expressed, as means ± S.E.M. The statistical analysis of the data was carried out by one-way ANOVA-followed by Tukey's test. In all comparisons, $P < 0.05$ was considered significant.

Results

The Effect of Acute and Chronic Intrahippocampal Microinjection of Ghrelin on the Latency to Seizure Onset, Duration of Seizures and the Total Seizure Score in Epileptic Rats

As shown in Figure 1, a one-way ANOVA indicated that latency to seizure onset after microinjection of single dose and 10-day ghrelin (0.3 nmol/µl/side), was not significant.

The effect of acute and chronic microinjection of ghrelin on duration of seizures was determined. Single dose of ghrelin 0.3 nmol/µl/side decreased the duration of seizures and it was extremely significant ($p < 0.001$) with respect to saline group. Animals treated with ghrelin 0.3 nmol/µl/side for 10 days had also significantly ($p < 0.01$) reduced duration. But the difference in duration of seizure between acute and chronic ghrelin was not significant (Figure 2).

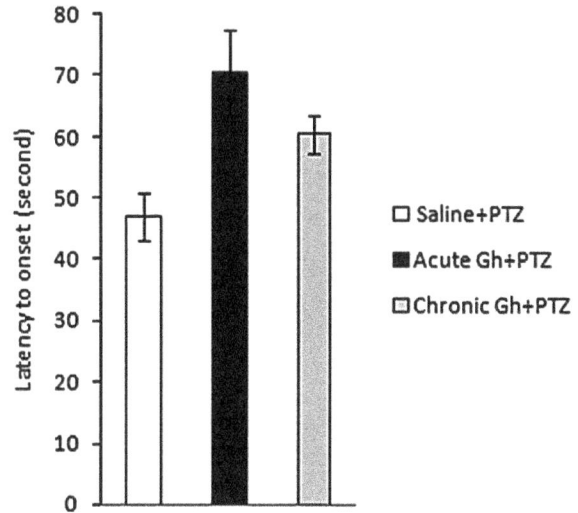

Figure 1. Effect of single dose and 10 days intrahippocampal microinjection of ghrelin (0.3 nmol/µl/side) on the latency to onset in PTZ-induced seizure. Results are expressed as mean ± SEM; n=10 animals per group.

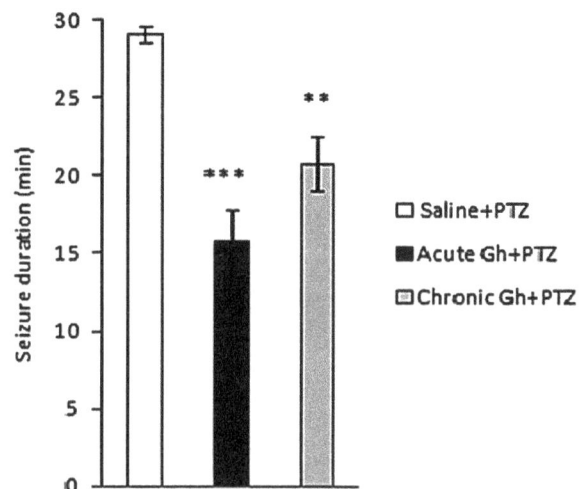

Figure 2. Effect of single dose and 10 days intrahippocampal microinjection of ghrelin (0.3 nmol/µl/side) on the duration in PTZ-induced seizure. Results are expressed as mean ± SEM; n=10 animals per group; ** $p < 0.01$, *** $p < 0.001$.

As illustrated in Figure 3, a repeated measure ANOVA revealed that ghrelin 0.3 nmol/µl/side could decrease total seizure score (scores during 30 minutes) significantly ($p < 0.001$) both in the single dose and 10 - day groups, compared with saline group.

The Effect of Intrahippocampal Microinjection of CGP35348 on the Latency to Seizure Onset, Duration of Seizures and Total Seizures Score in Epileptic Rats

Pre-treatment with CGP35348 (GABA$_B$ receptor antagonist), in dorsal hippocampus, 20 min prior to ghrelin administration reversed the antiepileptic effects of ghrelin. CGP35348 administration significantly prolonged duration of seizures ($p < 0.001$) (Figure 4) and intensified total seizure score ($p < 0.001$) (Figure 5). Intrahippocampal administration of CGP35347 alone did not induce convulsion (figure is not shown).

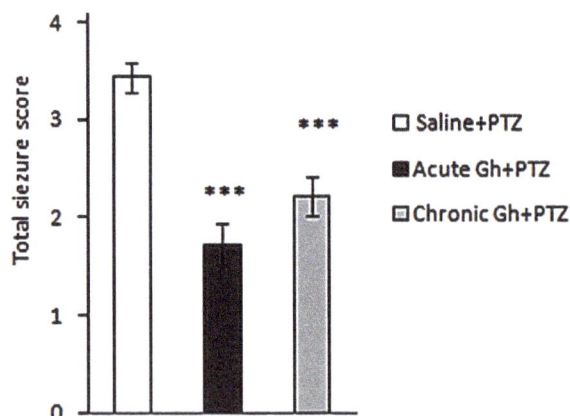

Figure 3. Effect of single dose and 10 days intrahippocampal microinjection of ghrelin (0.3 nmol/µl/side) on the total seizure score in PTZ-induced seizure. Results are expressed as mean ± SEM; n=10 animals per group, *** p<0.001.

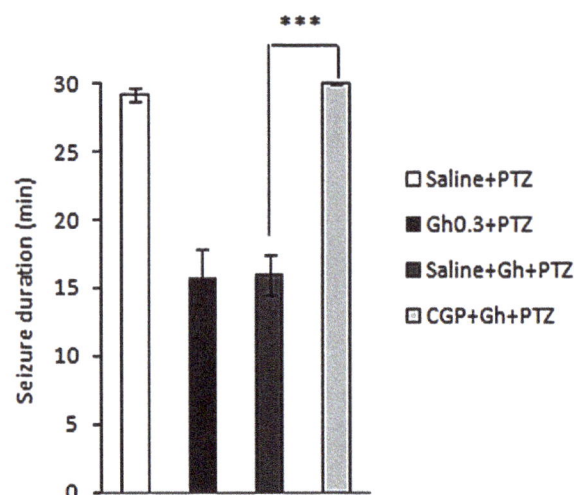

Figure 4. Effect of intrahippocampal injection of ghrelin preceded by CGP35348 (GABA$_B$ receptor antagonist) or saline on the duration of seizures during the 30-min post-PTZ behavior assessment. Results are expressed as mean ± SEM, n=10 animals per group; *** P<0.001.

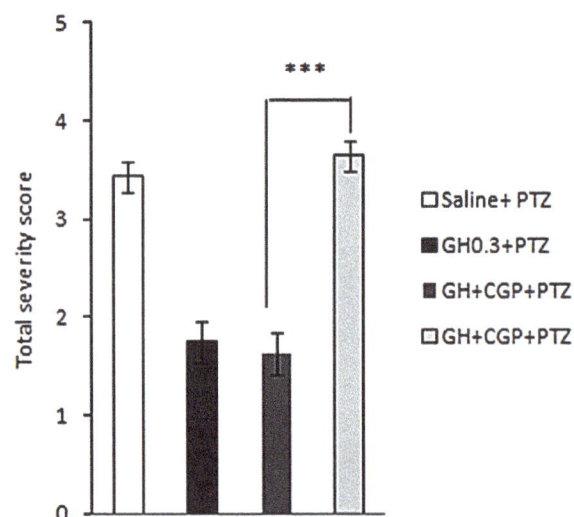

Figure 5. Effect of intrahippocampal injection of ghrelin preceded by CGP35348 (GABA$_B$ receptor antagonist) or saline on the total seizure score during the 30-min post-PTZ behavior assessment. Results are expressed as mean ± SEM, n=10 animals per group; *** P<0.001.

Discussion

In the present study, we assessed the antiepileptic effect of acute and chronic i.h. microinjection of ghrelin and one of the possible mechanisms of ghrelin action through GABA$_B$ receptors (CGP35348). To evaluate the contribution of specific receptor subtype to the anticonvulsant actions of ghrelin we used PTZ model of epilepsy. Our findings demonstrated that acute and chronic microinjection of ghrelin to dorsal hippocampus could significantly attenuate the severity and duration of seizures. In addition, our findings demonstrated that CGP35348, GABA$_B$ receptors antagonist, completely antagonized antiepileptic effects of ghrelin in the dorsal hippocampus.

Ghrelin is a peptide that expresses in a variety of tissues, and it plays a role in physiological and pathophysiological conditions.[4] Growth hormone release and stimulation of feeding] are the most known physiological functions for ghrelin.[6,10,24] Other findings indicate a role for ghrelin in mediating neuroprotective and behavioral responses. The neuroprotective action of ghrelin has been evidenced in different animal models of neuronal injury, such as cerebral ischemia/reperfusion neuronal loss, dopaminergic neurodegeneration and pilocarpine-induced hippocampal neuronal loss.[13,25] Ghrelin can also promote dendritic spine synapse formation and neurogenesis in adult rat.[7,26] Recently, it has been shown that ghrelin or its agonists have anti-epileptic action in rodents.[11,12,27] Our results in acute and chronic 10-day intrahippocampal administration of ghrelin are in accordance with Obay etal 2007 and Aslan etal 2009 studies. Therefore, ghrelin could be a potential benefit treatment for relieving the intensity of epilepsy and the hippocampal neuron demise caused by seizures.

A number of naturally occurring brain substances, such as GABA, adenosine, and the neuropeptides galanin and neuropeptide Y, may function as endogenous anticonvulsants and, in addition, may interact with the process of epileptogenesis. GABA is one of the main inhibitory neurotransmitters in the brain.[28] Focal augmentation of GABA in the limbic system is an obvious strategy for seizure control.[14]

GABA$_B$ receptors are G protein–linked receptors that hyperpolarize the neuron by increasing potassium conductance. GABA$_B$ receptors decrease calcium entry and have a slow inhibitory effect.[29] The involvement of GABA$_B$ receptors in controlling seizures has been reported in various models of epilepsy.[30] GABA$_B$ receptors are important in controlling partial or tonic – clonic seizures, despite their role in enhancing absence seizures.[31] Seizure disorders are often associated with a decreased efficacy of GABA receptor-mediated inhibition that is mainly mediated by two receptor subtypes (termed A and B) located pre- and postsynaptically on both interneurons and principal cells.[32] GABA$_B$ receptors are considered promising drug targets for the treatment of neurological and mental health disorders.[33] CGP 35348 is a selective

GABA$_B$ receptor antagonist and It is used as a tool in the studies of the role of GABA$_B$ receptors in brain.[34]

GABA mediates ghrelin action, in some areas of CNS. In mouse spinal cord slices, have been show that ghrelin significantly enhances inhibitory (GABAergic/glycinergic) neurotransmission.[35] In arcuate nucleus ghrelin hyperpolarizes POMC neurons that, likely mediated by the GABAergic NPY/AGRP neurons.[9] Circulating ghrelin enter the hippocampus, where specially has been shown to be a critical region for temporal lobe epilepsy, and bind to the hippocampal neurons.[3,13] It is possible that ghrelin affect epilepsy parameters through GABA$_B$ receptors.

Our findings showed that intrahippocampal administration of the GABA$_B$ receptor antagonist, CGP35348; prior to intrahippocampally administration of ghrelin antagonize the antiepileptic effect of ghrelin in PTZ-induced seizures in rats. Therefore, it is possible to speculate that ghrelin acts in the hippocampus to modulate seizures via GABA$_B$ receptor dependent mechanism. The anti-epileptiform effects of ghrelin may be due to the stimulation of GABA release. It is beneficiary to measure GABA level after ghrelin administration to prove that ghrelin acts through GABA release to control limbic seizures in dorsal hippocampus.

Conclusion

In conclusion in vivo, acute and repeated i.h. applications of ghrelin exert anticonvulsant properties on seizures of PTZ-induced model. The anti-epileptiform action of ghrelin was diminished by GABA$_B$ selective antagonist, CGP 35348. Therefore, these findings may imply on GABA$_B$ receptors participate in the anti-epileptiform activity of ghrelin.

Conflict of Interest

The authors report no conflicts of interest.

References

1. Strine TW, Kobau R, Chapman DP, Thurman DJ, Price P, Balluz LS. Psychological distress, comorbidities, and health behaviors among U.S. adults with seizures: results from the 2002 National Health Interview Survey. *Epilepsia* 2005;46(7):1133-9.
2. Luef G, Rauchenzauner M. Epilepsy and hormones: a critical review. *Epilepsy Behav* 2009;15(1):73-7.
3. Acharya MM, Hattiangady B, Shetty AK. Progress in neuroprotective strategies for preventing epilepsy. *Prog Neurobiol* 2008;84(4):363-404.
4. Leontiou CA, Franchi G, Korbonits M. Ghrelin in neuroendocrine organs and tumours. *Pituitary* 2007;10(3):213-25.
5. Kojima M, Kangawa K. Ghrelin: structure and function. *Physiol Rev* 2005;85(2):495-522.
6. Korbonits M, Goldstone AP, Gueorguiev M, Grossman AB. Ghrelin--a hormone with multiple functions. *Front Neuroendocrinol* 2004;25(1):27-68.
7. Diano S, Farr SA, Benoit SC, Mcnay EC, Da Silva I, Horvath B, et al. Ghrelin controls hippocampal spine synapse density and memory performance. *Nat Neurosci* 2006;9(3):381-8.
8. Carlini VP, Varas MM, Cragnolini AB, Schioth HB, Scimonelli TN, De Barioglio SR. Differential role of the hippocampus, amygdala, and dorsal raphe nucleus in regulating feeding, memory, and anxiety-like behavioral responses to ghrelin. *Biochem Biophys Res Commun* 2004;313(3):635-41.
9. Cowley MA, Smith RG, Diano S, Tschop M, Pronchuk N, Grove KL, et al. The distribution and mechanism of action of ghrelin in the CNS demonstrates a novel hypothalamic circuit regulating energy homeostasis. *Neuron* 2003;37(4):649-61.
10. Carlini VP, Monzon ME, Varas MM, Cragnolini AB, Schioth HB, Scimonelli TN, et al. Ghrelin increases anxiety-like behavior and memory retention in rats. *Biochem Biophys Res Commun* 2002;299(5):739-43.
11. Obay BD, Tasdemir E, Tumer C, Bilgin HM, Sermet A. Antiepileptic effects of ghrelin on pentylenetetrazole-induced seizures in rats. *Peptides* 2007;28(6):1214-9.
12. Portelli J, Aourz N, Ver Donck L, Michotte Y, Smolders I. Anticonvulsant effects of ghrelin receptor ligands against pilocarpine-induced limbic seizures. *Acta Physiologica* 2009;197:3.
13. Xu J, Wang S, Lin Y, Cao L, Wang R, Chi Z. Ghrelin protects against cell death of hippocampal neurons in pilocarpine-induced seizures in rats. *Neurosci Lett* 2009;453(1):58-61.
14. Boison D. Cell and gene therapies for refractory epilepsy. *Curr Neuropharmacol* 2007;5(2):115-25.
15. Bettler B, Kaupmann K, Mosbacher J, Gassmann M. Molecular structure and physiological functions of GABA(B) receptors. *Physiol Rev* 2004;84(3):835-67.
16. Sharma AK, Reams RY, Jordan WH, Miller MA, Thacker HL, Snyder PW. Mesial temporal lobe epilepsy: pathogenesis, induced rodent models and lesions. *Toxicol Pathol* 2007;35(7):984-99.
17. Riediger T, Traebert M, Schmid HA, Scheel C, Lutz TA, Scharrer E. Site-specific effects of ghrelin on the neuronal activity in the hypothalamic arcuate nucleus. *Neurosci Lett* 2003;341(2):151-5.
18. Chen HY, Trumbauer ME, Chen AS, Weingarth DT, Adams JR, Frazier EG, et al. Orexigenic action of peripheral ghrelin is mediated by neuropeptide Y and agouti-related protein. *Endocrinology* 2004;145(6):2607-12.
19. Abizaid A, Liu ZW, Andrews ZB, Shanabrough M, Borok E, Elsworth JD, et al. Ghrelin modulates the activity and synaptic input organization of midbrain

dopamine neurons while promoting appetite. *J Clin Invest* 2006;116(12):3229-39.

20. Paxinos G, Watson C. The Rat Brain in Stereotaxic Coordinates. 5th ed. Sydney: *Academic press;* 2004.

21. Ghahramanian Golzar M, Ataei Z, Babri S, Ebrahimi H, Mirzaie F, Mohaddes G. Effect of acute and chronic intrahippocampal microinjection of ghrelin on pentylenetetrazole-induced seizures in rats. *Pharm Sci* 2011;17(1):11-8.

22. Meurs A, Clinckers R, Ebinger G, Michotte Y, Smolders I. Seizure activity and changes in hippocampal extracellular glutamate, GABA, dopamine and serotonin. *Epilepsy Res* 2008;78(1):50-9.

23. Toscano CD, Ueda Y, Tomita YA, Vicini S, Bosetti F. Altered GABAergic neurotransmission is associated with increased kainate-induced seizure in prostaglandin-endoperoxide synthase-2 deficient mice. *Brain Res Bull* 2008;75(5):598-609.

24. Nakazato M, Murakami N, Date Y, Kojima M, Matsuo H, Kangawa K, et al. A role for ghrelin in the central regulation of feeding. *Nature* 2001;409(6817):194-8.

25. Guneli E, Onal A, Ates M, Bagriyanik HA, Resmi H, Orhan CE, et al. Effects of repeated administered ghrelin on chronic constriction injury of the sciatic nerve in rats. *Neurosci Lett* 2010;479(3):226-30.

26. Johansson I, Destefanis S, Aberg ND, Aberg MA, Blomgren K, Zhu C, et al. Proliferative and protective effects of growth hormone secretagogues on adult rat hippocampal progenitor cells. *Endocrinology* 2008;149(5):2191-9.

27. Aslan A, Yildirim M, Ayyildiz M, Guven A, Agar E. The role of nitric oxide in the inhibitory effect of ghrelin against penicillin-induced epileptiform activity in rat. *Neuropeptides* 2009;43(4):295-302.

28. Czapinski P, Blaszczyk B, Czuczwar SJ. Mechanisms of action of antiepileptic drugs. *Curr Top Med Chem* 2005;5(1):3-14.

29. Treiman DM. GABAergic mechanisms in epilepsy. *Epilepsia* 2001;42 Suppl 3:8-12.

30. Qu L, Boyce R, Leung LS. Seizures in the developing brain result in a long-lasting decrease in GABA(B) inhibitory postsynaptic currents in the rat hippocampus. *Neurobiol Dis* 2010;37(3):704-10.

31. Tsai ML, Shen B, Leung LS. Seizures induced by $GABA_B$-receptor blockade in early-life induced long-term GABA(B) receptor hypofunction and kindling facilitation. *Epilepsy Res* 2008;79(2-3):187-200.

32. Motalli R, D'antuono M, Louvel J, Kurcewicz I, D'arcangelo G, Tancredi V, et al. Epileptiform synchronization and GABA(B) receptor antagonism in the juvenile rat hippocampus. *J Pharmacol Exp Ther* 2002;303(3):1102-13.

33. Vigot R, Barbieri S, Brauner-Osborne H, Turecek R, Shigemoto R, Zhang YP, et al. Differential compartmentalization and distinct functions of $GABA_B$ receptor variants. *Neuron* 2006;50(4):589-601.

34. Olpe HR, Karlsson G, Pozza MF, Brugger F, Steinmann M, Van Riezen H, et al. CGP 35348: a centrally active blocker of $GABA_B$ receptors. *Eur J Pharmacol* 1990;187(1):27-38.

35. Ferrini F, Salio C, Lossi L, Merighi A. Ghrelin in central neurons. *Curr Neuropharmacol* 2009;7(1):37-49.

9

Synthesis, Characterization and Antimicrobial Activity of Certain Novel Aryl Hydrazone Pyrazoline-5-Ones Containing Thiazole Moiety

Maliki Reddy Dastagiri Reddy[1], Aluru Raghavendra Guru Prasad[2]*, Yadati Narasimha Spoorthy[1], Lakshmana Rao Krishna Rao Ravindranath[1]

[1] *Sri Krishnadevaraya University, Anantapur, A.P., India.*

[2] *ICFAI Foundation for Higher Education, Hyderabad, A.P., India.*

ARTICLE INFO

Keywords:
Pyrazoline-5-ones
Thiazole
Synthesis
Elemental analysis
Spectral analysis
Antimicrobial activity

ABSTRACT

Purpose: The aim of this article is to synthesize, characterize and evaluate the antimicrobial activity of certain novel 3-methyl-5-oxo-4-(phenyl hydrazono)-4,5-dihydro-pyrazol-1-yl]-acetic acid N^{l}-(4-substituted thiazol-2-yl)-hydrazides. *Methods*: The synthesized compounds were characterized by elemental analysis and IR, NMR and mass spectral data. The antimicrobial activity of novel compounds was evaluated by broth dilution method. *Results:* XVe, XVf and XVg have shown better antibacterial activity than other compounds of the series. XVa, XVc, XVd and XVe have shown better antifungal activity than the other compounds of the series. *Conclusion*: All compounds were found to exhibit fair degree of antimicrobial activity.

Introduction

Among nitrogen containing five membered heterocycles, pyrazolines and related heterocycles demonstrate various types of biological activities. The pharmaceutical importance of these compounds lies in the fact that they can be effectively utilized as antibacterial, antifungal, antidepressant, anti inflammatory, antioxidant, antiviral, antiparasitic, antitubercular and antitumor, insecticidal agents.[1-7] On the other hand the pharmacological properties of thiazoles have been well established. They also exhibit broad spectrum of chemotherapeutic properties such as antibacterial, antifungal and antitubercular, anti-HIV, anticonvulsant, anticancer, anti-inflammatory and analgesic.[8-14] Keeping in view the easily reproducible and feasible synthetic routes for synthesis and the importance of these two moieties namely, pyrazolines and thiazoles in the field of medicine, the authors have made an attempt to synthesize some novel compounds containing both these moieties and investigated for the possible antimicrobial activity.

Materials and Methods

All chemicals were obtained from Ranbaxy Laboratories Ltd, India. Nutrient broth, nutrient agar and 5 mm diameter antibiotic assay discs were obtained from Hi-Media Laboratories Limited, India. The standard bacterial and fungal strains were procured from National Centre for Cell Science (NCCS), Pune, India. UV/Visible Spectrophotometer manufactured by Shimadzu Corporation, Japan was used for absorption measurements.

General procedure for the synthesis of [3-methyl-5-oxo-4-(4^{l}-substituted aryl hydrazono)-4,5-dihydro-pyrazol-1-yl]- acetic acid N^{l}-(4-substituted thiazol-2-yl)-hydrazide XVa – h

Preparation of phenacyl bromides II a – g
Phenyl aryl bromides II a – g employed in the preparation of aryl hydrazono pyrazoline-5-ones containing substituted thiazole moiety XV were prepared by the reaction of various acetophenones I a – g with bromine in diethyl ether in presence of anhydrous aluminum chloride at 0 °C.

A solution of aromatic ketone I a–g (0.05 mole) in pure anhydrous diethyl ether (10 mL) was taken in a three necked flask fitted with mechanical stirrer and a thermometer. The solution was cooled to 0 °C and anhydrous aluminium chloride (50 mg) was added. Bromine (0.05 mole) was slowly added to the above solution. Excess of ether and hydrogen bromide were removed by applying suction. The solution was filtered and washed with petroleum ether. The crystals so obtained were washed with fresh portions of the solvent and recrystallized from minimum quantity of ethanol.

*Corresponding author: Aluru Raghavendra Guru Prasad, ICFAI Foundation for Higher Education, Hyderabad, A.P., India.
email:guruprasadar@yahoo.mail.com

Similar procedure was applied for the synthesis of other compounds II b – g of the series (Scheme 1). The substituted aryl bromides were characterized by their characteristic melting points reported in the literature.[15-19]

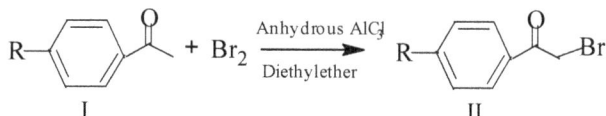

Scheme 1. Synthesis procedure of compounds II series. [R = H(IIa), -CH₃ (IIb), -OCH₃ (IIc), -OH (IId), -NO₂ (IIe), -Cl (IIf), -Br (IIg)]

Synthesis of 3-(4'-substituted phenyl)-4-bromoacetyl sydnone VIII a – c

Synthesis of N-substituted glycines (aniline acetic acid)[20,21] IV a – c: A mixture of substituted aniline (0.5 mole), ethylchloroacetate (73.0g) and anhydrous sodium acetate (49.2 g) in 120 mL of ethyl alcohol was refluxed on an oil bath (120 °C) for 6 hours. The reaction mixture was left overnight at room temperature and poured onto crushed ice. The precipitate formed was collected by filtration and dried. (ethyl ester of N-substituted glycine)

A mixture of ethyl ester of N-substituted glycine (0.4 mole) and sodium hydroxide (18 g) in 200 mL of water were refluxed for half an hour. The reaction mixture was cooled and acidified to a pH of 2 using hydrochloric acid. The precipitated N-substituted glycine was filtered, washed with cold water and recrystallized from ethyl alcohol.

Synthesis of N-nitroso-N-substituted glycines V a – c[20]: To a suspension of N-substituted glycine IV a–c (0.1 mole) in water (120 mL) at 0 °C, a solution of sodium nitrite (6.9 g, 0.1 mole) in water (24 mL) was added drop wise. After 2 hours, the reaction mixture was filtered and acidified with concentrated hydrochloric acid. The precipitate so formed was collected by filtration, washed with cold water, dried in air and recrystallized from aqueous alcohol.

Synthesis of 3-arylsydnone VI a – c[21]: N-nitroso-N-substituted glycine V a–c (0.1 mole) was heated with acetic anhydride (51 g) on a water bath for 3 hours. The reaction mixture was allowed to stand for 12 hours and poured into ice cold water, filtered and washed with water and then with 5% sodium bicarbonate solution. The solid obtained was washed with water, dried and recrystallized from benzene.

Synthesis of 4-acetyl-3-arylsydnone VII a – c[22]: To a suspension of phosphorous pentoxide (21.3 g, 0.15 mole) in thiophene (125 mL) taken in a three necked 500 mL round bottom flask fitted with reflux condenser equipped with a calcium chloride drying tube, 3-arylsydnone VI a – c (0.05 mole) was added. The magnetically stirred mixture was heated to reflux on a water bath. Glacial acetic acid (2.86 mL, 0.05 mole)

was added drop wise through a dropping funnel. The stirred reaction mixture was heated for 5 hours. The mixture was cooled to room temperature. Benzene present was decanted and the remaining black residue was washed with 20 mL of benzene. Washings and the decanted solution were evaporated to dryness to yield a pale yellow solid. The solid was recrystallized from ethyl alcohol.

Synthesis of 4-bromoacetyl-3-arylsydnones VIII a – c[23]: To a solution of 4-acetyl-3-arylsydnone VII a–c (0.01 mole) in 30 mL of chloroform, 1.6 mL (0.01 mole) of bromine was added under irradiation of visible light (40 Watt candle). After 15 minutes, solvent was removed under vacuum. The residue was recrystallized from ethyl alcohol.

The reaction sequence is shown in Scheme 2.

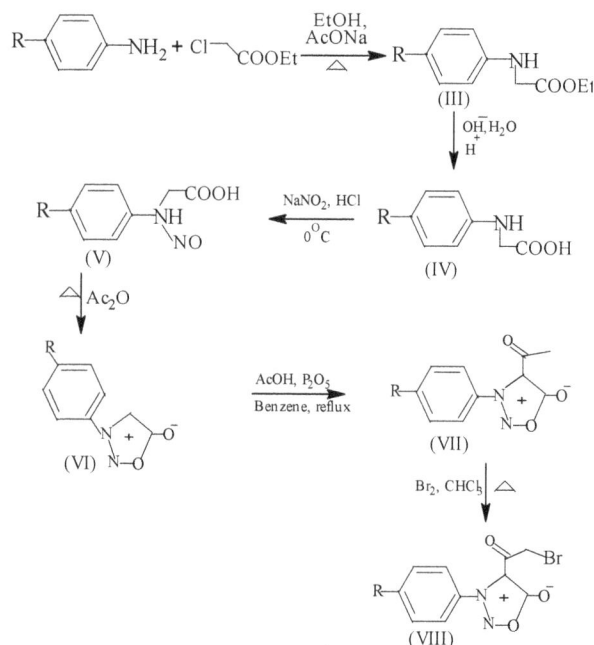

Scheme 2. Synthesis of 3-(4'-substituted phenyl)-4-bromoacetyl sydnone VIII. [R = -H(a), -CH₃(b), -OCH₃(c)]

Synthesis of 3-methyl-5-oxo-4-(phenyl hydrazono)-4,5-dihydro-pyrazol-1-yl]-acetic acid N'-(4-substituted thiazol-2-yl)-hydrazide XV a-h

Synthesis of substituted phenyl diazoniam chloride IX (A): The required primary amine was dissolved in a suitable volume of water containing 2.5 – 3.0 equivalents of hydrochloric acid (or sulphuric acid) by the application of heat if necessary. The solution obtained was cooled to 0°C to crystallize amine hydrochloride (or sulphate). An aqueous solution of sodium nitrite was added portion wise till there was free nitrous acid.

Synthesis of substituted phenyl diazonium ethyl acetoacetic ester (X): To a mixture of sodium acetate (1.0 g) in 100 mL of aqueous ethanol (50%) and a solution of ethylacetoacetate (0.1 mole) in 50 mL of ethanol at 0 °C, corresponding diazonium chloride was added slowly to get yellow crystals of X. The crystals were filtered, washed with water and dried.

Synthesis of 3-methyl-4-(phenyl hydrazono)-pyrozoline-5-one XI: Condensation of 4-substituted aryl hydrazono acetoacetic ester (X) and hydrazine in the presence of required amount of dimethyl formamide under microwave irradiation (microwave irradiation at 150W intermittently at 30 sec intervals for 2 minutes) led to the formation of 3-methyl-4-(4ᶦ-substituted arylhydrazono)-pyrozoline-5-one XI. After complete conversion as indicated by TLC, the reaction mixture was cooled by adding cold water. The precipitate XI was filtered and recrystallized from ethanol.

Synthesis of [3-methyl-5-oxo-4-(phenyl hydrazono)-4,5-dihydro-pyrazol-1-yl]-acetic acid ethyl ester XII: A mixture of XI, anhydrous K_2CO_3 and DMF was stirred at room temperature for 8 hours. The reaction mixture was diluted with ice cold water. The solid separated XII was filtered and recrystalized from ethanol.

Synthesis of [3-Methyl-5-oxo-4-(phenyl hydrazono)-4,5-dihydro-pyrazol-1-yl]-acetic acid hydrazide XIII: A solution of XII and hydrazine hydrate in ethanol were refluxed for five hours. The reaction mixture was cooled and poured onto ice cold water. The solid separated was filtered, washed with water and recrystallized from ethanol to give XIII.

Synthesis of thiosemicarbazone XIV: A mixture of [3-methyl-5-oxo -4-(phenyl hydrazono)-4,5-dihydro-pyrazol-1yl]-acetic acid hydrazide XIII (0.01 mole), potassium thiocyanate (0.02 mole), concentrated hydrochloric acid (1 mL), ethyl alcohol (10 mL) and water (20 mL) were refluxed for 3 hours. The solid obtained was filtered, washed with water, dried and recrystallized from ethanol-DMF mixture to give crystals of [3-methyl-5-oxo-4-(phenylhydrazono)-4,5-dihydropyrazol-1-yl]-acetothiosemicarbazone XIV.

Synthesis of [3-methyl-5-oxo-4-(phenyl hydrazono) 4,5-hydrazono)-4,5-dihydro-pyrazol-1-yl]-acetic acid Nᶦ-(4-substituted-thiazole-2-yl)-hydrazide XV: A mixture of [3-methyl-5-oxo-4-(phenyl hydrazono)-4,5-dihydro pyrazol-1-yl]-acetothiosemi-carbazone XIV (0.01 mole) in DMF (10 mL) and various bromoacetyl derivatives (0.01 mole) in ethanol (10 mL) was stirred at room temperature for about 2 hours. The solid separated was filtered, dried and recrystallized from ethanol-DMF mixture.
The above reaction of XIV with bromo acetophenone has been extended to *p*-tolyl, *p*-anisyl, *p*-hydroxy phenyl, *p*-nitrophenyl, *p*-chlorohphenyl, *p*-bromo phenyl, *N*-phenyl hydronyl, N-*p*-tolyl hydronyl, N-*p*-anisyl hydronyl substituents. The reaction sequence leading to the formation of these compounds is outlined in Scheme 3.

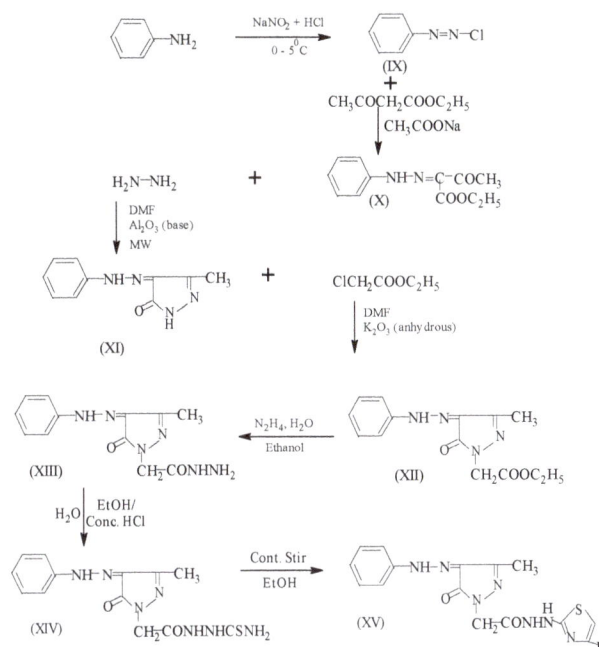

Scheme 3. Synthesis of [3-methyl-5-oxo-4-(phenyl hydrazono)-4,5-dihydro-pyrazol-1-yl]- acetic acid Nᶦ-(4-substituted thiazol-2-yl)-hydrazide XV. [R = Phenyl (XVA), *p*-Tolyl (XVb), *p*-Anisyl (XVc), *p*-Hydroxy phenyl (XVd), *p*-nitro phenyl (XVe), *p*-chloro phenyl (XVf), *p*-bromo phenyl (XVg), *p*-phenyl sydnonyl (XVh), *p*-tolyl sydnonyl (XVi), *N*-*p*-anisyl sydnonyl (XVj)]

Results and Discussion
The structure of critical intermediate compounds namely XIII, XIV and XV were characterized by elemental analysis and IR, NMR and mass spectra (Table 1).

Table 1. Characterization data of [3-methyl-5-oxo-4-(phenyl hydrazono)-4,5-dihydro-pyrayol-1-yl]-acetic acid hydrazide XIII.

Comp	MP (°C)	Yield (%)	Mol. formula	Found (%) (Cald)			
				C	H	N	O
XIII	152	65	$C_{12}H_{14}N_6O_2$	52.63 (52.55)	5.22 (5.14)	30.71 (30.64)	11.74 (11.67)

IR spectral details
The IR(KBr) spectra of [3-Methyl-5-oxo-4-(phenyl hydrazono)-4,5-dihydro-pyrazol-1-yl]-acetic acid hydrazide (XIII) showed absorption bands around 3445, 3425, (2 bands) 3305, 1620, 1665, 1460 and 1455 cm^{-1} due to – NH_2, >NH, exo >C = N, cyclic carbonyl and five membered heterocyclic ring respectively.
XIII: 3445, 3425 (NH_2), 3305 (NH), 1620 (C=N), 1665 (C=O).

¹H NMR spectral details
The ¹H NMR (200MHz) spectrum of [3-Methyl-5-oxo-4-(phenyl hydrazono)-4,5-dihydro-pyrazol-1-yl]-acetic acid hydrazide XIII was recorded in $CDCl_3$ + DMSO – d_6. The signal due to the methyl group appeared as a singlet at δ 1.0, integrating for three protons. The N-CH_2-CO protons came into resonance at δ3.85 as a singlet. The proton of NH-N = C has appeared as singlet at δ7.0. The NMR signal for CO-NH was

noticed at δ8.4 as a broad singlet. The NH_2 signal was observed at δ2.1 as a broad singlet. The aromatic protons of phenyl group have appeared at δ7.0 and δ7.14.

The characterization details of XIV are given below.

IR spectral details

The IR (KBr) spectra of XIV shows absorption bands around 3260, 1622, 1685, 1176, 2959 and 3180 cm^{-1} due to Ar-NH, C = N, C = O, C = S, C – H and NH functional groups respectively.

^{1}HNMR spectral details

The ^{1}HNMR (200MHz) spectra of XIV was recorded in CDCl$_3$+DMSO-d$_6$. The signals were noticed at δ2.29 (s, 3H, CH$_3$), δ δ3.3 (s, 2H, NH$_2$), δ4.80 (s, 2H, N-CH$_2$), δ 9.36 and δ 10.27 due to NH-NH group appeared as a two broad singlets, δ7.8 (s, 1H, Ar-NH), δ 7.4-7.6 (m, 5H, Ar-H).

Mass Spectral details

The mass spectrum of [3-methyl-5-oxo-4-(phenylhydrazono)-4,5-dihydro pyrazol-1-yl]-aceto thiosemicarbazone XIV exhibits the molecular ion peak (M$^+$) at m/z 347.

The fragmentation pattern noticed in mass spectrum of XIV is presented in Scheme 4. The molecular ion (M$^+$) was observed at m/z 347 (A, 23.7%). Disintegration (loss of NH$_2$ radical) of molecular ion (M$^{+\cdot}$) 'A' yielded the cation peak at m/z 331 (B, 15.7%). Elimination of CH$_3$CN molecule from molecular ion resulted in the fragment 'C' at m/z 306 (C, 31.5%). Expulsion of CSNH$_2$ radical from molecular ion 'A' produced the fragment 'D' at m/z 287 (D, 15.1%). Elimination of CSN$_3$H$_4$ radical afforded the cation 'E' at m/z 257 and was the base peak (100%). Disintegration (loss of C$_{11}$H$_{11}$N$_4$O radical) of molecular ion 'A' resulted in the cation 'F' at m/z 132 (F, 51.3%). The fragmentation pattern clearly supported the structure of XIV.

The characterization (Elemental analysis and spectral data) details of XV are given below.

IR spectral details

The IR (KBr) spectrum of 3-methyl-5-oxo-4-(phenyl hydrazono)-4,5-dihydro-pyrazol-1-yl]-acetic acid N$^|$-(4-phenyl thiazol-2-yl)-hydrazide XVa exhibited absorption band around 3230 cm^{-1} (C = Ostr), 1546 cm^{-1} (C = Nstr). Characterization data of compound XV is presented in Table 2.

IR Spectral data of [3-methyl-5-oxo-4-(phenyl hydrazono)-4,5-dihydro-pyrazol-1-yl]-acetic acid N$^|$-(4-substituted thiazol-2-yl)-hydrazide XV.

XVa: 3230 (NH), 2962 (CH), 1692 (C=O), 1546 (C=N)

XVc: 3240 (NH), 2868 (CH), 1687 (C=O), 1546 (C=N)

XVd: 3250 (NH), 2972 (CH), 1710 (C=O), 1552 (C=N)

XVe: 3260 (NH), 2980 (CH), 1720 (C=O), 1560 (C=N)

XVf: 3222 (NH), 2960 (CH), 1687 (C=O), 1548 (C=N)

XVh: 3276 (NH), 2930 (CH), 1690 (C=O), 1560 (C=N)

XVi: 3276 (NH), 2941 (CH), 1689 (C=O), 1559 (C=N) 1739 (sydnone C=O str).

XVj: 3269 (NH), 2910 (CH), 1681(C=O), 1541(C=N)

^{1}HNMR spectral details

The ^{1}HNMR (200MHz) spectra of [3-methyl-5-oxo-4-(phenyl hydrazono)-4,5-dihydro-pyrazol-1- yl]-acetic acid N$^|$-(4-substituted thiazol-2-yl)-hydrazide XV taken in CDCl$_3$ + DMSO-d$_6$ showed signals at δ2.23 (S, 3H.CH$_3$), δ4.90 (s, 2H, NCH$_2$CO), δ7.35 (s, H, thiazole, 4H), δ7.2 (s, H, Ar-NH), δ9.54 (s, H, NH), δ10.65 (s, H, CONH), δ7.2-7.4 (m, 10H, Ar-H).

^{1}HNMR spectral data of [3-methyl-5-oxo-1(phenyl-hydrazono)-4,5-dihydro-pyrazol-1-yl]-acetic acid N|-(4-substituted thiazol-2-yl)-hydrazide XV.

XVa: 2.23 (s, 3H, CH$_3$), 4.90 (s, 2H, NCH$_2$CO), 7.35 (s, H, thiazole-4H), 7.2 (s, H, Ar-NH), 9.54 (s, H, NH), 10.65 (s, H, CONH), 7.2-7.4 (m, 10H, Ar-H).

XVd: 2.27 (s, 3H, CH$_3$), 4.90 (s, 2H, NCH$_2$CO), 7.46 (d, 2H, o-protons of p-hydroxy phenyl), 7.60 (d,2H, m-protons of p-hydroxy phenyl), 7.36 (s, H, thiayole-4H), 7.4 (s, H, Ar-NH), 9.56 (s, H, NH), 10.67 (s, H, CONH, 7.2-7.4 (m, 5H, Ar-H)

XVf: 2.33 (s, 3H, CH$_3$), 4.95 (s, 2H, NCH$_2$CO), 7.59 (d, 2H, o-protons of p-hydroxy phenyl), 7.77 (d, 2H, m-protons of *p*-chloro phenyl), 7.37 (s, H, thiazole-4H), 7.8 (s, H, Ar-NH), 9.69 (s, H, NH), 10.71 (s, H, CONH), 7.4-7.6 (m, 5H, Ar-H)

XVh: 2.27 (s, 3H, CH$_3$), 4.66 (s, 2H, NCH$_2$CO), 7.26 (s, H, thiazole 4H), 7.98 (s, H, Ar NH), 9.85 (s, H, NH), 10.48 (s, H, CONH), 7.6-7.77 (m, 5H, Ar-H), 7.2 (d, 2H, Ar-H), 7.4 (d, 2H, Ar-H)

XVi: 2.26 (s, 3H, CH$_3$), 3.85 (s, 3H, OCH$_3$), 4.85 (s, 2H, N-CH$_2$-CO), 7.13 (d, 2H, o-protons of p-methoxy phenyl), 7.36 (d, 2H, m-protons of *p*-methoxy phenyl), 7.38 (s, H, thiazole-4H), 7.8 (s, H, Ar-NH), 9.52 (s, H, NH)

XVj: 2.48 (s, 3H, CH$_3$), 4.85 (s, 2H, NCH$_2$CO), 7.53-8.11 (m, 5H, aromatic protons of coumarin), 7.37 (s, H, thiazole 4H), 7.9 (s, H, Ar-NH), 10.13 (s, H, NH), 10.72 (s, H, CONH), 7.4-7.6 (m, 5H, Ar-H).

Mass spectral details

The mass spectrum of [3-methyl-5-oxo-4-(phenyl-hydrazono)-4,5-dihydro-pyrazol-1- yl]-acetic acid N$^|$-(4-phenyl thiazol-2-yl)-hydrazide XVa exhibited the molecular ion (M$^+$) peak at m/z 447 indicating the presence of odd number of nitrogens. The fragmentation pattern noticed in the mass spectrum of XVa is presented in Scheme 5. The molecular ion (M$^+$) was observed at m/z 447 (22.4%). Disintegration (loss of CH$_3$CN molecule) of molecular ion 'A' forms cation 'B' at m/z 406 (24.3%). Loss of C$_6$H$_5$ radical from molecular ion afforded cation 'C' at m/z 370 (31.2%). Expulsion of $C_9H_7N_2S$ radical from molecular ion 'A' produced the fragment 'D' at m/z 272 (11.4%). Loss of nitrogen radical from 'D' produced cation 'E' at m/z 258 (9.8%). The molecular ion on decomposition produces cation 'F' at m/z 246 (2.8%). Loss of $C_{10}H_{10}N_3S$ radical from molecular ion 'A' resulted in the cation 'G' at m/z 243 (16.4%). The fragmentation pattern clearly supported the structure of XVa.

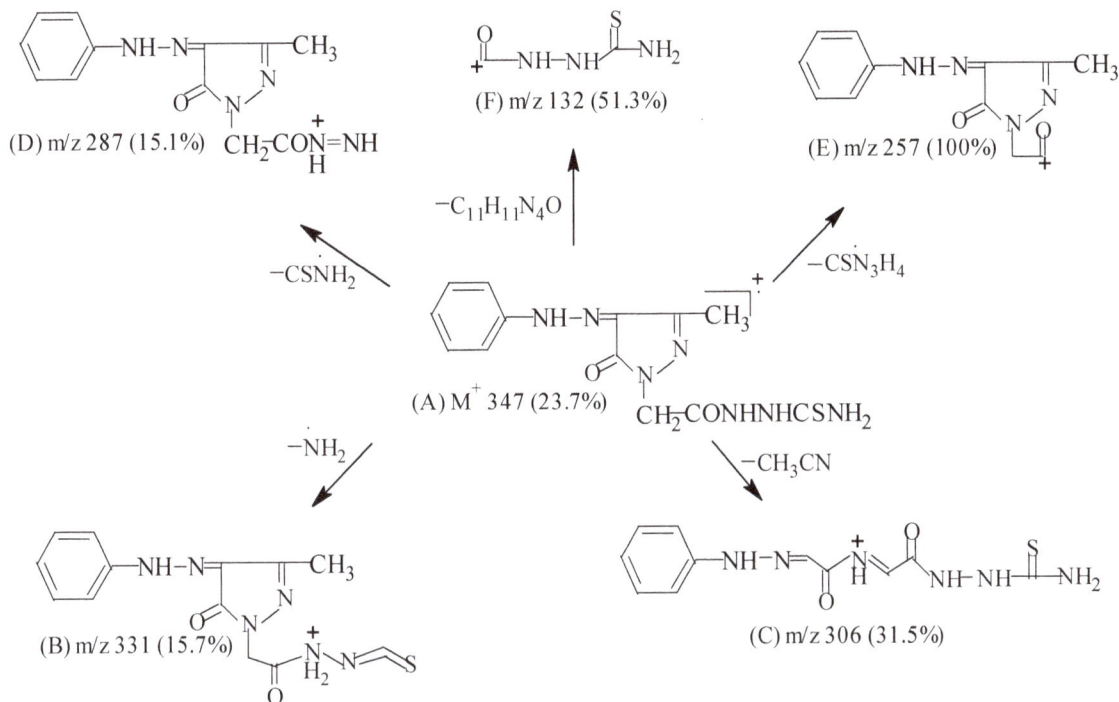

Scheme 4. Mass spectral fragmentation of [3-methyl-5-oxo-4-(phenyl hydrazono)-4,5-dihydro-pyrazol-1-yl]-aceto thiosemicarbazone XIV.

Table 2. Characterization data of [3-methyl-5-oxo-4-(phenyl hydrazono)-4,5-dihydro-pyrazol-1-yl]-acetic acid N^l-(4-substituted-thiazol-2-yl)-hydrazide. (XV)

Compd.	R	mp °C	Yield %	Mol. formula	Found (%) (calcd)						
					C	H	N	O	S	Cl	Br
XVa	phenyl	180	75	$C_{21}H_{28}N_8O_3S$	58.25 (58.18)	4.60 (4.42)	22.70 (22.62)	7.45 (7.38)	7.45 (7.40)		
XVb	p-tolyl	192	80	$C_{26}H_{28}N_8O_3S$	59.15 (59.05)	4.58 (4.47)	22.00 (21.91)	7.25 (7.15)	7.20 (7.17)		
XVc	p-anisyl	189	80	$C_{26}H_{28}N_8O_3S$	57.10 (57.01)	4.65 (4.57)	21.25 (21.15)	10.45 (10.36)	7.0 (6.92)		
XVd	p-hydroxy phenyl	185	75	$C_{26}H_{28}N_8O_3S$	56.24 (56.11)	4.35 (4.26)	21.90 (21.81)	10.78 (10.68)	7.25 (7.13)		
XVe	p-nitro phenyl	182	75	$C_{26}H_{28}N_8O_3S$	52.83 (52.71)	3.85 (3.79)	23.56 (23.42)	13.48 (13.38)	6.85 (6.70)		
XVf	p-chloro phenyl	183	76	$C_{26}H_{28}N_8O_3S$	54.00 (53.90)	3.98 (3.88)	21.02 (20.95)	7.01 (6.84)	7.05 (6.85)	7.62 (7.58)	
XVg	p-bromo phenyl	190	80	$C_{26}H_{28}N_8O_3S$	50.01 (49.23)	3.62 (3.54)	19.25 (19.14)	6.36 (6.25)	6.35 (6.26)		15.7 (15.59)
XVh	p-phenyl sydronyl	187	75	$C_{26}H_{28}N_8O_3S$	53.45 (53.38)	3.75 (3.67)	24.50 (24.37)	12.48 (12.37)	6.30 (6.18)		
XVi	N-p-tolyl sydronyl	186	75	$C_{26}H_{28}N_8O_3S$	54.35 (54.23)	4.08 (3.95)	23.85 (23.72)	12.25 (12.05)	6.20 (6.02)		
XVj	N-p-anisyl sydronyl	181	77	$C_{26}H_{28}N_8O_3S$	52.78 (52.65)	3.95 (3.83)	23.23 (23.03)	14.80 (14.62)	5.97 (5.85)		

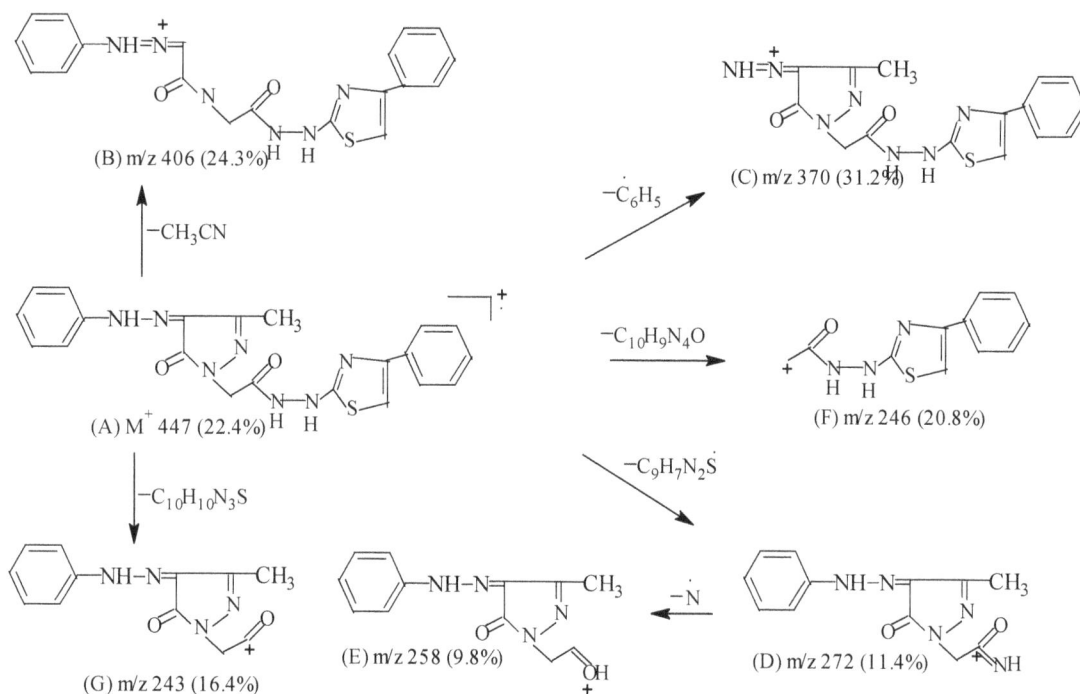

Scheme 5. Mass spectral fragmentation of 3-methyl-5-oxo-4-(phenyl hydrazono)-4,5-dihydro-pyrazol-1-yl]-acetic acid N$^{|}$-(4-phenyl thiazol-2-yl)-hydrazide XVa.

Antibacterial activity and Antifungal activity

The antibacterial activity of synthesized compounds was studied against certain pathogenic organisms. Th gram-positive bacterial screened were *Staphylococcus aureus* NCCS 2079 and *Bacillus cereus* NCCS 2106. The gram negative bacterial screened were *Escherichia coli* NCCS 265 and *Pseudomonas aeruginosa* NCCS2200.

The antifungal activity of synthesized compounds were studied against *Aspergillus niger* nccs 1196 and *Candida albicans* NCCS 3471.

The minimum inhibitory concentration (MIC) was found by broth dilution method. MIC was noted as the concentration of the test substance, which completely inhibits the growth of the microorganism i.e. 100% transparency (Table 3).

Table 3. Antimicrobial activity details of compounds synthesized

| | | | Zone inhibition in mm (concentration of the drug in µg/mL) | | | | | |
| | | | Bacteria | | | | Fungi | |
#	Compd.	-R	*Staphylococus aureus* NCCS 2079	*Bacillus Cereus* NCCS 2106	*Escherichia coli* NCCS 2065	*Pseudomanas aeruginos* NCCS 2200	*Aspergillus niger* NCCS 1196	*Candida albicans* NCCS 2106
1	XVa	phenyl	1.5 (44.27)	1.75 (46.23)	1.75 (46.23)	1.5 (45.18)	5.25 (31.2)	6.25 (30.25)
2	XVb	*p*-tolyl	1.25 (45.56)	1.5 (47.34)	1.5 (47.34)	1.75 (44.26)	4.5 (32.48)	5.5 (32.48)
3	XVc	*p*-anisyl	1.5 (39.57)	1.5 (43.85)	1.75 (41.79)	1.5 (42.38)	5.5 (31.58)	6.75 (31.58)
4	XVd	*p*-hydroxy phenyl	1.75 (36.14)	1.5 (38.59)	1.5 (38.59)	1.25 (40.34)	5 (32.59)	6 (33.57)
5	XVe	*p*-nitro phenyl	2.75 (29.21)	3 (28.42)	3.25 (27.5)	2.75 (29.21)	5 (29.21)	6 (28.42)
6	XVf	*p*-chloro phenyl	2.5 (30.13)	2.75 (29.45)	2.75 (29.45)	2.5 (30.13)	4.25 (29.45)	4.75 (29.45)
7	XVg	*p*-bromo phenyl	2.5 (29.56)	2.25 (31.28)	2.75 (29.56)	2.5 (30.13)	3.5 (29.56)	4.5 (29.56)
8	XVh	*p*- phenyl sydnonyl	1.5 (39.38)	1.75 (36.8)	1.75 (35.86)	1.75 (36.8)	4 (35.86)	4 (35.86)
9	XVi	*p*-tolyl sydnonyl	1.5 (40.68)	1.5 (37.83)	1.75 (36.62)	1.5 (37.83)	3.75 (37.83)	4.25 (37.83)
10	XVj	*N-p*-ansyl sydnonyl	1.25 (41.61)	1.5 (40.52)	1.75 (39.59)	1.5 (40.52)	4.25 (39.59)	3.75 (39.59)

Conclusion

A series of 10 novel pyrazoline-5-ones containing thiazole moiety were synthesized and characterized by elemental analysis, IR, NMR and mass spectral analysis. The antibacterial and antifungal activity of all compounds were evaluated and reported. From the study, it can be concluded that all the synthesized compounds demonstrated potential antimicrobial activity.

Conflict of Interest

There is no conflict of interest in this study.

References

1. Gokhan N, Yesilada A, Ucar G, Erol K, Bilgin AA. 1-N-substituted thiocarbamoyl-3-phenyl-5-thienyl-2-pyrazolines: Synthesis and evaluation as MAO inhibitors. *Arch Pharm (Weinheim)* 2003;336(8):362-71.
2. Palaska E, Aytemir M, Uzbay IT, Erol D. Synthesis and antidepressant activities of some 3,5-diphenyl-2-pyrazolines. *Eur J Med Chem* 2001;36(6):539-43.
3. Kucukguzel SG, Rollas S. Synthesis, characterization of novel coupling products and 4-arylhydrazono-2-pyrazoline-5-ones as potential antimycobacterial agents. *Farmaco* 2002;57(7):583-7.
4. Bekhit AA, Ashour HM, Guemei AA. Novel pyrazole derivatives as potential promising anti-inflammatory antimicrobial agents. *Arch Pharm (Weinheim)* 2005;338(4):167-74.
5. Hariraj N, Kannappan N. Synthesis of certain Pyrazolin-5-One Derivatives and Evaluation of Antibacterial and Antioxidant Activities. *J Sci Res Phar* 2012; 1(3): 112-4.
6. Taylor EC, Patel H, Kumar H. Synthesis of pyrazolo 3,4-d pyrimidine analogues of the potent agent N-4-2-2-amino-4 3H-oxo-7H-pyrrolo 2,3-d pyrimidin-5-yl ethylbenzoyl-L-glutamic acid (LY231514). *Tetrahedron* 1992; 48(37): 8089-100.
7. Arnold CG, Roelof VH, Kobus W. 1-Phenylcarbamoyl-2-pyrazolines, a new class of insecticides. 3. Synthesis and insecticidal properties of 3, 4-diphenyl-1-phenylcarbamoyl-2-pyrazolines. *J Agric Food Chem* 1979; 27(2): 406-9.
8. Abdel-Wahab BF, Abdel-Aziz HA, Ahmed EM. Synthesis and antimicrobial evaluation of 1-(benzofuran-2-yl)-4-nitro-3-arylbutan-1-ones and 3-(benzofuran-2-yl)-4,5-dihydro-5-aryl-1-[4-(aryl)-1,3-thiazol-2-yl]-1H-pyrazoles. *Eur J Med Chem* 2009;44(6):2632-5.
9. Bharti SK, Nath G, Tilak R, Singh SK. Synthesis, anti-bacterial and anti-fungal activities of some novel Schiff bases containing 2,4-disubstituted thiazole ring. *Eur J Med Chem* 2010;45(2):651-60.
10. Mallikarjuna BP, Sastry BS, Suresh Kumar GV, Rajendraprasad Y, Chandrashekar SM, Sathisha K. Synthesis of new 4-isopropylthiazole hydrazide analogs and some derived clubbed triazole, oxadiazole ring systems--a novel class of potential antibacterial, antifungal and antitubercular agents. *Eur J Med Chem* 2009;44(11):4739-46.
11. Rawal RK, Tripathi R, Katti SB, Pannecouque C, De Clercq E. Design, synthesis, and evaluation of 2-aryl-3-heteroaryl-1,3-thiazolidin-4-ones as anti-HIV agents. *Bioorg Med Chem* 2007;15(4):1725-31.
12. Agarwal A, Lata S, Saxena KK, Srivastava VK, Kumar A. Synthesis and anticonvulsant activity of some potential thiazolidinonyl 2-oxo/thiobarbituric acids. *Eur J Med Chem* 2006;41(10):1223-9.
13. Liu ZY, Wang YM, Li ZR, Jiang JD, Boykin DW. Synthesis and anticancer activity of novel 3,4-diarylthiazol-2(3H)-ones (imines). *Bioorg Med Chem Lett* 2009;19(19):5661-4.
14. Sondhi SM, Singh N, Lahoti AM, Bajaj K, Kumar A, Lozach O, Meijer L. Synthesis of acridinylthiazolino derivatives and their evaluation for antiinflammatory, analgesic and kinase inhibition activities. *Bioorg Med Chem* 2005; 13(13): 4291-9.
15. Greco CV, Tobias J, Keir LB. Acylation of 3-Phenylsydnone with carboxylic acid and phosporous pentoxide. *J Heterocycl Chem* 1967; 4: 160-7.
16. Garg LC, Atal CK. Evaluation of anthelmintic activity. *Indian J Pharm* 1969; 31: 104-5.
17. Seelay HW, Van Demark PJ. Microbes in Action, A laboratory Manual in Microbiology. 2nd ed. Bombay: D.B.Taraporewala Sons and Co; 1975.
18. Winter CA, Risley EA, Nuss GW. Carrageenin-induced edema in hind paw of the rat as an assay for antiiflammatory drugs. *Proc Soc Exp Biol Med* 1962;111:544-7.
19. Zav'yalov SI, Dorofeeva OV, Rumyantseva EE, Sitkareva IV, Zavozin AG. Br2-B(OMe)3-MeOH system for the α-monobromination of ketones. *Seriya Khimicheskaya* 1987; 10: 2224.
20. Porteili M, Bartolini G. Synthesis of N-substituted glycines. *Ann Chim* 1963; 53: 1180-1.
21. Gottleib OR, Mors WB. The chemistry of rosewood. III. Isolation of 5,6-Dehydrokavain and 4-Methoxyparacotoin from Aniba formula. *J Org Chem* 1959; 24: 17-8.
22. Koelsch CF. Bromonation of 3-Acetocoumarin. *J Am Chem Soc* 1950; 72: 2993-5.
23. Eade RA, Earl JC. The sydnones; a new class of compound containing two adjacent nitrogen atoms. *J Chem Soc* 1946:591-3.

10

Supplementary Health Benefits of Linoleic Acid by Improvement of Vaginal Cornification of Ovariectomized Rats

Saadat Parhizkar[1], Latiffah A Latiff[2]*

[1] Medicinal Plants Research Centre, Yasuj University of Medical Sciences (YUMS), Yasuj, Iran.

[2] Community Health Department, Faculty of Medicine and Health Sciences, University Putra Malaysia (UPM), Malaysia.

ARTICLE INFO

Keywords:
Estrogenic Effects
Gama-Linolenic acid
Linoleic acid
Ovariectomized Rats
Vaginal Cornification Assay

ABSTRACT

Purpose: This study aimed to evaluate the possible estrogenic activity of some ingredients of Nigella sativa including Linoleic acid and Gama-Linolenic acid by vaginal cornification assay. ***Methods:*** Forty ovariectomized (OVX) rats, aged 16 weeks were allotted randomly to five groups: negative control (taking 1 ml olive oil/ day); positive control (taking 0.2 mg/kg/day Conjugated Equine Estrogen-CEE); experimental groups (taking 50 mg/kg/day Linoleic acid or 10 mg/kg/day Gamma Linolenic acid or 15mg/kg/day Thymoquinone). All of supplements administered via intragastric gavage for 21 consecutive days. To assess estrogen like activity, vaginal smear was examined daily and serum estradiol was measured at baseline, after 10 days and at the end of experiment. ***Results:*** The significant occurrence of vaginal cornification cell ($p<0.05$) after Linoleic acid supplementation indicated estrogenic activity of Linoleic acid which was in consistency with serum estradiol level, but this effect was not as much as CEE. Gama-Linolenic acid also exist a few cornified cell in smear which was not significantly differ from those control group. ***Conclusion:*** Linoleic acid showed the beneficial effects on OVX rats' reproductive performance, thereby indicating its beneficial role in the treatment of the postmenopausal symptoms.

Introduction

Menopause is the period in a woman's life when hormonal changes cause menstruation to cease permanently[1] and it is a natural part of the aging process. The experience of menopause varies greatly from one woman to another. For some, it is completely symptom free. Others may require assistance to cope with physical and psychological effects of menopause including hot flashes, vaginal atrophy, reductions in cardiovascular health and enhanced risk for developing osteoporosis and Alzheimer's disease.[2] For women requiring assistance, a range of options and supports are available such as lifestyle changes, medical treatments such as Hormone replacement therapy (HRT) and complementary approaches.[3] Since some studies showed linkage between HRT use and some women cancers (e.g. Breast and endometrial cancer) and cardiovascular risk, therefore women tended to look for viable and safe alternatives.[4] In addition due to the fear of developing cancer and discomfort, many users of HRT exhibit poor compliance.[5] As a result, women frequently considered natural estrogenic alternatives for the treatment of menopausal pathologies and symptoms, because natural products offer the hope of improved safety and greater compliance.

Nigella sativa seeds have traditionally been used in Middle Eastern folk medicine as a natural remedy for various diseases as well as a spice for over 2000 years. The seeds of Nigella sativa have been subjected to a range of pharmacological, phytochemical and nutritional investigations in recent years.[6-8] It has been shown to contain more than 30% (w/w) of a fixed oil with 85% of total unsaturated fatty acid.[9] Nigella sativa oil is a rich source of linoleic acid (LA) an omega-6 fatty acid. Because estrogens have typically been used for the treatment of menopausal symptoms and because Nigella sativa have been shown to have a remarkable number of 23 sterols have been identified in the seed which can improve some symptoms associated with menopause, we investigated the potential estrogenic effects of some of its active ingredients. Although there have been no studies to determine the specific impact of LA and other principles of Nigella sativa on reproductive performance, previous studies have shown essential Fatty Acids (EFA) have been implemented as key nutrients in sustaining reproductive performance.[10] In the present study, we evaluated the potential of some active ingredients on Nigella sativa including Linoleic Acid (LA), Gamma-Linolenic Acid (GLA) and thymoquinone (TQ) to exhibit estrogenic effects using vaginal cornification assay.

*Corresponding author:** Latiffah A. Latiff, Community Health Department, Faculty of Medicine and Health Sciences, University Putra Malaysia (UPM), Malaysia, 43400 Serdang, Selangor, Darul Ehsan, Malaysia. E-mail: llatiffah@gmail.com

Materials and Methods

Experimental Design

In order to induce menopause and to investigate reproductive changes following supplementation with different ingredients of *Nigella sativa*, the rats were ovariectomized under a combination of xylazine and ketamine (10 mg/kg + 75 mg/kg, i.p. respectively) anesthesia. Bilateral ovariectomy was performed via a dorso-lateral approach with a small lateral vertical skin incision.[11] The ovariectomized animals were acclimatized at the Animal House of Faculty of Medicine and Health Sciences for one month prior to supplementation. Five experimental rat groups were established with 8 rats per group. The groups were as follows: group 1, negative control (1 ml Olive Oil), group 2, positive control (0.2mg/kg/day CEE diluted in distilled water), group 3 Linoleic acid (daily 50 mg/kg LA which calculated based on yielding *Nigella sativa* fixed oil (29%) and concentration of LA (57%) in fixed oil), group 4, Thymoquinone (daily 15mg/kg TQ which calculated based on yielding *Nigella sativa* fixed oil (29%) and concentration of TQ (16.1%) in fixed oil which analyzed and reported by Latiff et al.,[12] on the same plant source) and group 5, Gamma Linolenic acid (daily 10 mg/kg GLA which calculated based on yielding *Nigella sativa* fixed oil (29%) and concentration of GLA (2%) in fixed oil and probability of its production through conversion from LA). All ingredients were diluted in olive oil as vehicle. Dosage of the ingredients were selected based on the optimum desired effect of *Nigella sativa* and its extracts in the previous experiments,[13,14] which was at low dose (300mg/kg BW/day) and were administered by intra-gastric gavage for 3 weeks. Serum estradiol were measured at baseline (day 0), 11th days, and at the end of experiment (21st day) and vaginal epithelium was checked daily.

Animals

Forty female Sprague–Dawley rats weighing between 250 and 350g aged 4 months were used in this study. They were supplied by animal house of Faculty of Medicine and Health Sciences, University Putra Malaysia (Serdang, Selangor, Malaysia). Rats were individually housed in stainless steel cages in a well ventilated room with a 12/12h light/dark cycle at an ambient temperature of 29–32 °C and 50- 60 % relative humidity. Experiments were carried out according to the guidelines for the use of animals and approved by the Animal Care and Use Committee of the Faculty of Medicine and Health Sciences, University Putra Malaysia with UPM/FPSK/PADS/BR/UUH/F01-00220 reference number for notice of approval. They were fed standard rat chow pellets purchased from As-Sapphire (Selangor, Malaysia) and allowed to drink water ad libitum.

Chemicals

Linoleic Acid (95%), Gamma-Linolenic Acid and thymoquinone (99%) were obtained from Sigma-Aldrich Chemical Co. (St. Louis, MO, USA). Conjugated Equine Estrogen (0.625mg) was purchased from Wyeth, Montreal, Canada and prepared in a dosage of 0.2mg/kg[15-17] by dissolving it in distilled water,[13-15] and was used as a positive control for the purpose of comparison with the treated groups. All other reagents and chemicals were of analytical grade.

Blood collection

Fasting blood samples were collected under the deep ether anaesthesia by cardiac puncture using sterile disposable syringes at baseline (pre-treatment), day 11 (during treatment) and day 21 (after treatment). The blood samples were then centrifuged at 3000 rpm for 10 minutes to separate the serum. The serum was stored at -80°C until assays were carried out. Estradiol Radioimmunoassay (RIA) kit was purchased from Diagnostic Systems Laboratories (DSL), USA. The principle of the test is the competition of radioactive antigen and non-radioactive antigen for the fixed number of antibody binding sites. All tests were performed according to the manufacturer's instructions.

Vaginal Smear

Vaginal smears were carried out to monitor cellular differentiation and to evaluate the presence of leukocytes, nucleated epithelial cells, or cornified cells. Vaginal smear samples were collected between 08.00 and 10.00 am daily. The vaginal smears were prepared by washing with 10 µl of normal saline (NaCl 0.9%) and were then thinly spread on a glass slide. They were allowed to dry at room temperature and then stained using Methylene blue dripping. The slides were rinsed in distilled water after 30 minutes and allowed to dry. The smears were studied using the light microscope (40x) and the cell type and their relative numbers were recorded. Vaginal smear cell counts were performed on 100 cells randomly. The percentage of cornified cells was determined according to Terenius[18] using the following formula:

$$Percentage\ of\ Cornified\ Cells = \frac{Cornified\ Cells}{Cornified\ Cells + Nucleated\ Cells + Leucocytes} \times 100$$

Statistical Analysis

Data were expressed as means ± standard deviation. The data were analyzed using SPSS Windows program version 15 (SPSS Institute, Inc., Chicago, IL, USA) statistical packages. The One-Way Analysis of Variance (ANOVA) and General linear Model (GLM) followed by Duncan Multiple Range Test (DMRT) were used to determine which ingredients of *Nigella sativa* showed optimum effects. A p-value less than 0.05 ($p<0.05$) was considered to be significant.

Results

Serum estradiol

Over the period of treatment, all groups showed reduction in the level of estradiol except positive control (CEE) which significantly increased (p<0.05). OVX rats supplemented with CEE showed 359% elevation in the estradiol level at the end of experiment. The means of serum estradiol level were not significantly different at baseline (day 0) among groups. In the first 10 days of treatment, serum estradiol level tend to reduce in TQ, GLA and control groups compared to baseline while in LA and CEE groups, the levels increase. There was a significant difference between estradiol level in CEE and other groups. Instead of a tendency to decrease in estradiol levels, the value of serum estradiol in LA (15.74± 4.39) remained much higher than other groups except CEE (Table 1). There was also a significant effect for treatments and duration of treatment (p<0.05) and the interaction effect (p<0.05).

Table 1. Means of serum estradiol (pg/ml) of OVX rats supplemented with various ingredients of *Nigella sativa* or Conjugated Equine Estrogen.

Treatment	Day			Total
	0	11	21	
TQ	13.23± 4.09 [a]	9.84± 3.50 [a]	7.55± 3.73 [a]	9.93± 4.24 [A]
CEE	14.88± 12.11 [a]	15.89± 13.37 [a]	53.51± 34.77 [b]	28.09± 28.36 [B]
LA	16.45± 5.53 [a]	19.91± 2.68 [a]	15.74± 4.39 [a]	17.36± 4.54 [A]
GLA	12.77± 3.10 [a]	9.61± 2.07 [a]	5.87± 3.31 [a]	9.60± 4.00 [A]
C	11.72± 7.43 [a]	5.94± 4.15 [a]	6.26± 5.51 [a]	7.98± 6.22 [A]

Data are expressed as Mean ± SD.
Treatment TQ=Thymoquinone (15mg/kg/day); LA=linoleic Acid (50mg/kg/day); GLA= Gamma Linolenic Acid (10mg/kg/day); CEE= conjugated equine estrogen (0.2mg/kg/day); and C= control (1 ml Olive Oil/day)groups.
AB: Comparison of the means between rows within column with different superscripts are significantly different at p<0.05.
XY: Comparison of the means between columns within row with different superscripts are significantly different at p<0.05.
ab: Comparison of the means between column and between row with different superscripts are significantly different at p<0.05.

Vaginal epithelial cell cornification

There was no significant difference in the percentage of cornified cells between groups at baseline and results confirmed a menopausal pattern in OVX rats. However after treatment, cornification was observed in all treatment groups which was significantly different from those negative control group (p<0.05) which remained in an atrophic pattern as observed in the absence of estrogen (Figures 1-5). In the first 10 days of treatment, percentage of cornified cells increased significantly (p<0.05) in all groups except control group. Extending the supplementation period to 21 days, consistently increased percentage of cornified cells among LA and CEE groups until end of the treatment period, while control group remained unchanged until the end of the experiment.

Discussion

In the current study, we compared the possible beneficial effects of active ingredients of *Nigella sativa*, thymoquinone, linoleic acid and gamma linolenic acid on reproduction function in OVX induced rats. Results indicated that active ingredients of *Nigella sativa*, linoleic acid, had a weak estrogenic effect as shown in its effect in serum estrogen level and percent of cornified cells. The results, however, fail to show a linear consistent time dependent effect of linoleic acid on the parameter studied. In general the level of estradiol was much higher in linoleic acid group compare to control and other active ingredients.

Several studies have suggested that diet, particularly one enriched with either saturated or unsaturated fatty acids can alter serum steroid concentrations in a variety of species, including rodents and humans.[19-23] The mechanisms underlying diet-induced alteration of steroid concentration are likely complex. Dietary fat can influence the expression of enzymes that metabolize sex steroid hormones.[24,25] Adipose tissue is an important site of steroid hormone biosynthesis.[26,27] Moreover, ovarian derived Δ4 androstenedione and testosterone can be aromatized in adipose tissue to estrone and estradiol respectively.[28] An additional potential mechanism of dietary influence on sex steroid concentration relates to the status of cholesterol as a precursor to steroid hormones. Diet can influence serum cholesterol[29] and high cholesterol is correlated with high serum androgen and estrogen concentrations.[30,31] Past studies in rodents, cattle, and humans have indicated that diet might underpin changes in serum hormonal concentrations, including testosterone and estrogen.[20,22,32] Female rats fed a diet enriched with n-3 polyunsaturated fatty acids had a 48% increase in serum concentrations of 17β-estradiol compared with rats fed a diet enriched with n-6 fatty acids.[18] Similarly, female rats fed a low protein diet had a significant increase in 17β-estradiol compared with those fed a control diet.[32] A high saturated fat diet induces an increase in estrogen, estrone, and dehydroepiandrosterone sulfate concentrations in women.[33] A controlled clinical trial revealed that girls fed a low fat (LF) diet exhibited higher serum testosterone concentrations during the luteal phase of the cycle but lower estradiol concentrations.[22] In contrast, in other study there were no significant correlations between any measure of fat (total fat, saturated fat, and linoleic acid) and serum estrone and estradiol in 325 climacteric US women.[34]

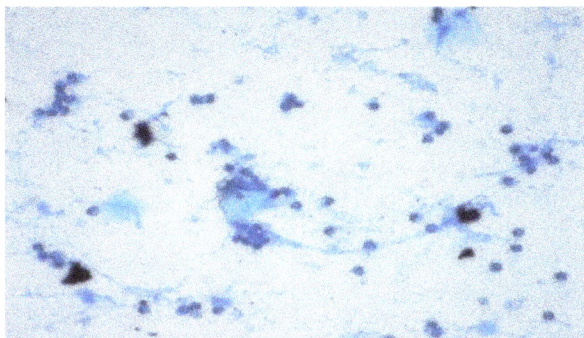

Figure 1. Vaginal smear of ovariectomized rat treated with thymoquinone (15mg/kg) for 3 weeks. A few number of cornified cells and also leukocytes are observed (methylene blue staining, 40x).

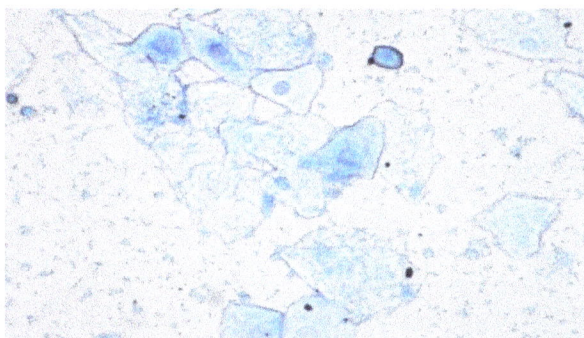

Figure 2. Vaginal smear of ovariectomized rat treated with conjugated equine estrogen (0.2 mg/kg) for 3 weeks. A great number of cornified cells and also nucleated epithelial cells are observed (methylene blue staining, 40x).

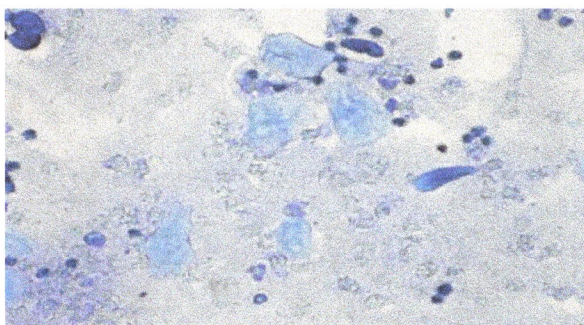

Figure 3. Vaginal smear of ovariectomized rat treated with linoleic acid (50mg/kg) for 3 weeks. A few number of cornified cells, nucleated epithelial cells and also leukocytes are observed (methylene blue staining, 40x).

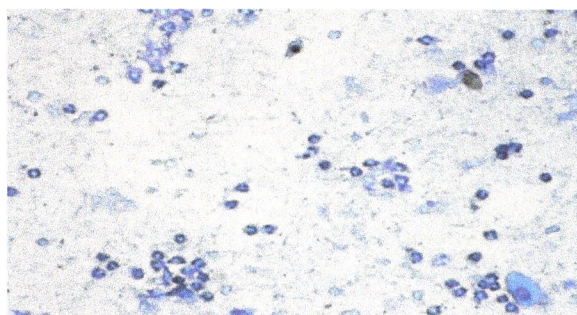

Figure 4. Vaginal smear of ovariectomized rat treated with gamma linoleic acid (10mg/kg) for 3 weeks. A few number of nucleated epithelial cells and also leukocytes are observed (methylene blue staining, 40x).

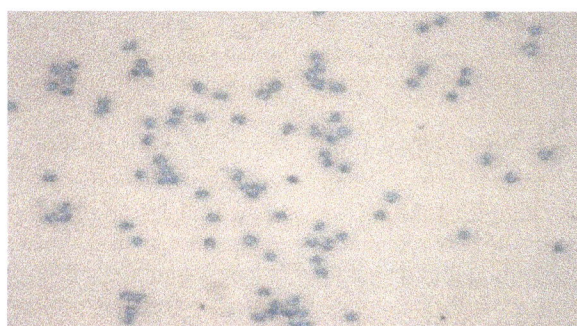

Figure 5. Vaginal smear of ovariectomized rat from control group treated with olive oil for 3 weeks. A great number of leukocytes are observed (methylene blue staining, 40x).

The insignificant change in the levels of estrogen in the present study suggests that linoleic acid may act directly on the estrogen receptors without enhancing the endogenous estrogen levels.

Linoleic acid is a fatty acid, which is ubiquitous in nature. Some fatty acids have been reported to bind noncompetitively or with mixed-competition to a variety of receptors most likely based on hypodrophobic interactions.[35-38] Arachidonic acid, palmitic acid, stearic acid, oleic acid, and docosahexaenoic acid have been reported to bind to the estrogen, progesterone, androgen, and glucocorticoid receptors at weak binding sites different from the endogenous steroid binding site.[35] Linoleic acid demonstrated the ability to interact with the opioid receptor and the nucleoside transport protein.[38]

The relationship between dietary fat and changes in reproductive function is not limited to affects on cholesterol and progesterone. Staples and Thatcher[39] proposed an elegant control feedback system that involves not only progesterone, but also affects prostaglandin synthesis and the role estrogen plays in biological (cellular) function as illustrated in Figure 6. Polyunsaturated fatty acids are proposed to decrease the release of prostaglandins that would augment the establishment of a pregnancy. In addition, the PUFA also decrease the effects of estradiol that enhance the action of prostaglandins.

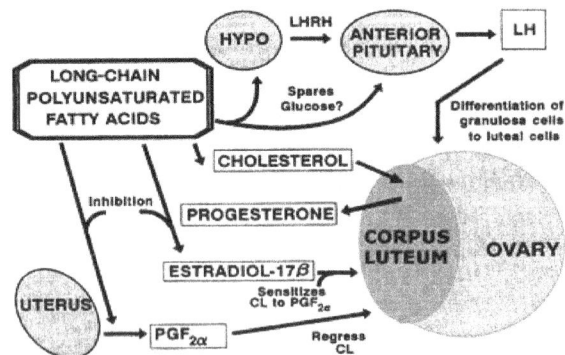

Figure 6. Possible mechanisms for the role of polyunsaturated fatty acids on reproductive function in dairy cows. (Staples and Thatcher, 1999).

Liu et al.,[40] reported the identification of linoleic acid as an estrogen receptor ligand capable of displacing estradiol from the ER and binding to the ligand binding domain of the protein using competitive binding assays and pulsed ultra filtration. They evaluated several other fatty acids for binding to the estrogen receptor. Among the 20 fatty acids tested, 13 bound to ER α and six bound to ER β. In general, fatty acids shorter than 16 carbons did not bind to the receptor; however, saturated acids had no obvious selectivity for the receptor compared with unsaturated acids.

Previous studies demonstrated the ability of conjugated linoleic acid to bind to PPAR gamma and alter the expression of some genes regulated by an estrogen response element (ERE).[41] Liu and his colleagues[40] reported that linoleic acid present in the fruits of V. agnus-castus can bind to estrogen receptors and induce certain estrogen inducible ER mRNA up-regulation. The interaction of linoleic acid with the estrogen receptor did increase the mRNA of estrogen inducible genes in Ishikawa and T47:A18 cells. These data suggest that the likely pathway for upregulation of genes regulated by ERE natural promoters, such as the ones reported in previous studies, is by linoleic acid binding to and activating estrogen receptors. Additional characterization must be completed to determine if *Nigella sativa* contains more compounds that interact with estrogen receptors and stimulate estrogen inducible genes. Functional assays should be used to determine if linoleic acid bound to nuclear receptors have any effect on the regulation of gene expression.

Conclusion

The observed estrogenic effect following linoleic acid treatment suggests that this fatty acid could possibly act on the estrogen receptors with enhancing the endogenouse estrogen levels. Linoleic acid showed the beneficial effects on OVX rats' reproductive performance, thereby indicating its beneficial role in the treatment of the postmenopausal symptoms.

Acknowledgements

The authors would like to thank University Putra Malaysia for its financial support of this research project.

Conflict of interest

The authors report no conflicts of interest.

References

1. Andrews WC. The transitional years and beyond. *Obstet Gynecol* 1995; 85(1):1-5.
2. Colditz GA, Hankinson SE, Hunter DJ, Willett WC, Manson JE, Stampfer MJ, et al. The use of estrogens and progestins and the risk of breast cancer in postmenopausal women. *New Engl J Med* 1995; 332: 1589-93.
3. Bones O. Menopause: What causes the menopause? Symptoms, Health risks. *Medical News Today* 17th July 2006.
4. Messina MJ, Persky V, Setchell KD, Barnes S. Soy intake and cancer risk: a review of the in vitro and in vivo data. *Nutr Cancer* 1994;21: 113-31.
5. De Lignieres B. Hormone replacement therapy: clinical benefits and side effects. *Maturitas* 1996; 23 Suppl: S31-6.
6. Coban S, Yildiz F. The effects of *Nigella sativa* on bile duct ligation induced-liver injury in rats. *Cell Biochem Funct* 2010; 28(1): 83-8.
7. Al-Nazawi MH, El-Bahr SM. Hypolipidemic and Hypocholestrolemic Effect of Medicinal Plant Combination in the Diet of Rats: Black Cumin Seed (*Nigella sativa*) and Turmeric (Curcumin). *J Anim Vet Adv* 2012;11: 2013-9.
8. Akhtar M, Maikiyo AM. Ameliorating effects of two extracts of *Nigella sativa* in middle cerebral artery occluded rat. *J Pharm Bioallied Sci* 2012;4(1): 70-5.
9. Houghton PJ, Zarka R, Heras BDL, Hoult JRS. Fixed oil of *Nigella sativa* and derived thymoquinone inhibit eicosanoid generation in leukocytes and membrane lipid peroxidation. *Planta Medica* 1994;61: 33-6.
10. Zeitlin L, Segev E, Fried A, Wientroub S. Effects of long-term administration of N-3 polyunsaturated fatty acids (PUFA) and selective estrogen receptor modulator (SERM) derivatives in ovariectomized (OVX) mice. *J Cell Biochem* 2003; 90(2): 347-60.
11. Parhizkar S, Rashid I, Latiffah AL. Incision Choice in Laparatomy: a Comparison of Two Incision Techniques in Ovariectomy of Rats. *World Appl Sci J* 2008;4(4): 537-40.
12. Latiffah AL, Hassanzadeh Ghahramanloo K, Hanachi P. Comparative analysis of essential oil composition of Iranian and Indian *Nigella sativa* extracted by using Supercritical Fluid Extraction (SFE) and solvent extraction. *Clin Biochem* 2011; 44(13):S20.
13. Parhizkar S, Latiff LA, Rahman SA, Dollah MA, Hanachi P. Assessing estrogenic activity of *Nigella sativa* in ovariectomized rats using vaginal

cornification assay. *Afr J Pharm Pharacol* 2011; 5(2):137-42.

14. Parhizkar S, Latiffah AL, Sabariah AR, Dollah MA. Preventive effect of *Nigella sativa* on metabolic syndrome in Menopause Induced Rats. *J Med Plants Res* 2011; 5(8):1478-84.

15. Genazzani AR, Stomati M, Bernardi F, Luisi S, Casarosa E, Puccetti S, et al. Conjugated equine estrogens reverse the effects of aging on central and peripheral allopregnanolone and beta-endorphin levels in female rats. *Fertil Steril* 2004;81(1): 757-66.

16. Oropeza MV, Orozco S, Ponce H, Campos MG. Tofupill lacks peripheral estrogen-like actions in the rat reproductive tract. *Reprod Toxicol* 2005;20:261-6.

17. Araujo LBF, Soares JM, Simoes RS, Santos RS, Calió PL, Oliveira-Filho, et al. Effect of conjugated equine estrogens and tamoxifen administration on thyroid gland histomorphology of the rat. *Clinics* 2006; 61: 321-6.

18. Terenius L. The Allen-Doisy test for estrogens reinvestigated. *Steroids* 1971;17:653-61.

19. Talavera F, Park CS, Williams GL. Relationships among dietary lipid intake, serum cholesterol and ovarian function in Holstein heifers. *J Anim Sci* 1985; 60: 1045-51.

20. Hilakivi-Clarke L, Cho E, Cabanes A, DeAssis S, Olivo S, Helferich W, et al. Dietary modulation of pregnancy estrogen levels and breast cancer risk among female rat offspring. *Clin Cancer Res* 2002;8:3601-10.

21. Woods MN, Barnett JB, Spiegelman D, Trail N, Hertzmark E, Longcope C, et al. Hormone levels during dietary changes in premenopausal African–American women. *J Natl Cancer Inst* 1996; 88:1369-74.

22. Dorgan JF, Hunsberger SA, McMahon RP, Kwiterovich PJ, Lauer RM, Van Horn L, et al. Diet and sex hormones in girls: findings from a randomized controlled clinical trial. *J Natl Cancer Inst* 2003; 95:132-45.

23. Whyte JJ, Alexenko AP, Davis AM, Ellersieck MR, Fountain ED, Rosenfeld CS. Maternal diet composition alters serum steroid and free fatty acid concentrations and vaginal pH in mice. *J Endocrinol* 2007;192:75-81.

24. Zhou Y, Lin S, Chang HH, Du J, Dong Z, Dorrance AM, et al. Gender differences of renal CYP-derived eicosanoid synthesis in rats fed a high-fat diet. *Am J Hypertens* 2005;18:530-7.

25. Dieudonne MN, Sammari A, Dos Santos E, Leneveu MC, Giudicelli Y, Pecquery R. Sex steroids and leptin regulate 11beta-hydroxysteroid dehydrogenase I and P450 aromatase expressions in human preadipocytes: sex specificities. *J Steroid Biochem Mol Biol* 2006; 99:189-96.

26. Belanger C, Luu-The V, Dupont P, Tchernof A. Adipose tissue intracrinology: potential importance of local androgen/estrogen metabolism in the regulation of adiposity. *Horm Metab Res* 2002;34: 737-74.

27. Simpson ER. Sources of estrogen and their importance. *J Steroid Biochem Mol Biol* 2003; 86:225-30.

28. Lambrinoudaki I, Christodoulakos G, Rizos D, Economou E, Argeitis J, Vlachou S, et al. Endogenous sex hormones and risk factors for atherosclerosis in healthy Greek postmenopausal women. *Eur J Endocrinol* 2006;154:907-16.

29. Menotti A. Diet, cholesterol and coronary heart disease. A perspective. *Acta Cardiol* 1999; 54:169-72.

30. Shelley JM, Green A, Smith AM, Dudley E, Dennerstein L, Hopper J, et al. Relationship of endogenous sex hormones to lipids and blood pressure in mid-aged women. *Ann Epidemiol* 1998;8:39-45.

31. Kumagai S, Kai Y, Sasaki H. Relationship between insulin resistance, sex hormones and sex hormone-binding globulin in the serum lipid and lipoprotein profiles of Japanese postmenopausal women. *J Atheroscler Thromb* 2001; 8:14-20.

32. Fernandez-Twinn DS, Ozanne SE, Ekizoglou S, Doherty C, James L,Gusterson B, Hales CN. The maternal endocrine environment in the low-protein model of intra-uterine growth restriction. *Br J Nutr* 2003;90:815-22.

33. Nagata C, Nagao Y, Shibuya C, Kashiki Y, Shimizu H. Fat intake is associated with serum estrogen and androgen concentrations in postmenopausal Japanese women. *J Nutr* 2005;135:2862-5.

34. Newcomb PA, Klein R, Klein BEK, Haffner S, Mares-Perlman J, Cruickshanks KJ, et al. Association of dietary and life-style factors with sex hormones in postmenopausal women. *Epidemiol* 1995;6:318-21.

35. Kato J. Arachidonic acid as a possible modulator of estrogen, progestin, androgen, and glucocorticoid receptors in the central and peripheral tissues. *J Steroid Biochem* 1989;34: 219-27.

36. Vallette G, Vanet A, Sumida C, Nunez EA. Modulatory effects of unsaturated fatty acids on the binding of glucocorticoids to rat liver glucocorticoid receptors. *Endocrinol* 1991;129: 1363-9.

37. Kang JX, Leaf A. Effects of long-chain polyunsaturated fatty acids on the contraction of neonatal rat cardiac myocytes. *Proc Natl Acad Sci USA* 1994;91: 9886-90.

38. Ingkaninan K, von Frijtag D, Kunzel JK, IJzerman AP, Verpoorte R. Interference of linoleic acid fraction in some receptor binding assays. *J Nat Prod* 1999; 62: 912-4.

39. Staples CR, Thatcher WW. Fat supplementation may improve fertility of lactating dairy cows. Proceedings of the Southeast Dairy Herd Management Conference. 1999. Macon, GA. 56.

40. Liu M, Xu X, Rang W, Li Y, Song Y. Influence of ovariectomy and 17β-estradiol treatment on insulin sensitivity, lipid metabolism and post-ischemic cardiac function. *Int J cardiol* 2004;97(3): 485-93.

41. Stoll BA. Linkage between retinoid and fatty acid receptors: Implications for breast cancer prevention. *Eur J Cancer Prev* 2002;11: 319-25.

11

HLA-G Expression Pattern: Reliable Assessment for Pregnancy Outcome Prediction

Elnaz Mosaferi[1,2], Jafar Majidi[1], Mozhdeh Mohammadian[3], Zohreh Babaloo[1], Amir Monfaredan[4], Behzad Baradaran[1]*

[1] Immunology Research Center, Tabriz University of Medical Sciences, Tabriz, Iran.

[2] Tabriz International University of Medical Sciences, Tabriz, Iran.

[3] Hematology and Oncology Research Center, Tabriz University of Medical Sciences, Tabriz, Iran.

[4] Department of Hematology, Faculty of Medicine, Tabriz Branch of Islamic Azad University, Tabriz, Iran.

ARTICLE INFO

Keywords:
HLA-G
Placenta
Recurrent miscarriage

ABSTRACT

Because mothers and fathers are more or less dissimilar at multiple HLA loci, mother considers her fetus as a semi-allograft. Mother's immune system may recognize paternal HLA as foreign antigen and may develop anti-paternal HLA antibodies and cytotoxic T lymphocyte. There are some mechanisms that modulate maternal immune responses during pregnancy, in order to make uterus an immune privileged site. This immunosuppression is believed to be mediated, at least partly, by HLA-G, non-classical class I human leukocyte antigen (HLA) molecule that is strongly expressed in cytotrophoblast and placenta. The major HLA-G function is its ability to inhibit T and B lymphocytes, NK cells and antigen-presenting cells (APC). Since HLA-G is expressed strongly at the maternofetal interface and has an essential role in immunosuppression, HLA-G polymorphism and altered expression of HLA-G seems to be associated with some complications of pregnancy, such as pre-eclampsia, recurrent misscariage and failure in IVF. This perspective discusses recent findings about HLA-G genetics, function, expression and polymorphism; and focus on HLA-G role in the etiology of recurrent miscarriage.

Introduction

Recurrent Miscarriage (RM) is referring to ≥3 consecutive fetus losses in first-trimester or ≥2 in second-trimester. By means of this definition, RM involves 1-2% of all couples trying pregnancy.[1] Although the frequency of 3 miscarriages accidentally is approximately 0.34%, the possibility of a spontaneous miscarriage is about 12–14%.[2-3] This discrepancy indicates that, besides accidental causes, risk of RM is increased in some couples pathologically as a result of genetic disorders or anatomical, infectious and endocrine complications. In about 50% of RM cases, the etiology still remains unknown.[4] Immunological factors play a significant role in RM etiology since the fetus and placenta are immunologically different from the mother.[5] Fetus is considered as a semiallograft for maternal immune system, and ordinarily, the mother would be expected to produce antibodies and CTL (cytotoxic T lymphocytes) to foreign paternal HLA or other antigens expressed by fetal cells.[6] Thus, particular mechanisms must modulate the maternal immune system in favor of

success of pregnancy, so that help fetus resides inside the uterus for 9 months.[7]

several mechanisms protect the semiallogeneic fetus from maternal graft rejection responses.[6] These strategies include lack of any physical connection between maternal and fetal tissues and fully separation of the blood circulations; lack of fetal antigens that could cause graft rejection; late appearance of transplantation antigens in the fetus; immunosuppression of leukocytes which present at the maternofetal interface; development of tolerance, build up the pregnant uterus as an immune privileged site by both the fetus and the mother.[6] Failure in these mechanisms may cause complications in pregnancy like maternal rejection of the embryo/fetus.[7]

Immunosuppression of leukocytes which present at the maternofetal interface is one of the mechanisms that might modulate maternal immune responses during pregnancy.[8] HLA-G, Non-classical class Ib human leukocyte antigen (HLA) molecules, is believed to be involved in this immunosuppression. As HLA-G is expressed on trophoblast cells in the placenta,[9] it seems

*Corresponding author: Behzad Baradaran, Faculty of Medicine and Immunology Research Center, Tabriz University of Medical Sciences, Tabriz, Iran. Email: behzad_im@yahoo.com

to be occupied in development of pregnant uterus as an immune privileged site.[6] Accordingly, diminished or aberrant HLA-G expression may involve in the etiology of immunological malfunction, like pre-eclampsia, recurrent miscarriage and implantation failure in IVF.[5,7]

HLA antigens are most powerful cause of graft rejection. Although anti-paternal HLA antibodies are detectable in pregnant women's sera, they do no damage and they are more tolerogenic rather than immunogenic.[7]

The human major histocompatibility complex (MHC) genes are located on the short arm of chromosome 6 and subdivided into class Ia, which includes HLA-A, -B, and -C, and class II, which includes HLA- DR, -DQ and -DP. The non-classical HLA class Ib genes encoding HLA-E, -G -H and –F that are clustered on chromosome 6p21 at the telomeric end of the MHC region. The HLA-G gene is located close to HLA-A and seems to have a close homology with that.[10]

HLA class Ib antigens are similar to the HLA class Ia antigens in some characteristics, but also differ from them in several major features, including: 1) HLA class Ia genes are highly polymorphic, with so many alleles, but HLA class Ib genes are distinguished by low numbers of alleles, for example HLA-G is almost monomorphic and has five alleles.[11] 2) All HLA class Ia antigens are membrane bound, but one member of the class Ib group has soluble isoforms too, for example HLA-G have seven alternatively spliced transcripts that encoded four membrane bound and three soluble proteins. 3) The expression of class Ia antigens is ubiquitous while expression of class Ib antigens is organ-specific and conditional.

Structural features of HLA-G is similar to other class I genes. It has eight exons; exon 1 encodes a signal peptide, exons 2, 3, and 4, encode external part (respectively α1, α2 and α3 domains), exon 5 encodes transmembrane domain and exons 6 and 7 encode intracellular domain.[12] α1 and α2 domains construct the peptide-binding cleft and α3 domain is binding site for leukocyte Ig-like receptor 1 and 2 (LIR-1 and LIR-2), which are inhibitory receptors. HLA-G has two unique characteristic; first, a stop codon in exon 6 cause a shortened cytoplasmic tail that results in the prolonged expression of HLA-G at the cell surface, and inefficient presentation of exogenous peptides.[10] Second, due to mRNA alternative splicing, HLA-G encodes multiple isoforms including four membrane-bound isoforms, HLA-G1 to -G4, and three soluble isoforms, HLA-G5 to -G7.[13,14]

Trophoblast cells, which originate from the fetus, regulate their expression of HLA genes and the production of their proteins. If these proteins recognize by maternal immune cells as foreign antigens, they would stimulate maternal CTL against fetal antigens, so destroy fetal cells which express HLA. In contrast, the antigens expressed in trophoblast cells induce tolerance in maternal leukocytes. A successful pregnancy is due

to Th2 cytokine profile that entitled 'Th2 phenomenon', while Th1 response may cause some complications of pregnancy, such as RM.[15]

Except HLA-C which may has weak expression on trophoblast cells, other HLA class Ia and II antigens are not expressed by these cells.[16] Hence, the fetal cells are not in direct contact with the maternal immune system. Although NK-cell will destroy cells that do not express MHC, the strong expression HLA-G on cytotrophoblast cells, in cooperation with the expression of HLA-E in the placenta, will prevent NK-mediated cell lysis.[7]

Even though HLA-G mRNA has been detected in various tissues, the HLA-G protein expression is restrictive and strongly expressed on invasive trophoblast cells of the placenta at the maternofetal interface.[7] IL-10 can up-regulate HLA-G expression.[15] The mouse monoclonal antibody W6/32 is used most regularly to identify HLA-G antigens.[6,17] sHLA-G can be detected in serum/plasma from both women and men.[18] Monocytes are the main source of sHLA-G in the blood of men and non-pregnant women.[7] Although sHLA-G can only be detected in some serum samples, it is detectable in all plasma samples from non-pregnant and pregnant women; hence plasma samples are preferred. HLA-G polymorphisms may effect the level, or even the presence, of sHLA-G in serum/plasma.[18]

HLA-E in another class Ib MHC that is expressed by trophoblasts.[10] Its binding site has a great affinity for the HLA-G signal peptide, and this binding plays an important role in HLA-E expression on the trophoblast cell surface.

The major function of HLA-G is not antigen presentation; it may play a significant role in immunosuppression and tolerance (Figure1).[9] Therefore, HLA-G is somehow essential to immune privilege in pregnancy.[6] HLA-G as an inhibitory ligand for natural killer cells and cytotoxic T-lymphocytes can inhibit CTL responses and NK functions,[19] both through direct interaction with the receptors LIR-1 and LIR-2 and with the killer Ig-like receptor 2 (KIR2),[20] hence may protect trophoblasts via these receptors.[21] Additionally, antigen-presenting cells (APC), which have been transfected with HLA-G, are able to inhibit the proliferation of CD4+ T cells that leads to suppression in T helpers.[22] Besides, soluble HLA-G (sHLA-G) can induce apoptosis in CD8+ T-cell.[23]

HLA-E is also help the fetus to avoid maternal immune surveillance, possibly by interacting with the CD94/NKG2A, NK-cell inhibitory receptor.[24] HLA-E is the most important ligand for the inhibition of NK cells.[10]

In contrast to the highly polymorphic HLA class Ia and II, the gene polymorphism of the HLA class Ib is very sparse as HLA-G proteins are almost monomorphic.[7] Most polymorphisms in the HLA-G gene do not alter the amino acid sequence; and some polymorphisms that do alteration are not change secondary structures.[11] However, some of these polymorphisms in regulatory regions of the HLA-G gene may influence transcription and mRNA abundance[25] and subsequently HLA-G expression.[18,26]

Some investigations carry out in order to find out if expression of HLA-G at the maternofetal interface in women with RM is different in comparison with normal pregnancies. Results indicated that expression pattern of HLA-G is associated with a risk of RM.[25] sHLA-G levels in the serum of women experiencing RM in comparison with serum sHLA-G concentration

of women with successful pregnancies were significantly lower.[18]

Although all evidences support the imperative role for HLA-G in maternal immunosuppression during pregnancy, in vivo experiments must be done to confirm this evidences. Since significance of HLA-G expression in pregnancy is proved, more research is needed to elucidate the molecular mechanisms associated with HLA-G expression and function.

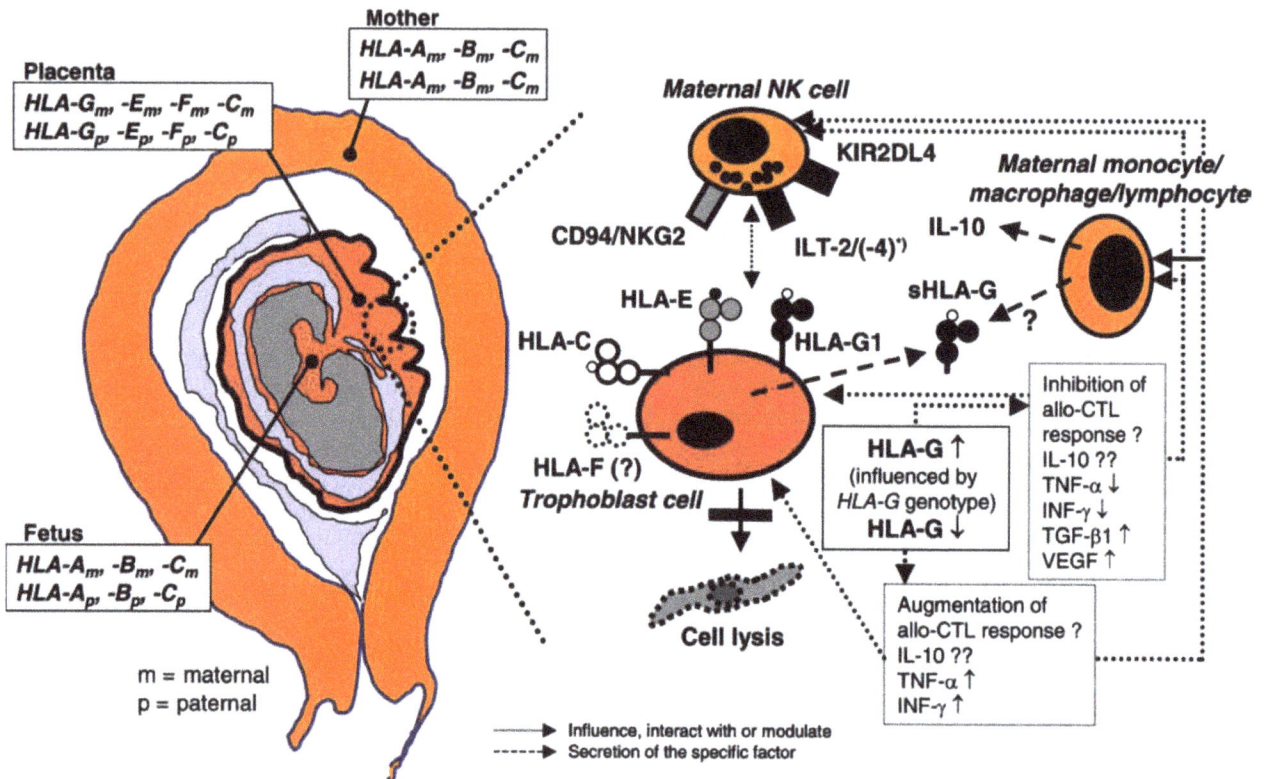

Figure 1. Expression HLA molecules during pregnancy and interactions between HLA class Ib molecules, natural killer (NK) receptors and cytokines at the feto–placental interface. The fetus inherits one *HLA* haplotype from the mother and one from the father and is thereby semiallogenic for the mother. However, the extreme polymorphic classical HLA class Ia and II antigens, HLA-A, -B and –DR, are not expressed by the trophoblast cells in the placenta. Instead, the nearly monomorphic non-classical HLA class Ib antigens, especially HLA-G, are expressed on the invasive cytotrophoblast cells. In this way, the trophoblast cells escape NK-cell-mediated lysis. Membrane-bound and soluble HLA-G (sHLA-G) can influence cytokine secretion and an allo-cytotoxic Tlymphocyte (CTL) response as described in detail in the text. *, ILT-4 is expressed on monocytes, macrophages and dendritic cells.[7]

According above, measuring of levels of HLA-G isoforms may be practical marker for the prediction of mother's capability to tolerate semiallograft fetus, success in IVF treatments and graft acceptance.

Conflict of Interest

The authors report no conflicts of interest.

References

1. Coulam CB. Epidemiology of recurrent spontaneous abortion. *Am J Reprod Immunol* 1991;26(1):23-7.
2. Stirrat G. Recurrent miscarriage. *Lancet* 1990;336:673-5.
3. Edmonds DK, Lindsay KS, Miller JF, Williamson E, Wood PJ. Early embryonic mortality in women. *Fertil Steril* 1982;38(4):447-53.
4. Lee RM, Silver RM. Recurrent pregnancy loss: summary and clinical recommendations. *Semin Reprod Med* 2000;18(4):433-40.
5. Bhalla A, Stone PR, Liddell HS, Zanderigo A, Chamley LW. Comparison of the expression of human leukocyte antigen (HLA)-G and HLA-E in women with normal pregnancy and those with recurrent miscarriage. *Reproduction* 2006;131(3):583-9.
6. Hunt JS, Petroff MG, Mcintire RH, Ober C. HLA-G and immune tolerance in pregnancy. *FASEB J* 2005;19(7):681-93.
7. Hviid TV. HLA-G in human reproduction: aspects of genetics, function and pregnancy complications. *Hum Reprod Update* 2006;12(3):209-32.
8. Loke YW, King A. Immunology of human placental implantation: clinical implications of our

current understanding. *Mol Med Today* 1997;3(4):153-9.

9. Ishitani A, Sageshima N, Lee N, Dorofeeva N, Hatake K, Marquardt H, et al. Protein expression and peptide binding suggest unique and interacting functional roles for HLA-E, F, and G in maternal-placental immune recognition. *J Immunol* 2003;171(3):1376-84.

10. Heinrichs H, Orr HT. HLA non-A,B,C class I genes: their structure and expression. *Immunol Res* 1990;9(4):265-74.

11. Ober C, Aldrich CL. HLA-G polymorphisms: neutral evolution or novel function? *J Reprod Immunol* 1997;36(1-2):1-21.

12. Park B, Lee S, Kim E, Chang S, Jin M, Ahn K. The truncated cytoplasmic tail of HLA-G serves a quality-control function in post-ER compartments. *Immunity* 2001;15(2):213-24.

13. Ishitani A, Geraghty DE. Alternative splicing of HLA-G transcripts yields proteins with primary structures resembling both class I and class II antigens. *Proc Natl Acad Sci U S A* 1992;89(9):3947-51.

14. Hviid TV, Moller C, Sorensen S, Morling N. Co-dominant expression of the HLA-G gene and various forms of alternatively spliced HLA-G mRNA in human first trimester trophoblast. *Hum Immunol* 1998;59(2):87-98.

15. Chaouat G, Ledee-Bataille N, Dubanchet S, Zourbas S, Sandra O, Martal J. TH1/TH2 paradigm in pregnancy: paradigm lost? Cytokines in pregnancy/early abortion: reexamining the TH1/TH2 paradigm. *Int Arch Allergy Immunol* 2004;134(2):93-119.

16. Hunt JS, Andrews GK, Wood GW. Normal trophoblasts resist induction of class I HLA. *J Immunol* 1987;138(8):2481-7.

17. Ober C, Aldrich C, Rosinsky B, Robertson A, Walker MA, Willadsen S, et al. HLA-G1 protein expression is not essential for fetal survival. *Placenta* 1998;19(2-3):127-32.

18. Hviid TV, Rizzo R, Christiansen OB, Melchiorri L, Lindhard A, Baricordi OR. HLA-G and IL-10 in serum in relation to HLA-G genotype and polymorphisms. *Immunogenetics* 2004;56(3):135-41.

19. Le Gal FA, Riteau B, Sedlik C, Khalil-Daher I, Menier C, Dausset J, et al. HLA-G-mediated inhibition of antigen-specific cytotoxic T lymphocytes. *Int Immunol* 1999;11(8):1351-6.

20. Ponte M, Cantoni C, Biassoni R, Tradori-Cappai A, Bentivoglio G, Vitale C, et al. Inhibitory receptors sensing HLA-G1 molecules in pregnancy: decidua-associated natural killer cells express LIR-1 and CD94/NKG2A and acquire p49, an HLA-G1-specific receptor. *Proc Natl Acad Sci U S A* 1999;96(10):5674-9.

21. Allan DS, Colonna M, Lanier LL, Churakova TD, Abrams JS, Ellis SA, et al. Tetrameric complexes of human histocompatibility leukocyte antigen (HLA)-G bind to peripheral blood myelomonocytic cells. *J Exp Med* 1999;189(7):1149-56.

22. Lemaoult J, Krawice-Radanne I, Dausset J, Carosella ED. HLA-G1-expressing antigen-presenting cells induce immunosuppressive CD4+ T cells. *Proc Natl Acad Sci U S A* 2004;101(18):7064-9.

23. Contini P, Ghio M, Poggi A, Filaci G, Indiveri F, Ferrone S, et al. Soluble HLA-A,-B,-C and -G molecules induce apoptosis in T and NK CD8+ cells and inhibit cytotoxic T cell activity through CD8 ligation. *Eur J Immunol* 2003;33(1):125-34.

24. Braud VM, Allan DS, O'callaghan CA, Soderstrom K, D'andrea A, Ogg GS, et al. HLA-E binds to natural killer cell receptors CD94/NKG2A, B and C. *Nature* 1998;391(6669):795-9.

25. Ober C, Aldrich CL, Chervoneva I, Billstrand C, Rahimov F, Gray HL, et al. Variation in the HLA-G promoter region influences miscarriage rates. *Am J Hum Genet* 2003;72(6):1425-35.

26. Hviid TV, Hylenius S, Rorbye C, Nielsen LG. HLA-G allelic variants are associated with differences in the HLA-G mRNA isoform profile and HLA-G mRNA levels. *Immunogenetics* 2003;55(2):63-79.

12

Effects of Zinc Supplementation on the Anthropometric Measurements, Lipid Profiles and Fasting Blood Glucose in the Healthy Obese Adults

Laleh Payahoo[1], Alireza Ostadrahimi[1]*, Majid Mobasseri[2], Yaser Khaje Bishak[1], Nazila Farrin[1], Mohammad Asghari Jafarabadi[3], Sepide Mahluji[1]

[1] Nutrition Research Center, Faculty of Health and Nutrition, Tabriz University of Medical Science, Tabriz, Iran.

[2] Department of Internal Medicine, Tabriz University of Medical Science, Tabriz, Iran.

[3] Tabriz Health Management Research Center, Faculty of Health and Nutrition, Tabriz University of Medical Science, Tabriz, Iran.

ARTICLE INFO

Keywords:
Anthropometric Measurements
Fasting Blood Glucose
Lipid Profile
Obesity

ABSTRACT

Purpose: The aim of this study was to assess the effects of zinc supplementation on anthropometric measures, improving lipid profile biomarkers, and fasting blood glucose level in obese people. *Methods:* This randomized, double- blind clinical trial was carried out on 60 obese participants in the 18-45 age range for one month. The participants were randomly divided into the intervention group, who received 30 mg/d zinc gluconate, and the placebo group who received 30mg/d starch. Anthropometric measurements (body mass index (BMI), weight and waist circumference) were recorded before and at the end of study. Lipid profile biomarkers and fasting blood glucose were determined using enzymatic procedure. Analysis of Covariance (ANCOVA) test was run to compare the post-treatment values of the two groups, and t-test was conducted to compare within group changes. *Results:* Serum zinc concentration was increased significantly in intervention group (p=0.024). BMI and body weight was significantly decreased (p=0.030 and p=0.020, respectively). Lipid profile biomarkers and fating blood glucose did not change significantly but triglyceride level was significantly decreased (p=0.006) in the intervention group. *Conclusion:* The obtained results indicate that zinc supplementation improves BMI, body weight, and triglyceride concentration without considerable effects on lipid profile and glucose level. Zinc can be suggested as a suitable supplementation therapy for obese people, but more studies are needed to verify the results.

Introduction

Obesity has become one of the major public-health concerns in the world[1] which is correlated with the incidence of many chronic diseases such as metabolic syndrome (MS), diabetes, cardiovascular diseases, certain cancers, respiratory disease, etc.[2-4] According to the World Health Organization (WHO) report, there are over 400 million obese and over 1.6 billion overweight adults in the world and it is estimated to be double by 2015. This concern is not restricted just to adults; at least 20 million children under the age of 5 were recognized as overweight in 2005.[5] The prevalence of obesity in Iran has been estimated to be 10.5% and 22.5% in men and women, respectively which indicates an obvious increase during a 14-year period.[6]

Obese people have high amounts of fat mass especially in adipose tissues. Plasma fatty acids are constantly influenced by adipose tissue fatty acids.[7] Plasma triacylglycerols are the major source of endogenous and exogenous fatty acids for the synthesis of complex lipids. The type of fatty acids in adipose tissue might exert a direct influence on serum lipids and the abnormality of serum lipids can affect the incidence of atherosclerosis, MS, and other chronic diseases. Therefore, adipose tissue region has an important role in the development of diseases. It has been suggested that intra-abdominal fat has a higher turnover rate than subcutaneous fat.[8] and it may have a greater influence on the plasma lipid profiles. Abdominal fat has been associated with insulin resistance, hyperlipidemia and hypertension, certain types of cancer and osteoporosis.[9] Recently, nutritional, hormonal, and biochemical status of obese patients are being attended by reserchers.[9-12] Overweight and obese individuals have lower blood level of vitamins and minerals compared to non-overweight and non-obese individuals.[13] zinc concentration in plasma, serum and erythrocytes of

*Corresponding author: Alireza Ostadrahimi, Nutrition Research Center, Faculty of Health and Nutrition, Tabriz University of Medical Science, Tabriz, Iran. Email: ostadrahimi@tbzmed.ac.ir

obese people is considered to be low.[14-15] Zinc, as an important micronutrient, plays a key role in macronutrient metabolism[16] as well as appetite control. In addition, zinc is involved in synthesis, storage, release, and action of insulin.[17,18] and its deficiency is associated with insulin resistance, impaired glucose tolerance and obesity.[19,20]

Weight loss is an effective approach in controlling obesity and it has been demonstrated that weight loss improves plasma concentration of glucose, insulin and lipids. Moreover, weight loss has a positive effect on increasing plasma zinc concentration.[21-23] The present study set out to investigate the effects of zinc supplementation on anthropometric measurements, lipid profiles and fasting blood glucose in healthy obese people.

Materials and Methods

This randomized, double- blind, placebo-controlled clinical trial was performed on 60 healthy obese participants. The research protocol was approved by regional Ethic Committee of Tabriz University in Medical Sciences. Clinical Trial Number was Irct ID: IRCT201112222017N5 with URL: www.irct.IR

Inclusion criteria were the age range of 18-45, nonsmoking, body mass index (BMI) between 30 and 40 (Kg/m^2), while exclusion criteria included pregnancy, breastfeeding and postmenopausal among women, as well as current clinical diseases specially gastrointestinal, liver and kidney, diabetes, and thyroid. Excluded from the study were also individuals who had defective immune systems, were using drugs that could interact with serum lipid profiles and weight loss, were consuming anti-coagulant drugs and beta blockers users, were taking mineral supplements such as zinc, Iron, calcium and vitamin A during the past 3 months, and finally those who were on a diet restriction. After explaining the nature of the study, a written informed consent was taken from the participants.

The eligible participants were randomly allocated to intervention-placebo groups based on random block procedure produced by Random Allocation Software (RAS).[24] Sample size was determined based on the information derived from the same study.[25] The confidence level was set at 95% and the formula N= [(Z1-α/2 + Z1-B)^2 (SD$_1^2$+SD$_2^2$)] /Δ^2 was used to calculate the 30 samples in each group. For one month, the Zinc group (n=30) had received a 30mg zinc gluconate tablet per day while the placebo group (n=30) had received 30mg placebo (starch) tablet per day. Tablets of the same color and shape were placed by a third person who labeled the bottles with 2 cods which remained unknown for the researchers until the end of the intervention. All the participants were asked not to change their usual dietary intakes during the study. To ensure that the participants would act in compliance with the prescriptions, they were weekly reached on phone and were required to return the tablet bottles at the end of the study so that the remainder of

the tablets could be checked. Subsequent statistical analysis was carried out based on the data obtained from the participants who had consumed more than 90% of the tablets.

Blood samples were taken in a 12 hour fasting state at the beginning and the end of study and were further frozen in -70 °C for biochemical analysis.

Demographic information was collected through questionnaires. Body weight was measured without shoes and light clothes by using a Seca scale (Seca, Hamburg, Germany). Height was also measured using a statiometer (Seca) without shoes. BMI was calculated as weight (in kilograms) divided by the square of height (in meters). Waist circumference (WC) was measured with a statiometer (Seca).

Serum zinc concentration was estimated by atomic absorption spectrometry (Chem Tech Analytical, CTA 2000, English).[26] Serum concentrations of triglyceride (TG), total cholesterol (TC), high-density lipoprotein cholesterol (HDL-C), and fasting blood glucose (FBS) were determined using kit (Parsazmon, Tehran, Iran) and enzymatic method. Low-density lipoprotein cholesterol (LDL-C) was calculated according to the procedure of Friede-Wald formula.

Statistical Analysis

The data were analyzed by SPSS software (version 16:0, Shikagho.IL, USA). Quantitative data were stated as mean ± standard deviation (SD) and qualitative data were presented as frequency (percentage). Normality of variables distribution was evaluated using Kolmogorov-Smirnov test. Paired t-test was used to compare within group changes before and after the intervention. Analysis of Covariance (ANCOVA) test was also run to compare post treatment variables after adjusting for baseline values in both groups. In addition, chi-square test was used to examine the differences in qualitative variables in both groups. Statistical significance was defined as p<0.

Results

Demographic Characteristics

Demographic characteristics of the participants are presented in Table 1. In this randomized, double-blind, placebo-controlled clinical trial, proportion of males and females was similar in both groups (p=0.559).

Table 1. Demographic characteristics of participated obese people

Characteristics		Intervention group (mean ± SD)	Placebo group (mean ± SD)	P value
Age (year)		31±8	33±8	0.502
Sex [N (%)]	Male	7(23.3%)	9 (30%)	0.559
	Female	23(76.7%)	21 (70%)	

Anthropometric Measurements

Paired T-test analysis showed that there is a significant reduction in anthropometric parameters in the intervention group (p<0.05). The changes in anthropometric parameters in the placebo group, however, were not significant (p>0.05). Regarding waist circumference, a significant reduction was also observed in the intervention group, but not in the placebo group (p<0.05).

Results obtained from the ANCOVA test (Table 2) indicate that there is significant differences in weight and BMI indexes between the intervention and the placebo groups after adjusting for baseline measurements (p<0.05). Nevertheless, reduction of waist circumference was not significant in the intervention group after adjusting for baseline values (p>0.05).

Table 2. Results of anthropometric measurements of zinc-supplemented obese people before and after intervention and between both groups.

Components	Intervention group		p^a	Placebo group		p^a	p^b
	before	after		before	after		
Weight (Kg)	90.4±15.4	88.7±15	0.014*	91.13±20.1	91.11±20	0.851	0.020*
Waist circumference (cm)	101.9±11.7	99.7±11.2	0.002*	100.2±11.8	99±11.2	0.058	0.319
BMI (kg/m^2)	35.4±4.3	34.7±3.9	0.015*	33.5±5.9	33.4±6.1	0.860	0.030*

*statistically significant, a: Paired *t*-test, b: ANCOVA test (between two groups with adjusting for baseline values)

Biochemical Markers

The participants' biochemical markers obtained at the onset of the study and at the end of it were further analyzed to compare the within-groups changes and the between-groups changes. The within-groups comparison of biochemical markers revealed no significant changes in serum FBS, TC, LDL-C and HDL-C levels after intervention (p>0.05), however, TG concentration represented significant reduction in the intervention group (p<0.05). Serum zinc concentration increased significantly in the intervention group at the end of study (p<0.05).

The between-groups comparison of biochemical markers at the end of the study indicated no significant change between groups in serum FBS, TC, LDL-C, TG and HDL-C levels. The increased level of serum zinc between groups was significant (p<0.05). Table 3 shows the results of biochemical markers.

Table 3. Results of biochemical markers of zinc-supplemented obese subjects before and after intervention and between two groups

Components	Intervention group (mean± SD)		p^a	Placebo group (mean± SD)		p^a	p^b
	before	after		before	after		
Fasting blood sugar (mg/dl)	96±9	94.9±13	0.535	86±3	90±4	0.210	0.103
Triglyceride (mg/dl)	146.4±6	131.4±5	0.006*	147±7	144±5	0.677	0.127
Total cholesterol (mg/dl)	185±30	182±34	0.472	153±39	156±35	0.648	0.489
Low density lipoprotein (mg/dl)	104±22	103±25	0.694	86±25	85±22	0.888	0.340
High density lipoprotein (mg/dl)	44±9	46±10	0.109	39±9	41±7	0.351	0.437
Serum zinc (μg/dl)	67±19	74.1±23	0.024*	40.8±19	45.8±17	0.054	0<001*

*statistically significant a: Paired t-test, b: ANCOVA test: between two groups with adjusting for baseline values

Discussion

Obesity is an important risk factor for metabolic abnormality and many chronic diseases.[4] In this study, the use of 30 mg/d zinc was higher than the recommended dose (DRIs 8-11 mg/day), and lower than the tolerable limit of highest intake (40 mg/day).[27] There were no significant changes in serum FBS, HDL-C, TC and LDL-C concentration at the end of the study but significant decrease was observed in serum TG. According to a Meta-analysis investigation results, regarding the effect of zinc supplementation on lipid profiles were inconsistent.[28] Afkhami-Ardekani et al.,[29] demonstrated that supplementation of forty diabetic patients with 660 mg zinc sulfate for six weeks resulted in a remarkable reduction in TG, TC and LDL-C concentrations, a non-significant increase in serum HDL-C concentration and non-significant reduction in

FBS at the end of the study. Samman et al.,[30] found that serum LDL-C, TC and TG concentration were unaffected by supplementation with up to 150 mg zinc per day. Hooper et al.,[31] assessed the effects of 440 mg/day zinc supplementation for five weeks and reported no significant changes in TC, TG and LDL-C concentration at the end of the study. However, TG concentration decreased in this study.

The present research findings were in line with of Roussel et al.,[32] and Fortes et al.[33] studies. Fortes et al.,[33] reported that 25 mg zinc sulphate for three months resulted in a decrease in plasma lipid peroxides. Mechanisms involved in improving lipid profiles and glucose concentration are not clearly identified yet. It has been stated that zinc can play an important role in enzymes involved in lipid and carbohydrate metabolism and similar action to insulin.[34-36] It has been suggested that higher doses of zinc and longer periods of supplementation can be effective in remarkably reduction in TG, TC, and LDL-C concentration.[30] Low doses of zinc over short periods of intervention may be main reasons for non-significant changes in lipid profiles and blood glucose concentration.

In this study, serum zinc concentration increased notably after intervention. Similar to our study's results, Christos et al.,[37] observed that supplementation with 30 mg elemental zinc/day (in zinc acetate form) for 12 weeks and 60 mg elemental zinc/day (as zinc acetate) for 6 to 8 weeks resulted in an increase in plasma zinc concentration. Gomez et al.,[38] reported a significant rise in serum zinc concentration in 14 obese male subjects supplemented with 100 mg/day oral zinc sulfate (p=0.001). In contrast, in the study done by Marreiro and coworkers[11] plasma zinc concentration did not increase significantly at the end of study.

Regarding the anthropometric measurements, there was a significant reduction in weight, waist circumference and BMI indices after intervention. These results are supported by Song et al. and Hashemipour et al. Song et al.,[21] demonstrated that supplementation of 30 obese male S-D rats divided in four groups of 5-6 rats with drinking (no additive, 10 mg zinc plus 1mg Cyclo-(His-Pro) CHP. L-1, 10 mg zinc plus 3mg CHP.L-1 and 10 mg zinc plus 6mg CHP.L-1) for 15 days resulted in a significant reduction in weight especially in rats that were receiving 10 mg zinc plus 3mg CHP.L-1 (p<0.01). Likewise, Hashemipour et al., found that supplementation with 20 mg elemental zinc in of 60 obese children aged between 6-10 for 8 weeks resulted in significant reduction of BMI and weight without changes in waist circumference.[39]

The effective mechanisms of zinc supplementation on weight loss can be due to 1) the role of zinc in appetite regulation through changes in hypothalamic neurotransmitter metabolism by affecting the leptin system and its receptors, although zinc can induce synthesis of leptin and prevention of hyperplasia[11] 2) preventive role of zinc in the gene mutation which can increase the risk of obesity[40] 3) similarity of zinc to insulin action and improving insulin sensitivity and insulin resistance.[36,41]

Conclusion

The results of this study indicated that one month supplementation of zinc gluconate (30 mg/day) in obese male and female adults resulted in a remarkable reduction in weight and BMI indices as well as an increase in serum zinc concentration. However, serum lipid profiles and fasting blood glucose with the exception of TG did not change noticeably. To the best of our knowledge, this was the first study in the region that investigated the effect of zinc supplementation on obese adults in both gender and it can be considered as the strength of the study. Nevertheless, there was limitations such as short period of follow-up. It can be

suggested that increasing the period of intervention and determining the safety and effectiveness of doses of zinc supplementation be considered in future studies.

Acknowledgments
The authors thank the Department of Nutrition, Faculty of Health and Nutrition. Nutrition Research Center supports thus study. This is a part of a database from thesis entitled Evaluation and comparison of zinc on leptin levels in obese peoples.

Conflict of Interest
The authors declare there is no Conflict of interest in the content of this study.

References
1. Malekzadeh R, Mohamadnejad M, Merat Sh, Pourshams A, Etemadi A. Obesity Pandemic: an Iranian perspective. *Arch Iranian Med* 2005;8(1):1–7.
2. Sola E, Jover A, Lopez-Ruiz A, Jarabo M, Vaya A, Morillas C, et al. Parameters of inflammation in morbid obesity: Lack of effect of moderate weight loss. *Obes Surg* 2009;19(5):571-6.
3. Ford ES. Prevalence of the metabolic syndrome defined by the international diabetes federation among adults in the U.S. *Diabetes Care* 2005;28(11):2745-9.
4. O'Kane JW, Teitz CC, Fontana SM, Lind BK. Prevalence of obesity in adult population of former college rowers. *J Am Board Fam Pract* 2002;15(6):451-6.
5. WHO. Obesity and overweight fact sheet [data base on the internet] UK: WHO Media centre; 2012; cited 2012 December; Available from: www.who.int/mediacentre/factsheets/fs311/en.
6. Ayatollahi SMT, Ghoreshizade Z. prevalence of obesity and overweight among adults in Iran. *Obesity Rev* 2010;10:335-7.
7. Lands WE. Long-term fat intake and biomarkers. *Am J Clin Nutr* 1995;61(3 Suppl):721S-5S.
8. Frayn KN. Visceral fat and insulin resistance--causative or correlative? *Br J Nutr* 2000;83 Suppl 1:S71-7.
9. Mataix J, Lopez-Frias M, Martinez-de-Victoria E, Lopez-Jurado M, Aranda P, Llopis J. Factors associated with obesity in an adult mediterranean population: Influence on plasma lipid profile. *J Am Coll Nutr* 2005;24(6):456-65.
10. Marreiro DN, Fisberg M, Cozzolino SM. Zinc nutritional status and its relationships with hyperinsulinemia in obese children and adolescents. *Biol Trace Elem Res* 2004;100(2):137-49.
11. Marreiro DN, Geloneze B, Tambascia MA, Lerario AC, Halpern A, Cozzolino SM. Effect of zinc supplementation on serum leptin levels and insulin resistance of obese women. *Biol Trace Elem Res* 2006;112(2):109-18.
12. Konukoglu D, Turhan MS, Ercan M, Serin O. Relationship between plasma leptin and zinc levels and the effect of insulin and oxidative stress on leptin levels in obese diabetic patients. *J Nutr Biochem* 2004;15(12):757-60.

13. Garcia OP, Long KZ, Rosado JL. Impact of micronutrient deficiencies on obesity. *Nutr Rev* 2009;67(10):559-72.

14. Richards BK, Steenhuis TS, Peverly JH, McBride MB, Perrone L, Gialanella G, et al. Zinc, copper, and iron in obese children and adolescents. *Nutr Res* 1998;18:183-9.

15. Chen MD, Lin PY, Sheu WH. Zinc status in plasma of obese individuals during glucose administration. *Biol Trace Elem Res* 1997;60(1-2):123-9.

16. Song Y, Wang J, Li XK, Cai L. Zinc and the diabetic heart. *Biometals* 2005;18(4):325-32.

17. Simon SF, Taylor CG. Dietary zinc supplementation attenuates hyperglycemia in db/db mice. *Exp Biol Med (Maywood)* 2001;226(1):43-51.

18. Chausmer AB. Zinc, insulin and diabetes. *J Am Coll Nutr* 1998;17(2):109-15.

19. Tallman DL, Taylor CG. Effects of dietary fat and zinc on adiposity, serum leptin and adipose fatty acid composition in c57bl/6j mice. *J Nutr Biochem* 2003;14(1):17-23.

20. Marreiro DN, Fisberg M, Cozzolino SM. Zinc nutritional status in obese children and adolescents. *Biol Trace Elem Res* 2002;86(2):107-22.

21. Song MK, Rosenthal MJ, Song AM, Uyemura K, Yang H, Ament ME, et al. Body weight reduction in rats by oral treatment with zinc plus cyclo-(his-pro). *Br J Pharmacol* 2009;158(2):442-50.

22. Jimenez J, Zuniga-Guajardo S, Zinman B, Angel A. Effects of weight loss in massive obesity on insulin and c-peptide dynamics: Sequential changes in insulin production, clearance, and sensitivity. *J Clin Endocrinol Metab* 1987;64(4):661-8.

23. Di Toro A, Marotta A, Todisco N, Ponticiello E, Collini R, Di Lascio R, et al. Unchanged iron and copper and increased zinc in the blood of obese children after two hypocaloric diets. *Biol Trace Elem Res* 1997;57(2):97-104.

24. Saghaei M. Random allocation software for parallel group randomized trials. *BMC Med Res Methodol* 2004;4(26):1-6

25. Dell RB, Holleran S, Ramakrishnan R. Sample size determination. *ILAR J* 2002;43(4):207-13.

26. Dabbaghmanesh MH, Kalantarhormozi MR, Soveid M, Sadeghalvad A, Ranjbar Omrani GR. Plasma zinc concentration in type 2 diabetic patients and control group in Shiraz city. *Iran J Diabetes Lipid Disorders* 2007;7(2):189-94.

27. Kathleen Mahan L, Escott-Stump S, Raymond JL, Krause MV. Krause's Food and the Nutrition Care Process. 13th ed. St. Louis: Elsevier Elsevier/Saunders; 2012.

28. Foster M, Petocz P, Samman S. Effects of zinc on plasma lipoprotein cholesterol concentrations in humans: A meta-analysis of randomised controlled trials. *Atherosclerosis* 2010;210(2):344-52

29. Afkhami Ardekani M, Karimi M, Mohammadi M, Nourani F. Effect of Zinc Sulfate Supplementation on Lipid and Glucose in Type 2 Diabetic Patients. *Pak J Nutr* 2008; 7(4): 550-3.

30. Hughes S, Samman S. The effect of zinc supplementation in humans on plasma lipids, antioxidant status and thrombogenesis. *J Am Coll Nutr* 2006;25(4):285-91.

31. Hooper PL, Visconti L, Garry PJ, Johnson GE. Zinc lowers high-density lipoprotein-cholesterol levels. *JAMA* 1980;244(17):1960-1.

32. Roussel AM, Kerkeni A, Zouari N, Mahjoub S, Matheau JM, Anderson RA. Antioxidant effects of zinc supplementation in tunisians with type 2 diabetes mellitus. *J Am Coll Nutr* 2003;22(4):316-21.

33. Fortes C, Agabiti N, Fano V, Pacifici R, Forastiere F, Virgili F, et al. Zinc supplementation and plasma lipid peroxides in an elderly population. *Eur J Clin Nutr* 1997;51(2):97-101.

34. Petering HG, Murthy L, O'Flaherty E. Influence of dietary copper and zinc on rat lipid metabolism. *J Agric Food Chem* 1977;25(5):1105-9.

35. Rogalska J, Brzoska MM, Roszczenko A, Moniuszko-Jakoniuk J. Enhanced zinc consumption prevents cadmium-induced alterations in lipid metabolism in male rats. *Chem Biol Interact* 2009;177(2):142-52.

36. Chen MD, Liou SJ, Lin PY, Yang VC, Alexander PS, Lin WH. Effects of zinc supplementation on the plasma glucose level and insulin activity in genetically obese (ob/ob) mice. *Biol Trace Elem Res* 1998;61(3):303-11.

37. Mantzoros CS, Prasad AS, Beck FW, Grabowski S, Kaplan J, Adair C, et al. Zinc May Regulate Serum Leptin Concentrations in Humans. *J Am Coll Nutr* 1998;17(3):270-5.

38. Gomez-Garcia A, Hernandez-Salazar E, Gonzalez-Ortiz M, Martinez-Abundis E. Effect of oral zinc administration on insulin sensitivity, leptin and androgens in obese males. *Rev Med Chil* 2006;134(3):279-84.

39. Kelishadi R, Hashemipour M, Adeli K, Tavakoli N, Movahedian-Attar A, Shapouri J, et al. Effect of zinc supplementation on markers of insulin resistance, oxidative stress, and inflammation among prepubescent children with metabolic syndrome. *Metab Syndr Relat Disord* 2010;8(6):505-10.

40. Prasad AS. Zinc in human health: Effect of zinc on immune cells. *Mol Med* 2008;14(5-6):353-7.

41. Haase H, Maret W. Protein Tyrosine Phosphatases as Targets of the combined insulinomimetric effects of zinc and oxidants. *Biometals* 2005;18(4):333-8.

13

Effect of Acute Administration of loganin on Spatial Memory in Diabetic Male Rats

Shirin Babri[1], Saeideh Hasani Azami[1], Gisou Mohaddes[2]*

[1]Neuroscience Research Center, Tabriz University of Medical Sciences, Tabriz, Iran

[2] Drug Applied Research Center, Tabriz University of Medical Sciences, Tabriz, Iran.

ARTICLE INFO	ABSTRACT
Keywords: Loganin Diabetes Spatial memory Rat	***Purpose:*** Diabetes is associated with memory and learning disorder. The purpose of this study is to determine the effect of acute oral administration of loganin on memory in diabetic male rats. ***Methods:*** 42 male Wistar rats (250-300 g) were divided into six groups: Control, Diabetic (1 week), Diabetic (12 weeks), Loganin, Diabetic (1 week) + Loganin, Diabetic (12 weeks) + Loganin. Diabetes was induced by IP injection of Streptozotocin (60 mg/kg). Loganin (40 mg/kg, po) was administrated 1 hour before test. Then, spatial memory was compared between groups with Morris Water Maze tests. ***Results:*** Administration of loganin during acquisition, significantly ($p<0.05$) decreased both escape latency and traveled distance to find hidden platform in 1 and 12 weeks diabetic rats. In evaluation of recall phase of memory, loganin significantly ($p<0.05$) increased time and distance spent in the target quadrant in 1 and 12 weeks diabetic rats. ***Conclusion:*** Acute administration of loganin could improve spatial memory in diabetic rats.

Introduction

Diabetes mellitus is a very common metabolic disorder characterized by hyperglycemia and insufficiency of secretion or action of endogenous insulin.[1] Diabetes causes complications affecting the retina, kidney, muscle and blood vessels, and the nervous system.[2] Many studies show that changes in cerebral structure and function in diabetes are related to hyperglycemia-induced end organ damage, macrovascular disease, hypoglycemia, insulin resistance, and amyloid lesions.[3] On the one hand, diabetes induces cytochrome c release from mitochondria into cytoplasm that may play a role in apoptosis of the CA1 pyramidal neurons.[4] On the other hand, diabetes causes a reduction in neurogenesis.[5]

There are also electrophysiological and structural abnormalities of the brain in diabetic patients providing good reasons to believe that cognitive functions may be impaired in diabetes mellitus.[6] Moreover, oxidative stress could contribute to learning and memory deficits in diabetes.[7]

Loganin as an iridoid glycoside first was found in Flos lonicerae, Fruit cornus, and Strychonos nux vomica.[8] It has been used as a traditional medicine in Japan and China.[9] According to one study, loganin has a plasma glucose lowering action in normal rats and regulates immune function and has anti-inflammatory, neuroprotective and anti-shock effects.[8,9]

In an Alzheimer's model of study, Kwon and colleagues proved that loganin could have anti-amnesic and anti acetylcholinesterase activity in the hippocampus and frontal cortex.[10] Furthermore, our recent studies showed that acute administration of loganin improves memory in passive avoidance tests and chronic application of it exhibits protective effect on spatial learning and memory in diabetic rats.[11,12]

In this study, we evaluated the effect of acute oral administration of loganin on learning and memory deficits in one and 12 weeks diabetic rats in the Morris water maze tasks.

Materials and Methods

Streptozotocin (STZ) was purchased from Tocris Bioscience (Bristol, UK) and dissolved in normal saline immediately before use. Loganin was purchased from Extrasynthese (France) and dissolved in normal saline.

Animals

Male Wistar rats, weighing (250–300) g, were used in the present experiment. All animals were maintained at a constant temperature (20±1) and on a 12 h light: 12 h dark cycle. They had free access to water and food ad libitum. The Regional Ethics Committee of Tabriz University of Medical Sciences approved all experimental procedures.

---

*Corresponding author: Gisou Mohaddes, Associate Professor, Drug Applied Research Center, Tabriz University of Medical Sciences, Tabriz, Iran.
E-mail: gmohades@yahoo.com

Experimental Design

Male Wistar rats ($n = 42$) were divided into six groups ($n = 7$ each): control, diabetic (1 week), diabetic (12 week), loganin, diabetic (1 week) + loganin, diabetics (12 week) + loganin. Experimental diabetes was induced by a single dose of STZ (60 mg/kg, intraperitoneal (ip)). Three days after STZ injection, fasting blood glucose levels were determined. Animals were considered diabetic if plasma glucose levels exceeded 300 mg/dl.[13] Loganin (40 mg/kg, po) was administrated once after confirming diabetes. Animals were tested for spatial memory 1 h after loganin treatment.[10]

Morris Water Maze Test

The Morris water maze was black circular pool (136 cm in diameter and 100 cm in height). The pool was filled to a depth of 60 cm with water (20 ± 1 °C) and divided into four quadrants of equal area (NE, SE, SW and NW). A platform (10 cm in diameter) was centered in one of the four quadrants of the pool and submerged 1 cm below the water surface so that it was invisible at water level. The swimming was monitored by a video camera, which was positioned directly above the center of the pool. The pool was located in a test room, which contained various prominent visual cues.[14]

One week after surgery, the rats were trained in the water maze. The single training session consisted of eight trials (in two blocks) with four different starting positions that were equally distributed around the perimeter of the maze. The task requires rats to swim to the hidden platform guided by distal spatial cues. After mounting the platform, the rats were allowed to remain there for 20 s, and then were placed in a holding cage for 30 s until the start of the next trial. Rats were given a maximum of 60 s to find the platform and if it failed to find the platform in 60 s, it was placed on the platform and allowed to rest for 20 s. Latency to platform and distance traveled were collected and analyzed later. After completion of the training, the animals were returned to their home cages until retention testing 24 h later. The probe trial consisted of 60 s free swim period without a platform and the time swum in the target quadrant was recorded.

In order to assess the possibility of drug interference with animal sensory and motor coordination or the animal motivation, the capability of rats to escape to a visible platform was tested in this study. The trained rats were given four trials for visuo-motor coordination on the visible platform.[15]

Statistics

SPSS 13.0 software was used for statistical comparisons of data, and data expressed as the means ± SEM. For comparisons between Block 1 and Block 2 in each group, a paired-sample T test was used. The statistical analysis of the data between groups was carried out by one-way ANOVA followed by Tukey

test. In all comparisons, $P<0.05$ was the criterion for statistical significance.

Results

In comparison of block 1 and block 2, diabetes increased escape latency and traveled distance (Figures 1, 2) in 1 and 12 weeks diabetic rats during acquisition phase. Loganin (40 mg/kg) significantly decreased latency time ($P<0.05$) and traveled distance ($P<0.05$) in 1 and 12 weeks diabetic rats.

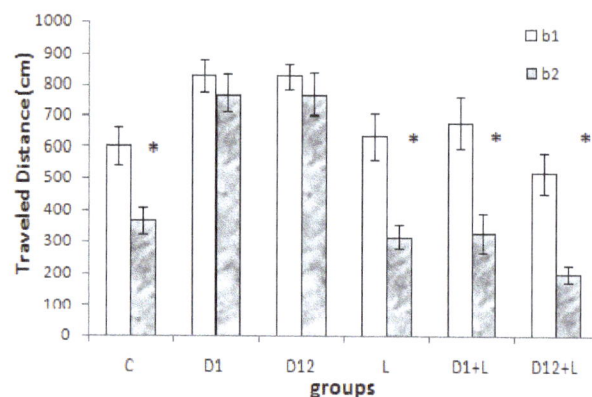

Figure 1. Effect of loganin on the traveled distance to find hidden platform in two consecutive blocks (b1 and b2). In the diabetic rats, loganin (40 mg/kg, po) were administered 60 min before the tests. Data represent means ± S.E.M. (n=7). *P<0.05, significantly different when compared with the b_1 same group.

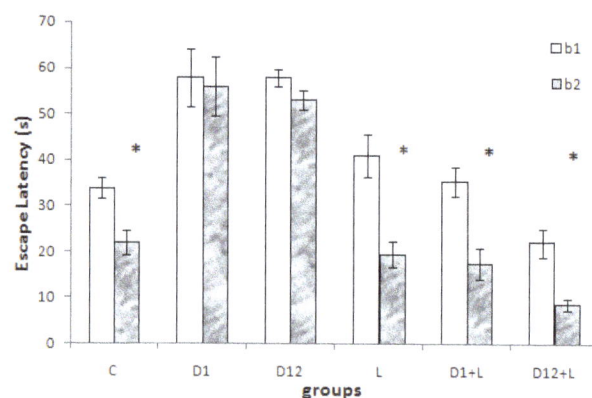

Figure 2. Effect of loganin on the escape latency to find hidden platform in two consecutive blocks (b1 and b2). In the diabetic rats, loganin (40 mg/kg, po) were administered 60 min before the tests. Data represent means ± S.E.M. (n=7). *P<0.05, significantly different when compared with the b_1 same group.

Probe test data were compared between groups. One-way ANOVA of the distance traveled in the target quadrant revealed significant differences ($P<0.05$) between groups. Loganin (40 mg/kg) increased the time and distance in the target quadrant after the platform was removed (Figures 3, 4). No treatments significantly changed swimming speed in the target quadrant (Figure 5). Loganin gavage 60 min before visual trial (visible platform) also showed no difference in escape latency and traveled distance to find the visible platform, compared to the control group (data are not shown).

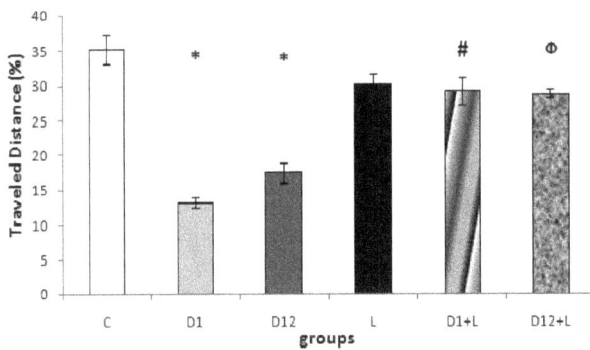

Figure 3. Effect of loganin on the traveled distance in trial sessions of the Morris water maze test. Data represent means± S.E.M. (n=7).
*P<0.05 significantly different when compared with the control group.
#P<0.05 significantly different when compared with the 1 week diabetic group.
ΦP<0.05 significantly different when compared with the 12 weeks diabetic group.

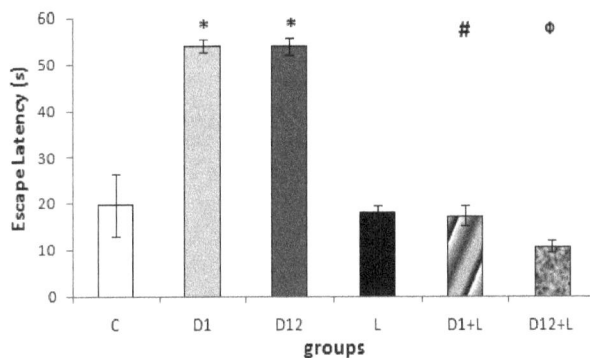

Figure 4. Effect of loganin on the escape latency in trial sessions of the Morris water maze test. Data represent means± S.E.M. (n=7).
*P<0.05 significantly different when compared with the control group.
#P<0.05 significantly different when compared with the 1 week diabetic group.
ΦP<0.05 significantly different when compared with the 12 weeks diabetic group.

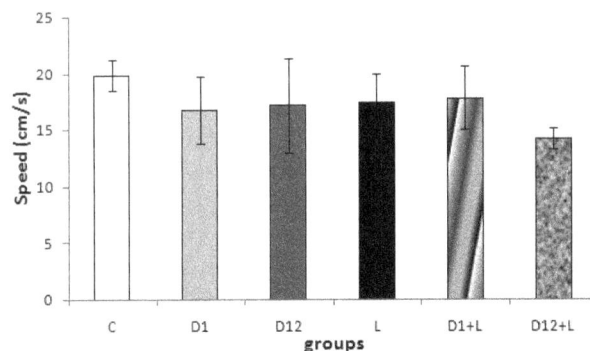

Figure 5. Effect of loganin on the swimming speed in trial sessions of the Morris water maze test. Data represent means± S.E.M. (n=7). Loganin did not change the swimming speed.

Discussion

In the present study, loganin was used for the first time in evaluating memory impairment of Streptozotocin-induced diabetes. Our results showed that diabetic (1, 12 weeks) rats had an increased escape latency time and traveled distance to find the hidden platform in a MWM task. Loganin administration with a dose of 40 mg/kg/po improved the acquisition and retrieval in diabetic rats. In addition, the results of the visible platform test suggest that loganin does not have an effect on mood or sensorimotor activity in rats; rather, it appears to shorten escape latency by enhancing memory due to the effect on brain areas involved in memory consolidation, such as the hippocampus.

Diabetes mellitus is a chronic disease characterized by widespread complications in CNS and PNS.[16] Learning and memory in animal model of diabetes are impaired.[17] Chronic hyperglycemia is associated with oxidative stress-induced neuronal and Schwann cell death and the reduction of neural size in the rat brain.[18,19] Also, learning deficits in diabetic rats have been associated with changes in hippocampal synaptic plasticity.[20]

As previously mentioned, loganin is an iridoid glycoside that is found in many traditional Chinese, Japan, and Korea herbs.[10] Loganin, is an active compound and was found to exhibit immune-regulating and anti-inflammatory activity.[21,22] It has hepato-protective, renal protective and neuroprotective effects.[8,23,24]

In addition Kwon and colleagues showed that loganin may have anti-amnesic activity in alleviating certain memory impairments observed in Alzheimer's disease.[10] Our recent study also showed that loganin improves passive avoidance learning in diabetic male rats.[11]

Although the exact mechanism of action of loganin on diabetic deficit of learning and memory is not clear, it may act by preventing oxidative stress, inhibiting acetyl cholinesterase activity in the hippocampus and inhibiting advanced glycation end product formation and NF-κB induced inflammation in the hepatic tissue.[10,25,26] Some other possible mechanisms of loganin action include inhibition of release of Cyt-c from mitochondria into cytoplasm of hippocampal pyramidal neurons and reduction of apoptosis levels and induction of neurogenesis and angiogenesis in the brain.[4,8,27]

Nevertheless, further studies are needed to increase the understanding of the physiological mechanisms leading to this memory enhancing effect of loganin.

Conclusion

In summary, our results suggested that loganin alleviates diabetes-induced memory impairments. Therefore, loganin could be used as an agent of treatment for the learning and memory-deficit cause by diabetes.

Acknowledgements
This study was financially supported by the Neuroscience Research Centre of Tabriz University of Medical Sciences. The article is derived from the MSc dissertation of Ms Saeedeh Hasani Azami entitled ''Effect of loganin on spatial memory and passive avoidance learning in diabetic male rats''.

Conflict of Interest
There is no conflict of interest in this study.

References

1. Maritim AC, Sanders RA, Watkins JB. Diabetes, Oxidative Stress, and Antioxidants: A Review. *J Biochem Mol Toxicol* 2003; 17(1): 24-38.
2. Sima AA, Kamiya H, Li ZG. Insulin, C-peptide, hyperglycemia, and central nervous system complications in diabetes. *Eur J Pharmacol* 2004; 490(1-3): 187-97.
3. Kodl CT, Seaquist ER. Cognitive Dysfunction and Diabetes Mellitus. *Endocr Rev* 2008; 29(4):494-511.
4. Ye L, Wang F, Yang RH. Diabetes impairs learning performance and affects the mitochondrial function of hippocampal pyramidal neurons. *Brain Res* 2011; 1411:57-64.
5. Jackson-Guilford J, Leander JD, Nisenbaum LK. The effect of streptozotocin-induced diabetes on cell proliferation in the rat dentate gyrus. *Neurosci Lett* 2000; 293(2): 91-4.
6. Gispen WH, Biessels GJ. Cognition and synaptic plasticity in diabetes mellitus. *Trends Neurosci* 2000; 23(11): 542-9.
7. Tuzcu M, Baydas G. Effect of melatonin and vitamin E on diabetes-induced learning and memory impairment in rats. *Eur J Pharmacol* 2006; 537(1-3):106-10.
8. Kwon SH, Kim JA, Hong SI, Jung YH, Kim HC, Lee SY, et al. Loganin protects against hydrogen peroxide-induced apoptosis by inhibiting phosphorylation of JNK, p38, and ERK 1/2 MAPKs in SH-SY5Y cells. *Neurochem Int* 2011; 58(4): 533-41.
9. Yamabe N, Kang KS, Goto E, Tanaka T, Yokozawa T. Beneficial effect of Corni Fructus, a constituent of Hachimi-jio-gan, on advanced glycation end-product-mediated renal injury in Streptozotocin-treated diabetic rats. *Biol Pharm Bull* 2007; 30(3):520-6.
10. Kwon SH, Kim HC, Lee SY, Jang CG. Loganin improves learning and memory impairments induced by scopolamine in mice. *Eur J Pharmacol* 2009; 619(1-3): 44-9.
11. Mohaddes G, Hasani Azami S, Babri Sh, Nikkar E, Ebrahimi H. The effect of loganin on passive avoidance learning in diabetic male rats. *Pharm Sci* 2012; 17(4): 219-24.
12. Mohaddes G, Ebrahimi H, Nikkar E, Hasani Azami S, Babri Sh. The effect of chronic oral administration of loganin on spatial memory in diabetic male rats. *Pharmaceut Sci* 2011; 17(3): 201-8.
13. Reisi P, Alaei H, Babri Sh, Sharifi MR, Mohaddes G. Effect of treadmill running on spatial learning and memory in streptozotocin-induced diabetic rats. *Neurosci Lett* 2009; 455(2): 79-83.
14. Moosavi M, Naghdi N, Maghsoudi N, Zahedi Asl S. The effect of intrahippocampal insulin microinjection on spatial learning and memory. *Horm Behav* 2006; 50(5): 748-52.
15. Mohaddes G, Rasi S, Naghdi N. Evaluation of the effect of intrahippocampal injection of leptin on spatial memory. *Afr J Pharm Pharmacol* 2009; 3(9): 443-8.
16. Grzeda E, Wisniewska RJ. Differentiations of the effect of NMDA on the spatial learning of rats with 4 and 12 week diabetes mellitus. *Acta Neurobiol Exp (Wars)* 2008; 68(3): 398-406.
17. Saberi M, Zarichi Baghlani K, Bahrami F, Zareie Mahmoodabadi A. Effect of diazinone-induced oxidative stressin neuroglial U373 MG cell line and its interaction with pyridpxine. *Kowsar Medical J* 2009; 14(1):25-9.
18. Vincent AM, Brownlee M, Russell JW. Oxidative stress and programmed cell death in diabetic neuropathy. *Ann N Y Acad Sci* 2002; 959:368-83.
19. Malone JI, Hanna S, Saporta S, Mervis R, Park CR, Chong L, et al. Hyperglycemia not hypoglycemia alters neuronal dendrites and impairs spatial memory. *Pediatr Diabetes* 2008; 9(6): 531-9.
20. Hasanein P, Shahidi S. Effects of combined treatment with vitamins C and E on passive avoidance learning and memory in diabetic rats. *Neurobiol Learn Mem* 2010; 93(4): 472-8.
21. Visen PKS, Saraswat B, Raj K, Bhaduri AP, Dubey MP. Prevention of galactosamine-induced hepatic damage by the natural product loganin from the plant Strychnos nux-vomica: studies on isolated hepatocytes and bile flow in rat. *Phytother Res* 1998; 12(6): 405-8.
22. Park CH, Tanaka T, Kim JH, Cho EJ, Park JC, Shibahara N, et al. Hepato-protective effects of loganin, iridoid glycoside from Corni Fructus, against hyperglycemia-activated signaling pathway in liver of type 2 diabetic db/db mice. *Toxicology* 2011; 290(1): 14-21.
23. Yokozawa T, Kang KS, Park CH, Noh JS, Yamabe N, Shibahara N, et al. Bioactive constituents of Corni Fructus: The therapeutic use of morroniside, loganin, and 7-*O*-galloyl-D-sedoheptulose as renoprotective agents in type 2 diabetes. *Drug Discov Ther* 2010; 4(4):223-34.
24. Jiang WL, Zhang SP, Hou J, Zhu HB. Effect of loganin on experimental diabetic nephropathy. *Phytomedicine* 2012; 19(3-4): 217-22.
25. Xu H, Shen J, Liu H, Shi Y, Li L, Wei M. Morroniside and loganin extracted from Cornus officinalis have protective effects on rat mesangial cell proliferation exposed to advanced glycation end

products by preventing oxidative stress. *Can J Physiol Pharmacol* 2006; 84(12):1267-73.

26. Yamabe N, Noh JS, Park Ch, Kang KS, Shibahara N, Tanaka T, et al. Evaluation of loganin, iridoid glycoside from Corni Fructus, on hepatic and renal glucolipotoxicity and inflammation in type 2 diabetic db/db mice. *Eur J Pharmacol* 2010; 648(1-3): 179-87.

27. Yao RQ, Zhang L, Wang W, Li L. Cornel iridoid glycoside promotes neurogenesis and angiogenesis and improves neurological function after focal cerebral ischemia in rats. *Brain Res Bull* 2009; 79(1): 69-76.

14

Percutaneous Absorption of Salicylic Acid after Administration of Trolamine Salicylate Cream in Rats with Transcutol® and Eucalyptus Oil Pre-Treated Skin

Paniz Sajjadi[1], Mohammad Javad Khodayar[2], Behzad Sharif Makhmalzadeh[3], Saeed Rezaee[3]*

[1] Department of Pharmaceutics, School of Pharmacy, Ahvaz Jundishapur University of Medical Sciences, Ahvaz, Iran.

[2] Department of Pharmacology and Toxicology, School of Pharmacy, Ahvaz Jundishapur University of Medical Sciences, Ahvaz, Iran.

[3] Nanotechnology Research Center, Ahvaz Jundishapur University of Medical Sciences, Ahvaz, Iran.

A R T I C L E I N F O

Keywords:
Trolamine salicylate
Transcutol
Eucalyptus oil
Transdermal absorption
Rat
Non-linear mixed effect modeling

A B S T R A C T

Purpose: This study was conducted to assess the effect of skin pre-treatment with Transcutol® and eucalyptus oil on systemic absorption of topical trolamine salicylate in rat. *Methods:* Pharmacokinetic parameters of salicylic acid following administration of trolamine salicylate on rat skin pre-treated with either Transcutol® or eucalyptus oil were determined using both non-compartmental and non-linear mixed effect modeling approaches and compared with those of control group. *Results:* Median (% of interquartile range/median) of salicylic acid AUC_{0-8hr} (ng/mL/hr) values in Transcutol® or eucalyptus oil treated rats were 2522(139%) and 58976(141%), respectively as compared to the 3023(327%) of the control group. Skin pre-treatment with eucalyptus oil could significantly decrease extravascular volume of distribution (V/F) and elimination rate constant (k) of salicylic acid. *Conclusion:* Unlike Transcutol®, eucalyptus oil lead to enhanced transdermal absorption of trolamine salicylate through rat skin.

Introduction

Delivery of pharmacological agents via the skin provides distinct benefits compared to other conventional routes of administration, such as minimizing adverse effects and toxicity due to a steady and optimum blood levels, bypassing intestinal and hepatic first pass effect, prevention of gastrointestinal irritation, etc.[1-3] However, transdermal absorption of most drugs often results in a low bioavailability because of the barrier nature of the skin. The most important reason of resistance to the passage of drugs through the skin is the stratum corneum, the outermost layer of the skin.[1,2,4,5] In order to enhance the permeability of drugs through the skin, many techniques have been employed to overcome stratum corneum impermeability. A popular applied technique is the use of penetration enhancers which reversibly decrease the barrier resistance of the skin.[3-5] These pharmacologically inactive chemical compounds tend to interact with the stratum corneum constituents to ease the absorption of drugs through the skin by temporarily increasing in skin permeability.[5] Trolamine salicylate is a topically applied salicylic acid derivative which is used for temporary relief of pain or inflammation in muscles, joints and other tissues below the skin.[6-10] As trolamine salicylate is an odor free compound and has no skin irritant properties[9], it can be a viable alternative to oral salicylate but is less permeable through skin compared with other salicylic acid derivatives like methyl salicylate.[11] Consequently, to achieve therapeutic concentrations of salicylic acid after transdermal administration of trolamine salicylate, the application of the penetration enhancers is needed.[12] A number of penetration enhancers have been used to evaluate their influence on the in vitro permeation of trolamine salicylate through the abdominal rat skin.

The results showed that the best enhancement of trolamine salicylate flux, was obtained from 12 hours skin pretreatment with Transcutol® (diethylene glycol monoethyl ether) and eucalyptus oil that were able to provide a near 12 and 10 fold increase in flux, respectively, in comparison with controls.[12] However, effect of skin pre-treatment with these enhancers on in vivo absorption of trolamine salicylate has not been investigated. Therefore, the aim of this study was to assess the influence of pre-treatment with Transcutol® and eucalyptus oil on percutaneous absorption of trolamine salicylate in rat. To do this, both non-compartmental and non-linear mixed effect modeling approaches were used to evaluate trolamine salicylate pharmacokinetics after its topical administration in rats with Transcutol® and eucalyptus oil pre-treated skin.

Corresponding author: Saeed Rezaee, Department of Pharmaceutics, School of Pharmacy, Ahvaz Jundishapur University of Medical Sciences, Ahvaz, Iran. Email: s.rezaee@ajums.ac.ir

Materials and Methods

Chemicals

Trolamine salicylate, potassium dihydrogen phosphate, perchloric acid and acetonitrile (HPLC-grade) were purchased from Merck, Germany. Eucalyptus oil, containing 70% 1,8 – cineole was from Barij Essence Company, Kashan, Iran . Transcutol®P (diethyleneglycol monoethyl ether) was kindly donated by Gattefosse, France.

Animal Experiments and Drug Administration

The study was approved by the ethics committee of the Vice Chancellor for Research and Technology of Ahvaz Jundishapur University of Medical Sciences. In vivo experiment was done on male wistar rats weighing 235 ± 20 g which supplied by Animals Care and Breeding Center of Ahvaz Jundishapur University of Medical Sciences. Twelve hours before application of penetration enhancers (one day prior to dosing), the hair of the abdominal region was removed with electric hair clippers. The rats were divided into three groups. In pre-treated groups Transcutol® (N=10) or eucalyptus oil (N=5) in the form of closed dressing were applied to the hairless surface of abdominal skin for 12 hours. Subsequently, the closed dressing was removed and the pre-treated site was carefully wiped clean 50 times with cotton to remove the excess solution and then 1 gram of 10% trolamine salicylate(PERRIGO®, USA) was applied to the pre-treated skin. In control group (N=7), trolamine salicylate was applied to the not-treated skin. Application area of depilated abdominal skin was 12 cm^2 (3 × 4 cm). Rats were under sleep condition with 140 mg/kg intra-peritoneal phenobarbital during the period of pretreatment, application of drug and blood sampling. Blood samples were collected from a heparinized catheter inserted into the tail vein at 0.5, 1, 2, 4, 6, 8 and 10 hours (when it was possible) after administration of drug. Plasma samples were immediately separated by centrifugation at 13,000 rpm for 5 minutes and were stored at -70 °C until the time of analysis.

Analytical Procedure

Salicylic acid concentration in rat plasma following topical administration of trolamine salicylate was determined using high-performance liquid chromatography (HPLC) with fluorescence detection as previously reported with some modifications.[13] The HPLC apparatus consisted of an Agilent 1260 Infinity quaternary pump and Agilent 1260 Infinity fluorescence detector (Agilent, USA) . An Alltech Altima® C18 column (150 mm × 2.1 mm, 5 µm particle size) (Grace Davison Discovery Sciences, USA) was used for the separation. The mobile phase consisted of acetonitrile: phosphate buffer (17: 83) (pH 3) delivered at a flow rate of 0.5 ml/min. Fluorescence detection was performed at 297 nm (excitation) and 407 nm (emission). Plasma samples (50 µL) were transferred into a 1.5-ml micro-centrifuge tubes and mixed with 100 µL of perchloric acid 35%. After vortex mixing for 1 min, 300 µL of acetonitrile was added to this solution. The contents were vortex mixed thoroughly for 2 minutes and centrifuged at 1500 g for 5 minutes. Twenty µL of the clear supernatant was injected onto the column.

Pharmacokinetic Analysis

Non-Compartmental Analysis

Area under the salicylic acid plasma concentration time curve between 0 and 8 hours post administration of trolamine salicylate ($AUC_{0-8 \ hr}$) was calculated using trapezoidal rule to compare the extent of absorption in rats with Transcutol® or eucalyptus oil pre-treated skin with that of the control group. Kruskal-Wallis test followed by pairwise multiple comparisons (SPSS Statistics 20, IBM, USA) was used to check any significant difference of AUC values between treatment groups.

Non-linear mixed effect modeling: Salicylic acid plasma concentration –time data were modeled by a one-compartment model with zero-order absorption input. The inter-animal error terms for all structural model parameters including Tk0 (duration of zero order absorption), k (first order elimination constant) and V/F (extravascular apparent volume of distribution) were assumed to be independently and log-normally distributed with mean zero and variance ω^2. A constant error model was used for the residual random variability. Covariate analysis was also done to assess the effect of skin pre-treatment on trolamine salicylate pharmacokinetics. Influence of pre-treatment on the pharmacokinetic parameters were modeled using the following general equation:[14]

$$ln \ P_{i,pre-treated} = lnP_{i,control} + \beta_{i,pre-treatment}$$

in which $P_{i, \ pre-treated}$ and $P_{i, \ control}$ are the population values of pharmacokinetic parameter i in each of pre-treated groups and control group, respectively. β_i is the pre-treatment effect for parameter i. Non-linear mixed effect analysis was carried out using Monolix 4.2.0 (Lixoft, France). Model selection was based on the significant reduction in minimum objective function(MOF) that is equal to -2×log likelihood value; parameter precision(expressed as relative standard errors of the estimated parameters) and visual inspection of goodness-of-fit plots including the prediction distribution graph. Discrimination between two nested models (e.g. with and without covariate effect) was carried out using log-likelihood ratio test assuming a chi-squared distribution for the difference between minimum objective function values. A significance level of 0.005 corresponding to a decrease of 7.879 (1 degree of freedom) in minimum objective function was considered.

Results and Discussion

Salicylic Acid Analysis Method

The linear dynamic quantitation range of the employed HPLC method was between 25(limit of quantitation) and 5000 ng/mL in rat plasma with a correlation coefficient of 0.999. The intra- and inter-day accuracy for salicylic acid over the above concentration range fell in the ranges of 99-100 % and 110-113%, respectively with the analytical recovery of greater than 85%. The intra- and inter-day precision were 5-6% and 3-13%, respectively.

Non-Compartmental Analysis

Plasma concentration time profiles of salicylic acid following topical administration of trolamine salicylate in different groups of rats with Transcutol®- or eucalyptus oil pre-treated skin in comparison to control group(without any skin pre-treatment) is presented in Figure 1. Median values of $AUC_{0-8 hr}$(% of interquartile range/median) were 2522(139%), 58976(141%), 3023(327%) ng/mL/hr for Transcutol®, eucalyptus oil and control groups, respectively. As could be seen from Figure 2, significant differences were observed between median value of $AUC_{0-8 hr}$ in rats which their skins were pre-treated with eucalyptus oil with those of Transcutol® (p =0.030) and control (p=0.004)groups. However, no statistically significant difference was detected between the median of $AUC_{0-8 hr}$ in control and Transcutol® pre-treated rats. Furthermore, the inter-animal variability in $AUC_{0-8 hr}$ was lower in rats with either Transcutol® or eucalyptus oil pre-treated skin as compared to control group.

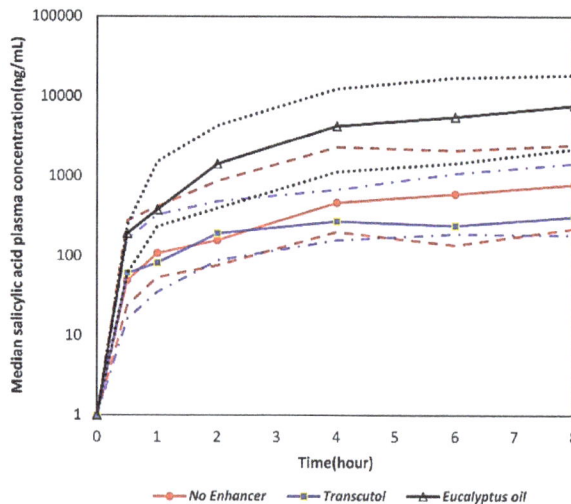

Figure 1. Median plasma concentration-time profile of salicylic acid following topical administration of trolamine salicylate in different groups of rats with Transcutol- or eucalyptus oil pre-treated skin in comparison to control group (dashed lines with the same color represent 95 % confidence around the median values).

Non-Linear Mixed Effect Modeling

Any attempt to estimate salicylic acid elimination rate constant (k) with enough precision was unsuccessful that could be related to insufficient plasma concentration-time data of the elimination phase in the majority of the rats under investigation. Therefore, the population value of k was fixed to 0.105 hr^{-1} which has been reported by Varma et al in a group of male rats

with the same range of age and weight.[15] Parameters of the base population model (model without including any covariates) are presented in Table 1. *Bayesian* individual rats' estimates of pharmacokinetic parameters were used for covariate screening. As could be seen from Figure 3, statistically significant differences were observed between the median of individual estimates of the pharmacokinetic parameters in eucalyptus oil pre-treated rats with both Transcutol pre-treated and control groups. So, the influence of pre-treatment on the pharmacokinetic parameters of salicylic acid was further assessed by including it as a categorical covariate in the population model. Results of covariate analysis are shown in Table 2. Although, inclusion of both pre-treatments(with Transcutol and eucalyptus oil) as an influential covariate on all pharmacokinetic parameters led to statistically significant reductions in MOF values, the estimated β coefficients were not enough precise(p-values greater than 0.05). In case of model with pre-treatment effect on Tk0 alone (second model in Table 2), the estimated values of Tk0 did not make sense (4 hour for control group).

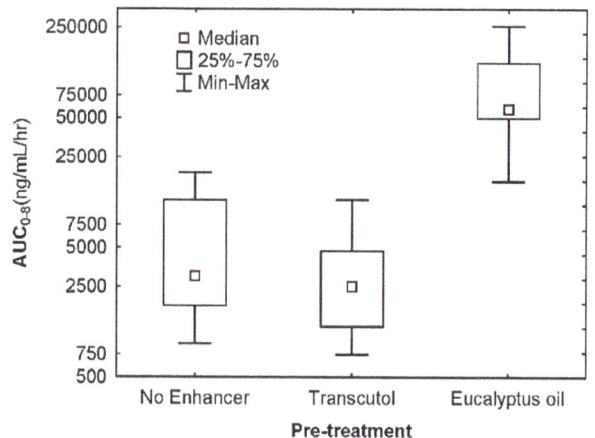

Figure 2. Comparison of area under the salicylic acid plasma concentration-time curve up to 8 hours (AUC_{0-8hr}) post administration of 100 mg trolamine salicylate (1g of 10% cream) in rats with untreated, Transcutol or eucalyptus oil pre-treated skin.

Table 1. Pharmacokinetic parameters of salicylic acid base population model (model without pre-treatment effect as a categorical covariate) following topical administration of trolamine salicylate in rats with Transcutol- or eucalyptus oil pre-treated skin and control group.

Parameter	Value	[a]SE	Relative SE (%)
Tk0(hr)	13.8	3.1	23
V/F(mL)	13.2	4.5	35
[b]*k(hr⁻¹)*	0.105	-	-
[c]ω_{Tk0}	0.53	0.17	32
[c]ω_V	1.13	0.26	23
[c]ω_k	2.55	0.56	22
Residual error(ng/mL)	413	24	6

[a] Standard error of estimate
[b] Not estimated
[c] Inter-individual variability of pharmacokinetic parameters in log-normal domain

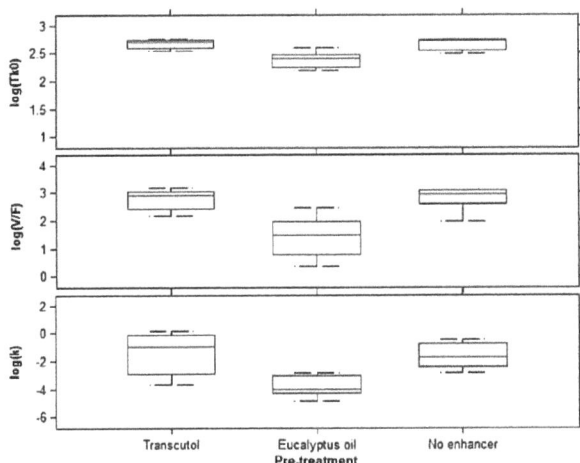

Figure 3. Comparison of base model (without pre-treatment effect as a covariate) individual estimates of salicylic acid pharmacokinetic parameters after topical administration of trolamine salicylate between different groups of rats with and without skin pre-treatment. Box and horizontal line inside it represents 25 - 75 percentile range and median, respectively. Non-outlier minimum and maximum observed values are shown by whiskers.

As could be seen from Table 2, effect of skin pre-treatment with Transcutol on pharmacokinetic parameters of salicylic acid was not statistically significant. Therefore, in the next step of covariate analysis, Transcutol® and control group rats were pooled into one group as not-treated with eucalyptus oil. The final selected covariate model (shown in italic letters) was the one that assumes a significant effect of skin pre-treatment with eucalyptus oil on extravascular volume of distribution and elimination rate constant of salicylic acid. Considering a covariance between Tk0 and V/F resulted in better estimates of all parameters. Prediction distribution of salicylic acid plasma concentration by the final population model along with the observed data are shown in Figure 4. The majority of the observed concentration data lie within the 90 percent confidence interval of the model prediction.

Table 2. Comparison of different models with skin pre-treatment as a covariate (levels of significant difference of the β parameters are given in parenthesis).

Model	-2log-likliehood ([a] MOF)	[b] ΔMOF	[c] β₁	[d] β₂	[e] β₃	[f] β₄	[g] β₅	[h] β₆
Base model(no-covariate effect)	2870.56	-	-	-	-	-	-	-
Effect of pre-treatment on Tk0	2833.61	-36.95	2.19 (0.0019)	0.74 (<0.0001)	-	-	-	-
Effect of pre-treatment on V/F	2844.93	-25.63	-	-	0.12 (0.75)	-2.02 (<0.0001)	-	-
Effect of pre-treatment on k	2853.97	-16.59	-	-	-	-	-0.70 (0.53)	-1.73 (0.0014)
Effect of pre-treatment on Tk0 and V/F	2840.70	-29.86	0.70 ([i] -)	0.07 (0.87)	-0.22 (0.69)	-1.98 (<0.0001)	-	-
Effect of pre-treatment on Tk0 and k	2846.82	-23.74	1.39 (0.0520)	1.13 (0.11)	-	-	-2.86 (0.77)	-1.53 (0.0001)
Effect of pre-treatment on V/F and k	2834.02	-36.54	-	-	0.36 (0.21)	-1.83 (<0.0001)	-1.99 (0.65)	-1.16 (<0.0001)
Effect of pre-treatment on Tk0 , V/F and k	2831.93	-38.63	1.32 (1)	-0.24 (0.71)	-0.52 (0.63)	-1.79 (<0.0001)	-.53 (0.63)	-1.26 (<0.0001)
[j] *Effect of eucalyptus oil on Tk0*	2860.15	-10.41	-	-1.48 (0.021)	-	-	-	-
[j] *Effect of eucalyptus oil on V/F*	2844.56	-26.00	-	-	-	-2.01 (<0.0001)	-	-
[j] *Effect of eucalyptus oil on k*	2853.51	-17.05	-	-	-	-	-	-1.89 (0.0005)
[j] *Effect of eucalyptus oil on V/F and k*	2834.62	-35.94	-	-	-	-1.98 (<0.0001)	-	-1.96 (0.012)
[j] *Effect of eucalyptus oil on Tk0 and V/F*	2841.62	-28.94	-	-0.11 (0.84)	-	-2.03 (<0.0001)	-	-
[j] *Effect of eucalyptus oil on Tk0 and k*	2849.24	-21.32	-	-1.73 (0.007)	-	-	-	-1.48 (<0.0001)
[j] *Effect of eucalyptus oil on Tk0, V/F and k*	2832.75	-37.81	-	-0.46 (0.42)	-	-1.85 (<0.0001)	-	-1.31 (0.0001)
[j, k] *Effect of eucalyptus oil on V/F and k assuming a covariance between Tk0 and V/F*	*2833.48*	*-37.08*	-	-	-	*-2.20 (<0.0001)*	-	*-1.63 (0.0015)*

[a] Minimum objective function; [b] in comparison to the base model; [c] coefficient of the effect of Transcutol pre-treatment on Tk0; [d] coefficient of the effect of eucalyptus oil pre-treatment on Tk0; [e] coefficient of the effect of Transcutol pre-treatment on V/F; [f] coefficient of the effect of eucalyptus oil pre-treatment on V/F; [g] coefficient of the effect of Transcutol pre-treatment on k; [h] coefficient of the effect of eucalyptus oil pre-treatment on k; [i] could not be calculated; assuming no difference between pharmacokinetic parameters of rats in Transcutol and control groups and putting them into one group as not0treated with eucalyptus oil; [k] final selected model

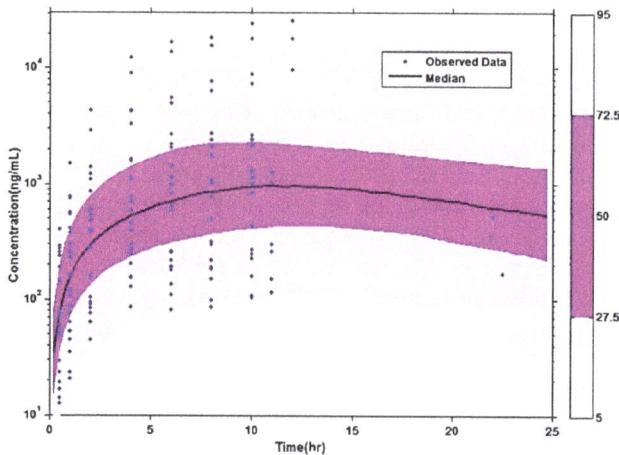

Figure 4. Prediction distribution of salicylic acid plasma concentration following administration of trolamine salicylate to rats by the final population model including skin pre-treatment with eucalyptus oil as an influential covariate (color bands represent different prediction percentiles)

Parameters of the final selected model are presented in Table 3. Results indicated that inclusion of pre-treatment with eucalyptus oil could lead to substantial reduction in inter-animal variability of pharmacokinetic parameters.

Table 3. Pharmacokinetic parameters of salicylic acid final population model (model including pre-treatment with eucalyptus oil as a categorical covariate) following topical administration of trolamine salicylate in rats with Transcutol- or eucalyptus oil pre-treated skin and control group.

Parameter	Value	[a] SE	Relative SE (%)
$Tk0(hr)$	17.3	3.0	17
$V/F(mL)$	24.0	4.1	17
[b] $\beta_{eucalyptus\ oil\ effect\ on\ V/F}$	-2.2	0.25	11
[c] $k(hr^{-1})$	0.105	-	-
[d] $\beta_{eucalyptus\ oil\ effect\ on\ k}$	-1.63	0.51	31
[e] ω_{Tk0}	0.64	0.13	21
[e] $\omega_{V/F}$	0.41	0.11	26
[e] ω_{k}	0.70	0.34	49
correlation between Tk0 and V/F	0.81	0.17	21
$V/F_{eucalyptus\ oil\ group}(mL)$	2.7	0.5	18
$V/F_{other\ groups}(mL)$	24.0	4.1	17
$k_{eucalyptus\ oil\ group}(hr^{-1})$	0.021	0.01	51
$k_{other\ groups}(hr^{-1})$	0.105	-	-
Residual error(ng/mL)	416	24	6

[a] Standard error of estimate

[b] Significant at p <0.0001

[c] Not estimated

[d] Significant at p = 0.0015

[e] Inter-animal variability of pharmacokinetic parameters in log-normal domain

Lower extravascular apparent volume of distribution in rats with eucalyptus oil pre-treated skin as compared to other groups, might be due to the enhanced bioavailability (increase in F) of trolamine salicylate.

On the other hand, a considerable decrease in elimination rate constant of the eucalyptus oil group rats, could be attributed to the saturation of salicylic acid elimination pathways due to the high plasma concentration of salicylic acid achieved following application of eucalyptus oil as transdermal penetration enhancer.[16,17]

Tk0 is not affected by pre-treatment, therefore the zero order absorption rate is not different among three groups of rats.

Permeation Enhancing Effect of Transcutol® and Eucalyptus Oil

The results of the present study show that eucalyptus oil created an appreciable increase in transdermal absorption of trolamine salicylate through rat skin compared with the control while Transcutol® did not have any significant enhancing effect on trolamine salicylate permeation.

The inability of Transcutol® to promote transdermal permeation of trolamine salicylate in the present study is inconsistent with the finding of in vitro study of Sharif Makhmalzade and Hasani.[12] In their experiments Transcutol® was found to cause the best enhancement of trolamine salicylate flux (12 fold) followed by eucalyptus oil (10 fold) in comparison to control. Such a lack of correlation between in vitro and in vivo permeability of triethanolamine salicylate was also reported by Cross et al during their study on topical penetration of salicylate esters and salts using human isolated skin and clinical microdialysis technique. They suggested that there is a possibility that in vivo salicylate in the epidermis could not be released as quickly as in vitro because of differences in sink condition or some sorts of strong binding to tissue constituents.[18]

According to the contradictory results that have been published in the literature, Transcutol® can increase or decrease transdermal delivery of topically applied compounds. It has been reported that prostaglandin[19] and theophylline[20] in vitro skin permeability was increased by the presence of Transcutol® due to its solubilizing effect that increases the solubility of drug in the skin, thus provides a raising in drug partitioning.[21] However, other researchers found that Transcutol® was not able to show any significant enhancing effect on the percutaneous absorption of morphine,[22] salicylic acid[23] and melatonin.[24]

It has been suggested that Transcutol® can lead to formation of cutaneous depot of drugs due to its ability to cause intercellular lipids swelling, thereby associated with drug entrapment in the skin.[25-27] In addition, high molecular weight of some drugs have been suggested to be one of the restrictions for Transcutol® effectiveness.[28]

1, 8 Cineol (eucalyptol) is the principal chemical component of eucalyptus oil. Cineol is a cyclic ether and tend to be more effective on hydrophilic drug (like salicylates) permeation. This penetration enhancer affects the lipid bilayer structure by forming liquid pools in those region. Thus cineol increases skin permeability by disrupting the lipid structure of the stratum corneum.[5,29,30]

Conclusion

Unlike eucalyptus oil, skin pre-treatment with Transcutol® could not lead to enhancement of trolamine salicylate transdermal absorption in rat. Eucalyptus oil could result in more than 20 fold increase in systemic absorption of trolamine salicylate through rat skin as compared to control group.

Acknowledgments

This paper was extracted from Pharm.D thesis no. 812 that submitted in School of Pharmacy of Ahvaz Jundishapur University of Medical Sciences and financially supported by grant no. N-27 from Nanotechnology Research Center of the same university. The authors also would like to thank Fratein Co.S.K for supplying Transcutol from Gattefosse company.

Conflict of Interest

There is no conflict of interest to be reported.

References

1. Hadgraft J. Skin, the final frontier. *Int J Pharm* 2001;224(1-2):1-18.
2. Prausnitz MR, Langer R. Transdermal drug delivery. *Nat Biotechnol* 2008;26(11):1261-8.
3. Barry BW. Dermatological formulations: Percutaneous absorption. Newe York: M. Dekker; 1983.
4. Finnin BC, Morgan TM. Transdermal penetration enhancers: Applications, limitations, and potential. *J Pharm Sci* 1999;88(10):955-8.
5. Williams AC, Barry BW. Essential oils as novel human skin penetration enhancers. *Int J Pharmaceut* 1989;57(2):R7-R9.
6. Algozzine GJ, Stein GH, Doering PL, Araujo OE, Akin KC. Trolamine salicylate cream in osteoarthritis of the knee. *JAMA* 1982;247(9):1311-3.
7. Baldwin JR, Carrano RA, Imondi AR. Penetration of trolamine salicylate into the skeletal muscle of the pig. *J Pharm Sci* 1984;73(7):1002-4.
8. Hill DW, Richardson JD. Effectiveness of 10% trolamine salicylate cream on muscular soreness induced by a reproducible program of weight training. *J Orthop Sports Phys Ther* 1989;11(1):19-23.
9. Rothacker D, Difigilo C, Lee I. A clinical trial of topical 10% trolamine salicylate in osteoarthritis. *Curr Therap Res* 1994;55(5):584-97.
10. Rothacker DQ, Lee I, Littlejohn TW, 3rd. Effectiveness of a single topical application of 10|x% trolamine salicylate cream in the symptomatic treatment of osteoarthritis. *J Clin Rheumatol* 1998;4(1):6-12.
11. Baldwin J, Carrano R, Imondi A. Penetration of trolamine salicylate into the skeletal muscle of the pig. *J Pharm Sci* 1984;73(7):1002-4.
12. Makhmal Zadeh BS, Hasani MH. The effect of chemical and physical enhancers on trolamine salicylate permeation through rat skin. *Trop J Pharm Res* 2010;9(6):541-8
13. Megwa SA, Benson HA, Roberts MS. Percutaneous absorption of salicylates from some commercially available topical products containing methyl salicylate or salicylate salts in rats. *J Pharm Pharmacol* 1995;47(11):891-6.
14. Lavielle M. Monolix user's guide. 4.2 ed: The monolix team; 2012.
15. Varma DR, Yue TL. Influence of age, sex, pregnancy and protein-calorie malnutrition on the pharmacokinetics of salicylate in rats. *Br J Pharmacol* 1984;82(1):241-8.
16. Cao Y, Dubois DC, Almon RR, Jusko WJ. Pharmacokinetics of salsalate and salicylic acid in normal and diabetic rats. *Biopharm Drug Dispos* 2012;33(6):285-91.
17. Patel DK, Notarianni LJ, Bennett PN. Comparative metabolism of high doses of aspirin in man and rat. *Xenobiotica* 1990;20(8):847-54.
18. Cross SE, Anderson C, Roberts MS. Topical penetration of commercial salicylate esters and salts using human isolated skin and clinical microdialysis studies. *Br J Clin Pharmacol* 1998;46(1):29-35.
19. Watkinson AC, Hadgraft J, Bye A. Aspects of the transdermal delivery of prostaglandins. *Int J Pharm* 1991;74(2-3):229-36.
20. Touitou E, Levi-Schaffer F, Shaco-Ezra N, Ben-Yossef R, Fabin B. Enhanced permeation of theophylline through the skin and its effect on fibroblast proliferation. *Int J Pharm* 1991;70(1-2):159-66.
21. Harrison JE, Watkinson AC, Green DM, Hadgraft J, Brain K. The relative effect of Azone and Transcutol on permeant diffusivity and solubility in human stratum corneum. *Pharm Res* 1996;13(4):542-6.
22. Rojas J, Falson F, Couarraze G, Francis A, Puisieux F. Optimization of binary and ternary solvent systems in the percutaneous absorption of morphine base. *STP Pharma Sci* 1991;1(1):70-5.
23. Smith JC, Irwin WJ. Ionisation and the effect of absorption enhancers on transport of salicylic acid through silastic rubber and human skin. *Int J Pharm* 2000;210(1-2):69-82.
24. Kikwai L, Kanikkannan N, Babu RJ, Singh M. Effect of vehicles on the transdermal delivery of melatonin across porcine skin in vitro. *J Control Release* 2002;83(2):307-11.
25. Panchagnula R, Ritschel WA. Development and evaluation of an intracutaneous depot formulation of corticosteroids using transcutol as a cosolvent:

In-vitro, ex-vivo and in-vivo rat studies. *J Pharm Pharmacol* 1991;43(9):609-14.

26. Du Plessis J, Weiner N, Müller DG. The influence of in vivo treatment of skin with liposomes on the topical absorption of a hydrophilic and a hydrophobic drug in vitro. *Int J Pharmaceut* 1994;103(2):R1-5.

27. Godwin DA, Kim NH, Felton LA. Influence of transcutol CG on the skin accumulation and transdermal permeation of ultraviolet absorbers. *Eur J Pharm Biopharm* 2002;53(1):23-7.

28. Bonina FP, Montenegro L. Effects of some non-toxic penetration enhancers on in vitro heparin skin permeation from gel vehicles. *Int J Pharmaceut* 1994;111(2):191-6.

29. Moghimi HR, Williams AC, Barry BW. Enhancement by terpenes of 5-fluorouracil permeation through the stratum corneum: Model solvent approach. *J Pharm Pharmacol* 1998;50(9):955-64.

30. Williams AC, Barry BW. Penetration enhancers. *Adv Drug Deliv Rev* 2004;56(5):603-18.

15

Comparison of Inhibitory Effect of Curcumin Nanoparticles and Free Curcumin in Human Telomerase Reverse Transcriptase Gene Expression in Breast Cancer

Fatemeh Kazemi-Lomedasht[1,2], Abbas Rami[2], Nosratollah Zarghami[1]*

[1] *Drug Applied Research Center, Tabriz University of Medical Sciences, Tabriz, Iran.*

[2] *Pasteur Institute of Iran, Tehran, Iran.*

ARTICLE INFO

Keywords:
Anti cancer drug
Target therapy
Telomerase
Breast cancer
Drug delivery

ABSTRACT

Purpose: Telomerase is expressed in most cancers, including breast cancer. Curcumin, a polyphenolic compound that obtained from the herb of Curcuma longa, has many anticancer effects. But, its effect is low due to poor water solubility. In order to improve its solubility and drug delivery, we have utilized a β-cyclodextrin-curcumin inclusion complex. ***Methods***: To evaluate cytotoxic effects of cyclodextrin-curcumin and free curcumin, MTT assay was done. Cells were treated with equal concentration of cyclodextrin-curcumin and free curcumin. Telomerase gene expression level in two groups was compared by Real-time PCR. ***Results***: MTT assay demonstrated that β-cyclodextrin-curcumin enhanced curcumin delivery in T47D breast cancer cells. The level of telomerase gene expression in cells treated with cyclodextrin-curcumin was lower than that of cells treated with free curcumin (P=0.001). ***Conclusion***: Results are suggesting that cyclodextrin-curcumin complex can be more effective than free curcumin in inhibition of telomerase expression.

Introduction

Telomerase activity is observed in more than 85% in the most cancer cells.[1] Telomerase is active in 74% of breast Carcinomas[2,3] Therefore, targeting the telomerase in this cancer could be promising step in its treatment.[4] For this purpose it is better to use natural compounds such as Curcumin (CUR). Curcumin (commonly known as turmeric) is obtained from Curcuma longa.[5] Curcumin has many pharmacological applications such as anticancer, with low or no intrinsic toxicity.[6] Despite all these, curcumin suffers from low water solubility and bioavailability.[7] To improve its solubility, β-Cyclodextrin was used for encapsulation of curcumin. β-Cyclodextrin is a semi-natural compound with low toxicity, which could enhance drug bioavailability.[7] To the best of our knowledge, comparison of inhibitory effect of free CUR and CD-CUR on hTERT gene expression in T47D cell line has never been done so far. Anti-telomerase effect of curcumin has been studied previously in lung cancer cell line[8,9] and preparation of β-cyclodextrin-curcumin inclusion complex for improvement of curcumin stability and solubility has been studied.[7] In our previous study we showed the inhibitory effect of β-Cyclodextrin-curcumin in telomerase gene expression in breast cancer cell line.[10] Rajeswari *et al* reported that cyclodextrin enhance the bioavailability of insoluble drugs by increasing the drug solubility.[11] Yadav and coworkers showed that Cyclodextrin-complexed curcumin had superior attributes compared with free curcumin for cellular uptake.[12] Murali *et al* found that CD-CUR inhibit the growth of prostate cells higher than free curcumin.[9] Therefore in this study we investigated the effect of β-Cyclodextrin-curcumin (CD-CUR) and free CUR (CUR) on human telomerase reverse transcriptase (hTERT) gene expression. Anticancer effect of free CUR and CD-CUR in breast cancer cell line, T47-D was compared. The level of telomerase gene expression after 24 h exposure was measured by Real-time PCR.

Materials and Methods

Cell culture and cell line

T47D cell line (breast cancer epithelial like cell line) was prepared from Pasteur Institute cell bank of Iran, code: C203. This cell line was cultured in RPMI1640 (Gibco, Invitrogen, UK) supplemented with 10% heat-inactivated fetal bovine serum (FBS) (Gibco, Invitrogen, UK), 2 mg/ml sodium bicarbonate, 0.05 mg/ml penicillin G (Serva co, Germany), 0.08 mg/ml streptomycin (Merck co, Germany) and incubated in 37°C with humidified air containing 5% CO_2.

In vitro cytotoxicity (MTT assay)

Cells in the exponential phase of growth were exposed to CD-CUR inclusion complex or free CUR. Cytotoxic

Corresponding author: Nosratollah Zarghami, Drug applied Research center, Tabriz University of Medical Sciences Tabriz, Iran.
E-mail : zarghami@tbzmed.ac.ir

effect of CD-CUR inclusion complex and free CUR was studied by 24, 48 and 72 h MTT assay. 2×10^3 cell/well was plated in a 96-well plate (Coastar from Corning, NY). After 24 h incubation, cells were treated with different concentrations (5-100 μM) of CD-CUR and free CUR for 24, 48 and 72 h in the quadruplicate manner. Media containing equivalent amounts of CD in PBS or DMSO was used as control. After different exposure duration, medium was removed and then fed of the cells with 200 μL of fresh medium. Cells were incubated for 24 h, then 50 μL of 2 mg/ml MTT (Sigma co, Germany) dissolved in PBS was added to each well and plats were covered with aluminum foil and incubated for 4 h. In the next step, wells' content was removed and 200 μL pure DMSO and 25 μL Sorensen's glycine buffer were added. Finally amount of formazan was determined by measuring the absorbance at 570 nm using an ELISA plate reader (with a reference wavelength of 630 nm).

Cell treatment

After determining of IC_{50}, 2.5×10^5 cells in 25 cm² flasks were treated with 3 concentrations lower than IC_{50} of 24h CD-CUR (5, 10 and 15 μM). Culture flasks were incubated for 24 h. For control cells, the same volume of 10%DMSO without CUR and CD-CUR was added to flask of control cells. An equivalent amount of CD in PBS was used as another control. Culture flasks were incubated in 37°C containing 5% CO2 with humidified atmosphere incubator for 24 h exposure duration.

Real-Time PCR (qRT-PCR) Assay

After the RNA extraction (by the TRIZOL kit, Cinnagene, Iran), cDNA synthesized according the instructions (First Strand cDNA Synthesis Kit fermentase, K1622).

For real-time PCR, according to our previous study[10], hTERT primers (Genbank accession: NM_198255, bp 2165-2362) and beta actin primers (Genbank accession: NM_001101, bp 787-917) were used. For hTERT, a 198 bp amplicon and for beta actin a 131 bp amplicon were generated in a 25 μl reaction mixture that contained: 5 pmole of the forward and reverse PCR primers of hTERT (5'CCGCCTGAGCT-GTACTTTGT3', 5' CAGGTGAGCCACGAACTGT3' respectively) or for beta actin (5'TCCCTGGAGAAGAGCTACG3', 5'GTAGTTT-CGTGGATGCCACA3' respectively), 2X PCR Master Mix Syber Green I, and 2μl of the cDNA was used. Each DNA sample was divided so that hTERT and beta actin could be amplified, in parallel, and in duplicated from equal amounts of starting cDNA separately. 25 μl reactions contained the following final concentrations: 1X of MaximaTM SYBR Green/ROX qPCR Master Mix (including Maxima TM Hot start Taq Polymerase, Maxima TM SYBR Green qPCR Buffer, SYBR Green I and ROX Passive reference dye), 5pmole of each primer and 2μl of the cDNA. Negative controls were

prepared each time, consisting of 2 μl ddH₂O instead of the cDNA template. The sample tubes were placed into the (Rotor-Gene 6000, Corbet) with the following settings as manufacture protocol.

Results and Discussion
Cell toxicity studies

In this study to evaluate the cytotoxic effect (MTT assay) of CD-CUR and free CUR, T47D breast cancer cell line were treated with different concentration (5-100μM) of CD-CUR and free CUR for 24, 48 and 72h. IC_{50} after 24 h treatment with CD-CUR and CUR was 18 μM and 22 μM respectively (Figure 1). Drug free CD as well as DMSO 2% showed an absorbance value equivalent of 90 and 92% of control respectively suggesting that CD and DMSO 2% have low effect on the cells. Cells treated with concentrations more than 60 μM of CD-CUR and free CUR for 48 and 72h were died completely. IC_{50} after 48 h treatment with CD-CUR and CUR was 13 and 17μM respectively (Figure 2 and 3). Considering the fact that IC_{50} values for different treatment durations are not similar, it might be concluded that the effect of CD-CUR and CUR on T47D cell line is time-depending. Moreover IC_{50} show that effect of CD-CUR on cells is more than free CUR, Demonstrating the enhanced uptake of CD-CUR with respect to CUR.

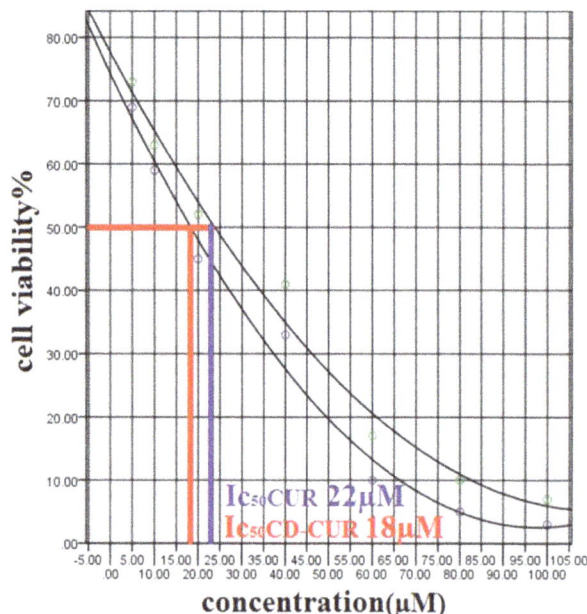

Figure 1. MTT assay graph of 24 h cell treatment with CD-CUR and CUR.

Real-time PCR

Figure 4 and 5 demonstrate the results of telomerase gene expression study at T47D breast cancer cell line after 24 h of CD-CUR and free CUR exposure. β-Cyclodextrin-curcumin suppresses cell proliferation in T47D breast cancer cells. Cells were treated with curcumin (CUR) or CD-CUR for 24 h. Cell proliferation was determined by MTT assay and normalized to cells treated with equivalent amounts of respective controls (DMSO for curcumin and cyclodextrin for CD-CUR). The level of hTERT mRNA was normalized to mRNA levels of the housekeeping gene, Beta actin, within each sample. The differences of $2^{-\Delta\Delta Ct}$ values were calculated. Increasing $2^{-\Delta\Delta Ct}$ amount resulted in enhanced expression of mRNA levels. Data analyses of real-time PCR showed that with increasing the concentration of CD-CUR and free CUR, a decreasing trend is observed in mRNA levels of hTERT. Compared to CUR, in the same concentration, CD-CUR resulted in a lower mRNA level of hTERT and lower level of hTERT mRNA expression (Figure 5). The difference between two groups was statistically significant (p=0.001, n=4) (Figure 6).

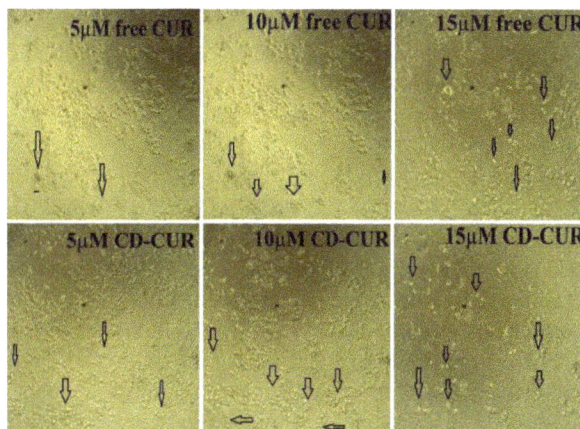

Figure 4. β-Cyclodextrin-curcumin and free curcumin treatment cells (Images were taken by Phase contrast microscope).

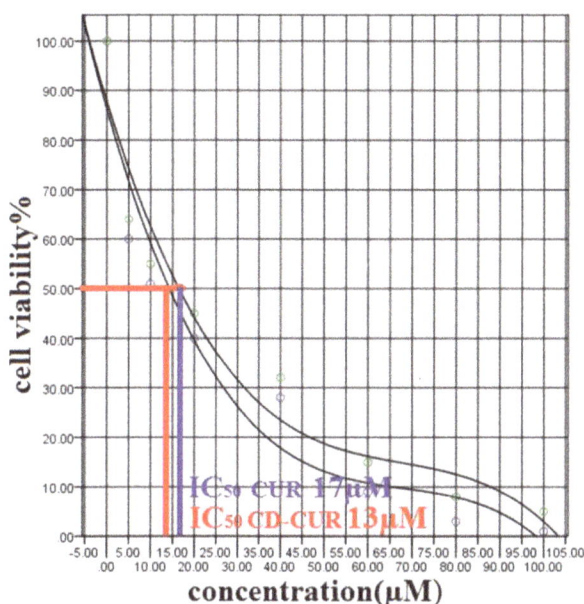

Figure 2. MTT assay graph of 48 h cell treatment with CD-CUR and CUR.

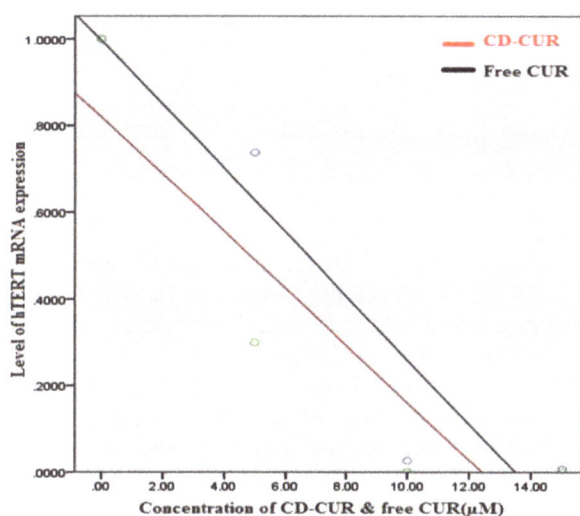

Figure 5. Level of hTERT mRNA expression in cells treated with CD-CUR or free CUR.

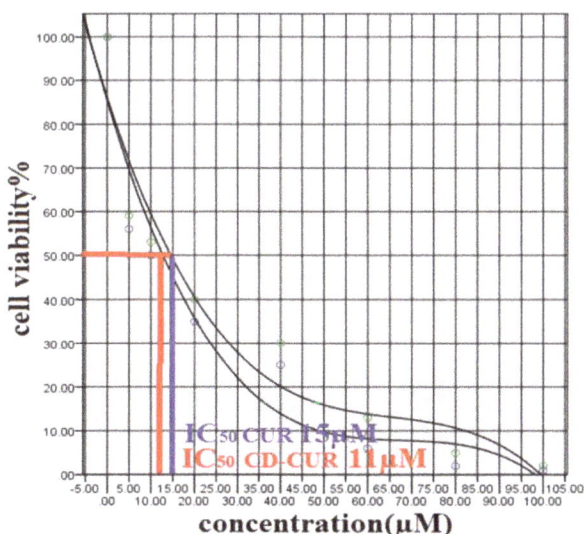

Figure 3. MTT assay graph of 72 h cell treatment with CD-CUR and CUR.

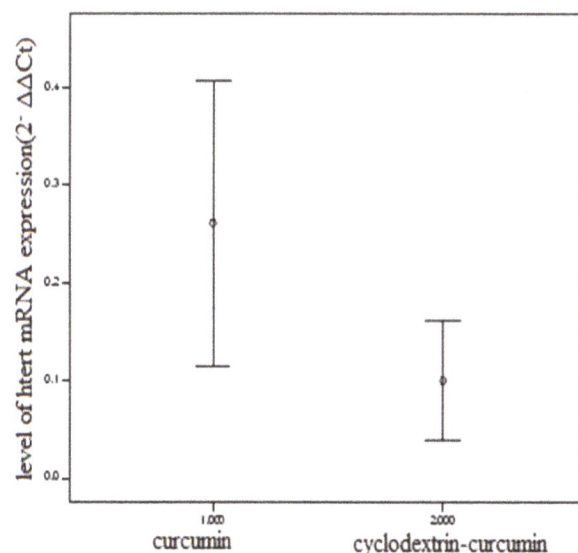

Figure 6. comparision of hTERT mRNA expression in curcumin as well as cyclodextrin-curcumin treated cells. The difference between two groups was statistically significant (p=0.001, n=4).

Conclusion
Our results showed that CD-CUR and free CUR had inhibitory effect on T47D breast cancer cell line. This inhibition was time and dose dependent. β-cyclodextrin-curcumin resulted in higher cell toxicity than free curcumin in breast cancer cell line. There was a significant difference between cells treated with CD-CUR and cells treated with free CUR in the levels of telomerase gene expression. The quantity of telomerase was decreased in the cells treated with CD-CUR in comparison to cells treated with free CUR (P=0.001). It may be concluded that relative to free CUR, CD-CUR inclusion complex inhibit the telomerase gene expression in T47D cell line more effectively.

Acknowledgements
This study was supported by grants from Drug Applied Research Center of Tabriz University of Medical Sciences. We thank thereby Drug Applied Research Center of Tabriz University of Medical Sciences for funding this research.

Conflict of interest
There is no conflict of interest in this study.

References
1. Tarkanyi I, Aradi J. Pharmacological intervention strategies for affecting telomerase activity: Future prospects to treat cancer and degenerative disease. *Biochimie* 2008;90(1):156-72.
2. Kirkpatrick KL, Ogunkolade W, Elkak AE, Bustin S, Jenkins P, Ghilchick M, et al. hTERT expression in human breast cancer and non-cancerous breast tissue: correlation with tumour stage and c-Myc expression. *Breast Cancer Res Treat* 2003;77(3):277-84.
3. Tian N, Gaines Wilson J, Benjamin Zhan F. Female breast cancer mortality clusters within racial groups in the united states. *Health Place* 2010;16(2):209-18.
4. Nicole MB. Targeting telomerase and telomeres with small molecule anticancer compounds. *MMG 445 Basic Biotechnology eJournal* 2008;4:72-9.
5. Daybe FV. Uber Curcumin. *Den Farbstoff der Curcumawurzzel Ber* 1870;3:609.
6. Kunnumakkara AB, Anand P, Aggarwal BB. Curcumin inhibits proliferation, invasion, angiogenesis and metastasis of different cancers through interaction with multiple cell signaling proteins. *Cancer Lett* 2008;269(2):199-225.
7. Aggarwal BB, Sundaram C, Malani N, Ichikawa H. Curcumin: The indian solid gold. *Adv Exp Med Biol* 2007;595:1-75.
8. Sharma RA, Gescher A, Steward WP. Curcumin: the story so far. *Eur J Cancer* 2005; 41(13): 1955-68.
9. Yallapu MM, Jaggi M, Chauhan SC. Beta-Cyclodextrin-curcumin self-assembly enhances curcumin delivery in prostate cancer cells. *Colloids Surf B Biointerfaces* 2010;79(1):113-25.
10. Kazemi F, Zarghami N, Fekri-aval S, Monfaredan A. β-Cyclodextrin-curcumin complex inhibit telomerase gene expression in T47-D breast cancer cell line. *Afr J Biotechnol* 2011; 83(10): 19481-88.
11. Challa R, Ahuja A, Ali J, Khar RK. Cyclodextrins in drug delivery: An updated review. *AAPS PharmSciTech* 2005;6(2):E329-57.
12. Yadav R, Sahdeo P, Ramaswamy K, Javaraj R, Chaturvedi M, Lauri V, et al. Cyclodextrin-complexd curcumin exhibits antiinflamatory and anti proliferative activity. *Biochem pharmacol* 2010; 80(7): 1021-32.

Effects of Enzyme Induction and/or Glutathione Depletion on Methimazole-Induced Hepatotoxicity in Mice and the Protective Role of N-Acetylcysteine

Reza Heidari[1,2], Hossein Babaei[1,2], Leila Roshangar[3], Mohammad Ali Eghbal[1,2]*

[1] Drug Applied Research Center, Tabriz University of Medical Sciences, Tabriz, Iran.

[2] Pharmacology and Toxicology Department, Faculty of Pharmacy, Tabriz University of Medical Sciences, Tabriz, Iran.

[3] Anatomical Sciences Department, Faculty of Medicine, Tabriz University of Medical Sciences, Tabriz, Iran.

ARTICLE INFO

Keywords:
Enzyme induction
Glutathione
Hepatotoxicity
Methimazole
Mice
N-acetylcysteine

ABSTRACT

Purpose: Methimazole is the most convenient drug used in the management of hyperthyroid patients. However, associated with its clinical use is hepatotoxicity as a life threatening adverse effect. The exact mechanism of methimazole-induced hepatotoxicity is still far from clear and no protective agent has been developed for this toxicity.

Methods: This study attempts to evaluate the hepatotoxicity induced by methimazole at different experimental conditions in a mice model. Methimazole-induced hepatotoxicity was investigated in different situations such as enzyme-induced and/or glutathione-depleted animals.

Results: Methimazole (100 mg/kg, i.p) administration caused hepatotoxicity as revealed by increase in serum alanine aminotransferase (ALT) activity as well as pathological changes of the liver. Furthermore, a significant reduction in hepatic glutathione content and an elevation in lipid peroxidation were observed in methimazole-treated mice. Combined administration of L-buthionine sulfoximine (BSO), as a glutathione depletory agent, caused a dramatic change in methimazole-induced hepatotoxicity characterized by hepatic necrosis and a severe elevation of serum ALT activity. Enzyme induction using phenobarbital and/or β-naphtoflavone beforehand, deteriorated methimazole-induced hepatotoxicity in mice. N-acetyl cysteine (300 mg/kg, i.p) administration effectively alleviated hepatotoxic effects of methimazole in both glutathione-depleted and/or enzyme-induced animals.

Conclusion: The severe hepatotoxic effects of methimazole in glutathione-depleted animals, reveals the crucial role of glutathione as a cellular defense mechanism against methimazole-induced hepatotoxicity. Furthermore, the more hepatotoxic properties of methimazole in enzyme-induced mice, indicates the role of reactive intermediates in the hepatotoxicity induced by this drug. The protective effects of N-acetylcysteine could be attributed to its radical/reactive metabolite scavenging, and/or antioxidant properties as well as glutathione replenishment activities.

Introduction

Methimazole is a worldwide used anti-hyperthyroidism drug, which its clinical use is associated with hepatotoxicity.[1] Although the exact mechanism that methimazole causes hepatotoxicity through it is not clearly understood yet, but some investigations revealed that cellular glutathione reservoirs has a fundamental role in preventing methimazole-induced damage.[2-5] Furthermore, the importance of glutathione in methimazole-induced cytotoxicity was shown previously in our laboratory in an *in vitro* model of isolated rat hepatocytes.[6] Previous studies proposed the role of reactive metabolites in methimazole-induced toxicity.[7,8] It has been shown that N-methylthiourea as a suspected reactive intermediate of methimazole is produced at *in vitro* models.[8,9] N-methylthiourea is further metabolized by cytochrome (CYP) and/or flavin monooxygenase (FMO) enzymes to sulfenic acid species.[8,10] Sulfenic acids are reactive electrophilic metabolites[11] and could interact with different intracellular targets, which might consequently encounter toxicity.[11] In a study on methimazole-induced toxicity in rat olfactory mucosa, it has been shown that the metabolic pathways and CYP enzymes play a major role in the toxicity induced by this drug.[5] In addition, glyoxal as another metabolite of methimazole[8], might plays a role in methimazole-induced hepatotoxicity.[6]

*Corresponding author: Mohammad Ali Eghbal, Tabriz University of Medical Sciences, Pharmacology and Toxicology Department, Faculty of Pharmacy, Tabriz, Iran. Email: m.a.eghbal@hotmail.com

This study attempted to evaluate the role of hepatic glutathione reservoirs in methimazole-induced hepatotoxicity. In addition, the role of N-acetyl cysteine (NAC) as a protective agent in this situation was studied. To investigate the effect of metabolism and metabolic pathways, the adverse effects of methimazole was studied in enzyme-induced animals and the protective role of NAC was also evaluated in this situation.

Serum alanine amino transferase (ALT) levels, lipid peroxidation, hepatic glutathione (GSH) contents, and liver histopathological changes were assessed in different conditions after methimazole administration alone and/or in combination with NAC.

Materials and Methods
Chemicals
Methimazole was purchased from Medisca pharmaceutique (Montreal, Canada). 5,5′-dithionitrobenzoic acid (DTNB) and L-buthionine sulfoximine (BSO) were purchased from Sigma-Aldrich (St. Louis, USA). Thiobarbituric acid (TBA) was obtained from SERVIA (Heidenberg, New York). Trichloro acetic acid (TCA), β-naphtoflavone, Sodium dodecyl sulfate (SDS), Phenobarbital, and Hydroxy methyl amino methane (Tris) were purchased from Merck (Dardamstd, Germany). The kit for alanine aminotransferase (ALT) analysis was obtained from Pars Azmun Company (Tehran, Iran). All salts for preparing buffer solutions were of the highest grade commercially available.

Animals
Male Swiss albino mice, 6 weeks old (25-40 g weight), were obtained from Tabriz University of Medical Sciences (Tabriz, Iran). Mice were housed in cages on wood bedding at a temperature of 25±3 °C. Unless otherwise stated, mice had free access to food and water. The animals were handled and used according to the animal handling protocol approved by the Tabriz University's ethics committee.

Animals were randomly divided equally into eleven groups of five animals. The treatments were as follows: Group A (control): vehicle (0.9% saline solution) only. Group B: 100 mg/kg methimazole (i.p, dissolved in 0.9% saline). Group C: 100 mg/kg methimazole + BSO (1 g/kg, i.p). Group D: 100 mg/kg methimazole + BSO (1 g/kg) + NAC (300 mg/kg, i.p). Group E: β-naphtoflavone-induced animals + methimazole 100 mg/kg. Group F: β-naphtoflavone-induced animals + methimazole 100 mg/kg + NAC 300 mg/kg. Group G: Phenobarbital-induced animals + methimazole 100 mg/kg. Group H: Phenobarbital-induced animals + methimazole 100 mg/kg + NAC 300 mg/kg. There was no significant differences between groups; I (BSO-treated animals), J (β-naphtoflavone-induced animals), and group K (Phenobarbital-induced animals), and the control (vehicle-treated) animals in the parameters assessed in this study.

Glutathione-depleted animals
Mice were treated with buthionine sulfoximine (BSO) (1 g/kg) as a model for hepatic glutathione depletion in animals.[12] One hour later, BSO-treated animals were given methimazole (100 mg/kg i.p). Food was removed at 15 hours before dosing with BSO and supplied again at 2 hours after methimazole administration.[3]

Enzyme-induced mice
β-naphtoflavone-induced animals were treated with β-naphtoflavone (40 mg/kg, i.p) for three consecutive days.[13] Phenobarbital-induced animals were treated with 80 mg/kg of phenobarbital (i.p injection for three days) before the experiments.[13] At the forth day, animals were treated with methimazole (100 kg/kg, i.p).

Serum biochemical analysis and liver histopathology
Blood was collected from the abdominal vena cava under pentobarbital anesthesia, and the liver was removed. The blood was allowed to clot at 25°C, and serum was prepared by centrifugation (1000 g, for 20 minutes).[14] Serum alanine transaminase (ALT) activities were measured with a commercial kit. For histo-pathological evaluation, samples of liver were fixed in formalin (10%). Paraffin-embedded sections of liver were prepared and stained with haematoxylin and eosin (H&E) before light microscope viewing.[14]

Liver glutathione content
The excised livers were immediately frozen at -70° C and analyzed for glutathione (GSH) within 24 hours. Briefly, samples of liver (200 mg) were homogenized in 8 ml of 20 mM EDTA. The GSH contents were assessed by determining non-protein sulphydryl contents with the Ellman reagent.[15]

Lipid peroxidation
Level of lipid peroxidation was measured in different experimental groups. Briefly, reaction mixture consist of 0.2 ml 8% SDS, 1.5 ml 20% trichloro acetic acid, and 0.6 ml distilled water. 0.2 ml of tissue homogenate was added to the reaction mixture. Reaction was initiated by adding 1.5 ml of 1% thiobarbituric acid (TBA) and terminated by 10% trichloroacetic acid (TCA). Samples were centrifuged (3000 g for 5 minutes) and the absorbance of developed color was read at 532 nm using an Ultrospec 2000® UV spectrophotometer.[16]

Statistical analysis
Results are shown as Mean±SE. Comparisons between multiple groups were made by a one-way analysis of variance (ANOVA) followed by Turkey's *post hoc* test. Differences were considered significant when P<0.05.

Results
Mice were treated with 100 mg/kg of methimazole, which was reported as a hepatotoxic dose of this drug in previous investigations.[3] Serum alanine aminotransferase (ALT) and liver histopathological changes were used as

Effects of Enzyme Induction and/or Glutathione Depletion on Methimazole-Induced Hepatotoxicity...

91

indicators for occurrence of hepatotoxicity induced by methimazole. Serum ALT levels were measured in different time points after methimazole administration (Figure 1). It was found that the maximum serum ALT levels occurred at 5 hours after drug administration (Figure 1), and gradually declined within the next 24 hours (Figure 1). Hence, all experiments (Serum transaminase levels in other groups, hepatic glutathione contents, lipid peroxidation, and histopathological evaluation of liver) were carried out five hours after methimazole administration to mice.

glutathione content (GSH) was depleted with BSO,[12] then the toxicity profile of methimazole was investigated in glutathione-depleted animals. The liver/animal weight ratio was assessed in different experimental groups (Table 1). When glutathione-depleted animals were treated with methimazole, a dramatic elevation in serum ALT levels was observed (Figure 2) (P<0.05). NAC (300 mg/kg) administration effectively reduced (P<0.05) methimazole-induced ALT elevation in both intact and/or glutathione-depleted animals (Figure 2).

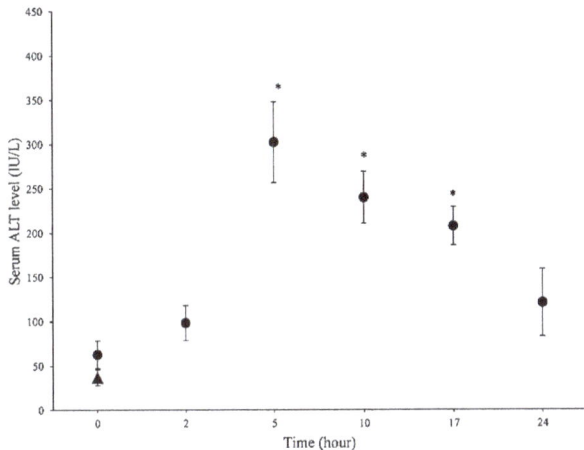

Figure 1. Serum ALT levels after methimazole (100 mg/kg) administration to mice. The peak serum ALT level was observed at 5 hours after methimazole administration.

▲: Control (vehicle-treated) animals. •: Methimazole-treated animals.

Data are expressed as Mean±SE for at least five animals.

* Significantly higher than control levels (P<0.05).

Methimazole (100 mg/kg) caused a significant elevation in serum ALT levels (P<0.05) as compared with the control animals (Figure 2). This might indicate the liver damage caused by this drug. To investigate the impact of glutathione reservoirs as a basic defense mechanism against xenobiotics-induced hepatic damage, hepatic

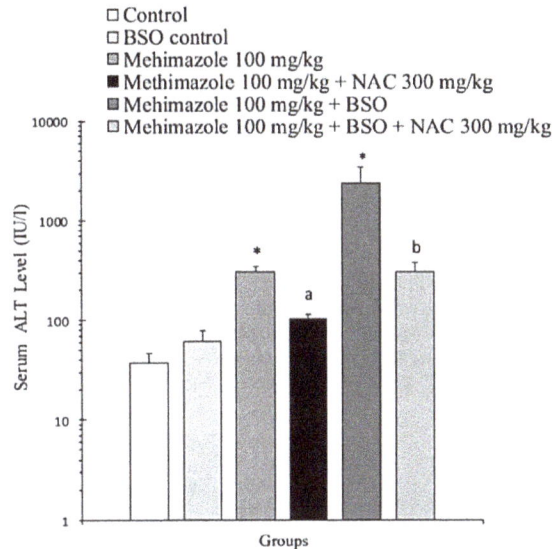

Figure 2. The effect of methimazole (100 mg/kg) on serum ALT level in mice. The role of glutathione reservoirs and protective effects of NAC administration.
BSO: L-buthionine sulfoximine. NAC: N-acetylcysteine.
Data are given as Mean±SE for five animals as measured after 5 hours of drug administration.
* Significant difference as compared to the control animals (P<0.05).
a Significant difference as compared to the methimazole-treated animals (P<0.05).

Table 1. Liver/Animal weight in the study on methimazole-induced hepatotoxicity.

Groups	Parameters assessed		
	Animal weight (gram)	Liver weight (gram)	Liver/animal weight Ratio (%)
Control (Vehicle-treated animals)	38±0.77	2.46±0.13	6.45±0.31
+ Methimazole 100 mg/kg	36±1.34	2.25±0.12	6.38±0.50
+ L-buthionine sulfoximine (BSO) 1 g/kg [§]	35±1.80	1.64±0.27	4.77±0.29
+ Methimazole 100 mg/kg	35±2.30	1.27±0.86	3.90±0.33
+ β-naphtoflavone (Enzyme-induced animals) [§§]	35±0.38	3.24±0.30*	9.27±1.04*
+ Methimazole 100 mg/kg [▲]	35±0.24	3.36±0.23*	9.72±0.71*
+ Phenobarbital (Enzyme-induced animals) [#]	37±2.50	2.85±0.32	7.70±0.39
+ Methimazole 100 mg/kg	38±2.32	2.5±0.42	6.60±0.92

Data are given as Mean±SE for at least five animals.
* Significantly different from control group (P<0.05).
[§] Mice were treated with BSO (1g/ kg, i.p).One hour later; the BSO-treated animals were given methimazole (100mg/kg i.p). Food was removed at 15 hours before dosing with BSO, and supplied again at 2 hours after methimazole administration.
[▲] Three out of five animals were death when they were treated with methimazole (100 mg/kg, i.p).
[§§] Mice were pre-treated with β-naphtoflavone (40 mg/kg, i.p) for three consecutive days. On the 4th day, animals were given methimazole (100mg/kg i.p) and the mentioned parameters were measured after five hours.
[#] Mice were pre-treated with phenobarbital (80 mg/kg, i.p) for three consecutive days. On the 4th day, animals were given methimazole (100mg/kg i.p) and parameters were measured after five hours.

To evaluate the role of reactive metabolites, the effect of enzyme-induction on methimazole-induced hepatotoxicity was investigated using serum ALT levels as an indicator. It was found that methimazole (100 mg/kg) caused a dramatic raise (P<0.05) in serum ALT activities in β-naphtoflavone treated animals as compared to the control groups (Figure 3). Three out of five animals were death after methimazole administration in β-naphtoflavone treated group (Table 1). Moreover, phenobarbital-induced animals showed higher serum ALT activity when treated with methimazole (Figure 3) (P<0.05). These findings might reveal the role of metabolic pathways and reactive intermediary metabolites in methimazole-induced hepatotoxicity. NAC (300 mg/kg) administration alleviated serum ALT elevation in enzyme-indiced animals, which were treated with methimazole (P<0.05) (Figure 3).

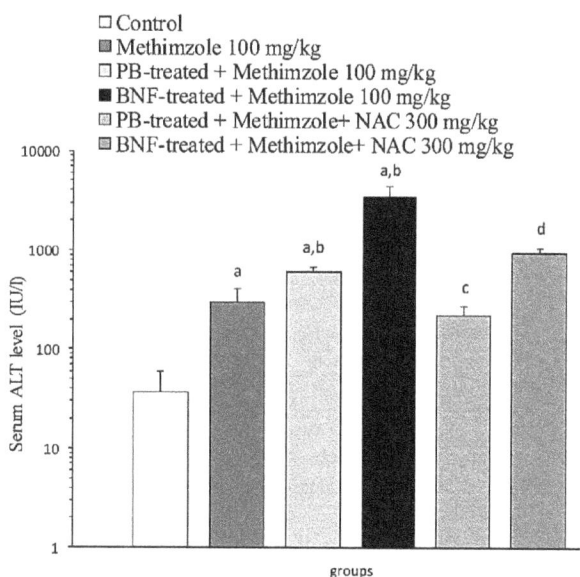

Figure 3. The effect of methimazole (100 mg/kg) on serum ALT level in mice. The role of enzyme-induction. BNF: β-naphtoflavone, PB: Phenobarbital.
Data are expressed as Mean±SE for five animals.
[a] Significantly higher than control animals (P<0.05).
[b] Significantly higher than methimazole-treated animals (P<0.05).
[c] Significantly lower than phenobarbital-induced animals which were treated with methimazole (P<0.05).
[d] Significantly lower than β-naphtoflavone-induced animals which were treated with methimazole (P<0.05).

As methimazole caused more ALT elevation in glutathione-depleted animals (Figure 2), hepatic glutathione levels were assessed to investigate the effect of methimazole on hepatic glutathione reservoirs. It was found that, methimazole (100 mg/kg) administration caused a decrease in hepatic glutathione (GSH) contents (P<0.05) as compared with control groups (Figure 4). When enzyme-induced mice were treated with methimazole the decline in glutathione reservoirs was more significant (P<0.05) (Figure 4). These findings might indicate that methimazole metabolites conjugated with glutathione in mice liver.

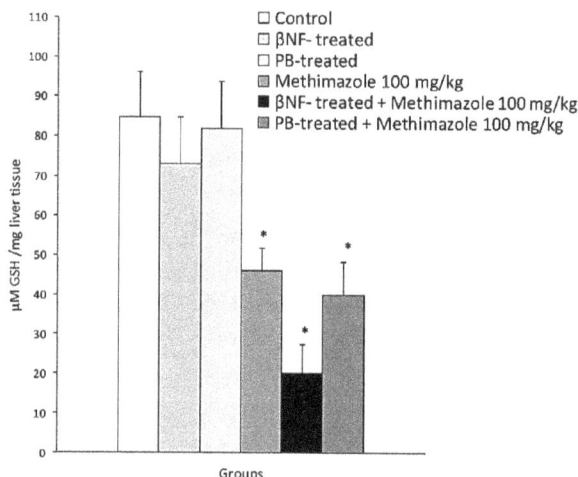

Figure 4. Methimazole-induced reduction in hepatic glutathione (GSH) content in mice.
Data are showed as Mean±SE for at least five animals. BNF: β-naphtoflavone, PB: Phenobarbital.
Significantly lower than control animals (P<0.05).

The probability of lipid peroxidation in liver tissue was investigated. We found that methimazole caused increase in thiobarbituric acid reactive substances (TBARS) in mice liver (Figure 5) (P<0.05), which indicates the occurrence of lipid peroxidation. Methimazole-induced lipid peroxidation was more severe in glutathione-depleted (BSO-treated) animals (P<0.05) (Figure 5). NAC administration effectively reduced methimazole-induced lipid peroxidation in intact and/or glutathione-depleted mice (Figure 5) (P<0.05). Enzyme induction using β-naphtoflavone and/or phenobarbital deteriorated (P<0.05) methimazole-induced lipid peroxidation (Figure 6), which might indicate the role of reactive metabolites. NAC (300 mg/kg) reduced (P<0.05) the level of methimazole-induced lipid peroxidation in enzyme-induced animals (Figure 6) (P<0.05).

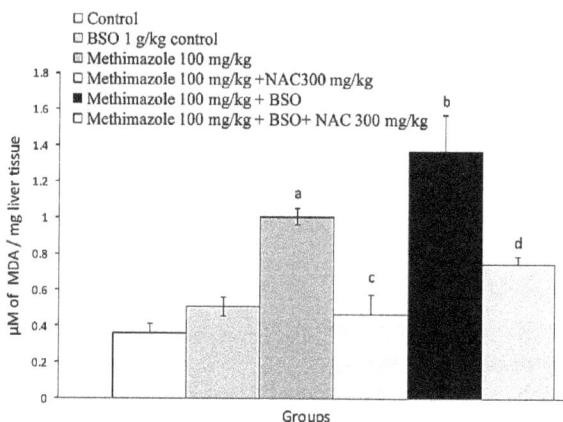

Figure 5. Methimazole-induced lipid peroxidation: the role of glutathione reservoirs and the effect of NAC administration. BSO: L-buthionine sulfoximine; NAC: N-acetyl cysteine.
Data are given as Mean±SE for five animals.
[a] Significantly higher than control animals (P<0.05).
[b] Significantly higher than methimazole-treated animals (P<0.05).
[c] Significantly lower than methimazole-treated animals (P<0.05).
[d] Significantly lower than methimazole-treated animals which were depleted of glutathione (P<0.05).

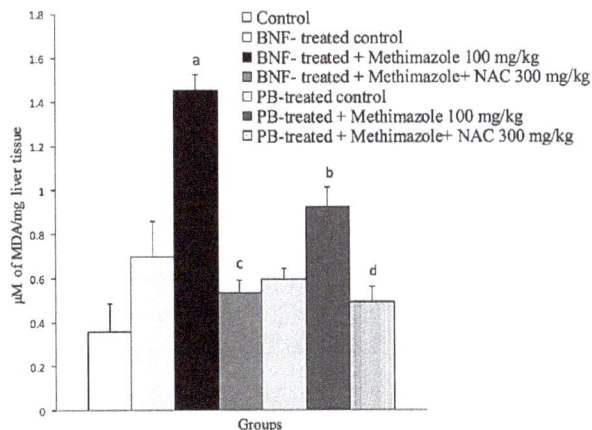

Figure 6. The effect of Enzyme induction on methimazole-induced lipid peroxidation in mice liver.
Data are expressed as Mean±SE for five animals.
[a] Significantly higher than control (BNF-treated) animals (P<0.05).
[b] Significantly higher than methimazole-treated animals (P<0.05).

Histopathological evaluation of mice liver revealed that methimazolecaused a mild inflammatory cell infiltration (Figure7, Part C). When glutathione-depleted animals were treated with methimazole (100 mg/kg), a severe inflammatory cells infiltration, and widespread bridging necrosis of liver was observed after 5 hours of drug administration (Figure 7, Part D).

The effect of enzyme-induction on mice liver pathology was studied. Histologically, the enzyme induction was evident as an expansion of the surface area of hepatocytes (Figure 8, Parts C&D). It was seen that, when enzyme-induced animals were treated with methimazole, the extensive necrosis of liver parenchymal cells and inflammatory cells infiltration was occurred (Figure 8, Parts C&D). The adverse effect of methimazole in β-naphtoflavone-induced animals seems to be more severe than phenobarbital-induced ones (Figure 8, Part C). The protective effects of NAC against methimazole-induced hepatotoxicity and its role in alleviating pathologic lesions were evaluated (Figure 7 and 8). It was found that NAC alleviated methimazole-induced histopathological changes in mice liver, even in glutathione depleted (Figure 7, Parts E & F) and/or enzyme-induced (Figure 8, Parts E & F) animals.

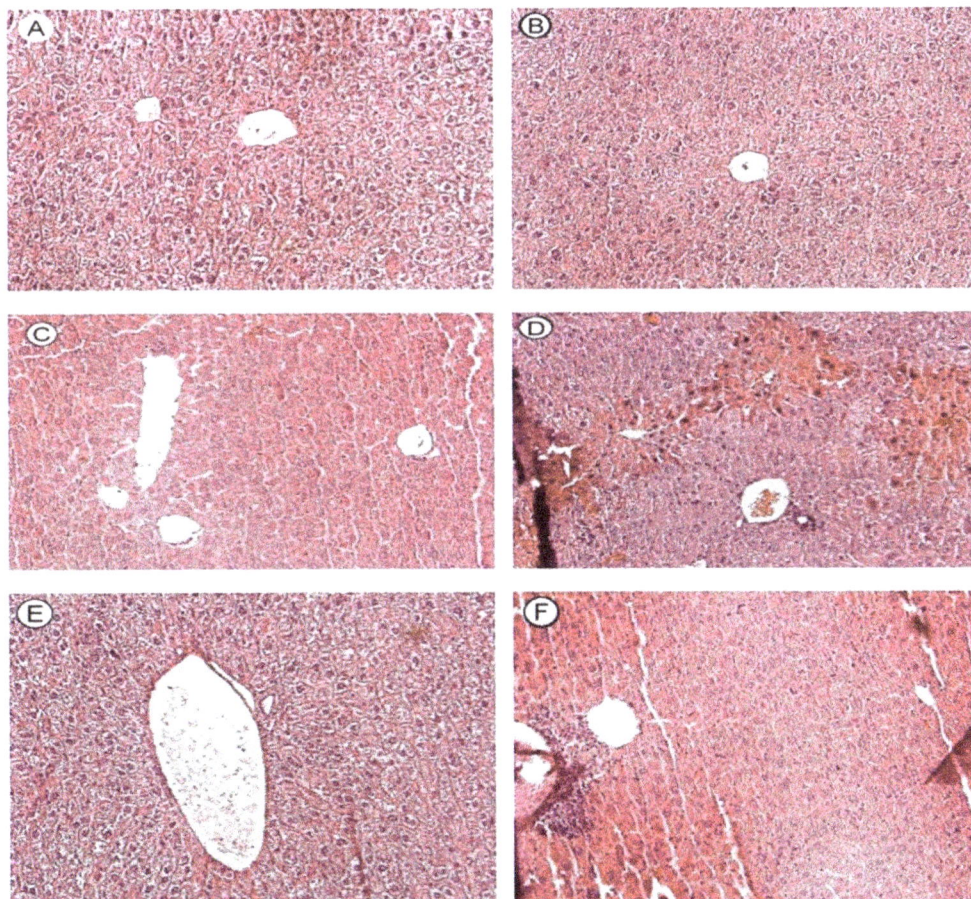

Figure 7. Histopathological evaluation of mice liver treated with methimazole (100 mg/kg). The effect of glutathione reservoirs depletion on methimazole-induced hepatotoxicity. Hematoxylin and eosin (H&E) staining. **A**: Control, **B**: BSO (1g/kg) control, **C**: Methimazole (100 mg/kg), **D**: Methimazole (100 mg/kg) + BSO (1g/kg), **E**: Methimazole (100 mg/kg) + NAC (300 mg/kg), **F**: Methimazole (100mg/kg) + BSO (1g/kg) + NAC (300 mg/kg). Methimazole caused a mild Inflammatory cell infiltration (**C**). A severe inflammatory cells infiltration, and widespread bridging necrosis of liver (**D**) was occurred when glutathione-depleted animals were treated with methimazole. NAC (300 mg/kg) administration, alleviated methimazole-induced changes in normal (**E**) and/or glutathione-depleted (**F**) animals.

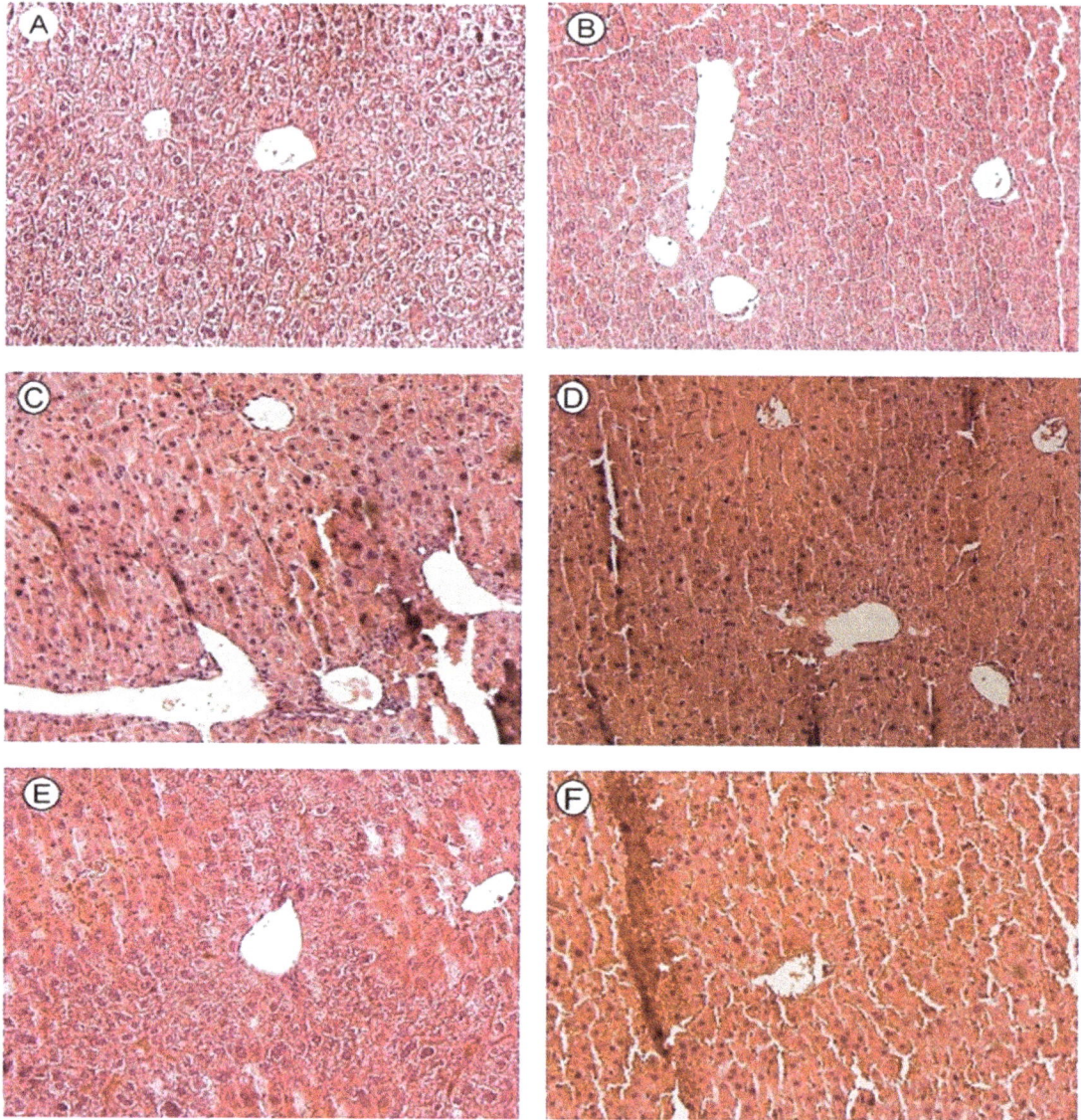

Figure 8. Effect of enzyme-induction on mice liver histopathological changes, caused by methimazole (100 mg/kg). **A**: normal control, **B**: Methimazole (100 mg/kg), **C**: BNF-induced + Methimazole (100 mg/kg), **D**: Phenobarbital-induced + Methimazole (100 mg/kg), **E**: BNF-induced + Methimazole (100 mg/kg) + NAC (300 mg/kg), **F**: Phenobarbital-induced + Methimazole (100 mg/kg) + NAC (300 mg/kg). When enzyme-induced animals were treated with methimazole a severe and widespread necrosis of liver parenchymal cells and inflammatory cells infiltration was occurred (**C & D**), mitigation of methimazole-induced changes in enzyme-induced animals was observed by NAC (300 mg/kg) administration, which reduced necrosis and inflammatory cells infiltration (**E&F**).

Discussion

Methimazole (100 mg/kg) caused hepatotoxicity in mice as revealed by elevation in serum ALT activities, a decrease in liver glutathione (GSH) reservoirs, lipid peroxidation, and histopathological changes of the liver. The toxic effects of methimazole toward mice liver were more severe in glutathione-depleted and/or enzyme-induced animals. NAC (300 mg/kg) administration effectively ameliorated all aspects of methimazole-induced hepatotoxicity in different conditions such as intact, glutathione-depleted, and/or enzyme-induced animals.

It has been shown in previous studies that cellular glutathione play a fundamental role in preventing the adverse effects of methimazole even in olfactory mucosa[4] and/or liver.[3,6] Our study on methimazole in glutathione-depleted animals is in line with previous investigations. Furthermore, in this study we showed that a significant amount of lipid peroxidation and a considerable reduction in hepatic glutathione (GSH) content was occurred as a consequence of methimazole administration.

Lipid peroxidation and/or serum ALT activities were more severe in glutathione-depleted animals which are another indicator that endorses the pivotal role of glutathione in preventing methimazole-induced toxicity. The role of glutathione in methimazole-induced hepatotoxicity might predict the risk of hepatotoxicity induced by this drug in human cases. Hence, in clinical situations where liver glutathione reservoirs are interrupted for example in malnutrition[17] or alcoholism,[18] the risk of hepatotoxicity induced by methimazole might be highest.

NAC, a protective agent which replenish glutathione reservoirs[19] and/or directly scavenges reactive species,[20] could protect mice liver against methimazole-induced hepatotoxicity in different situations. Furthermore, we previously showed the protective role of NAC against methimazole-induced cytotoxicity in a model of isolated rat hepatocytes.[21] These findings might suggest this protective agent as a potential therapeutic choice in methimazole-induced hepatotoxicity cases in humans.

The role of metabolic pathways and reactive intermediates in methimazole-induced hepatotoxicity was evaluated by investigating the effects of this drug in enzyme-induced animals. Methimazole showed a severe hepatotoxic profile in β-naphtoflavone-induced animals. Phenobarbital-induced animals showed an enhanced profile of toxicity too. These findings revealed that metabolism and reactive metabolites formation play an important role in methimazole-induced hepatotoxicity.

Different CYP450 types[5,8] as well as flavin containing monooxygenase (FMO)[2,8] are involved in methimazole metabolism and converting it to reactive intermediates. As previously proposed, N-methylthiourea is suspected to be the reactive and toxic metabolite of methimazole,[3,8,22] but in an *in vitro* study on methimazole-induced cytotoxicity toward isolated rat hepatocytes,[6] we showed that in addition than N-methylthiourea, glyoxal as another metabolite of methimazole,[8,22] might had a role in the hepatotoxic effects of this drug. A part of the protective effects of NAC on methimazole-induced hepatotoxicity might be attributed to the glyoxal trapping properties of N-acetyl cysteine.[23] However, other properties of NAC such as its glutathione replenishment activity might be included.

β-naphtoflavone induces different CYP enzymes, mainly CYP1A family.[24] Phenobarbital causes different type of CYP enzyme induction such as CYP 2C9 and 1AC.[25] Since a wide range of metabolic enzymes are induced by these agents, it is difficult to distinguish the specific enzyme which is involved in methimazole metabolism. Hence, more investigations are needed to elucidate the role of the exact CYP and/or other enzymes, which are responsible for converting methimazole to its reactive metabolites. Furthermore, using other glyoxal trapping agents such as metformin and/or aminoguanidine[23] against methimazole-induced hepatotoxicity could be the subject of future investigations.

Conclusion

Methimazole-induced hepatotoxicity seems to be mediated through its reactive intermediary metabolites. Hepatic glutathione reservoirs play a critical role in preventing methimazole-induced hepatotoxicity. NAC as a thiol containing hepatoprotective agent alleviated methimazole-induced hepatotoxicity in mice due to its effects on reactive metabolites.

Acknowledgments

This study was carried out at Drug Applied Research Center of Tabriz University of Medical Sciences. The authors thank Drug Applied Research Center for providing financial supports and facilities to carry out this investigation. Students' research committee in Tabriz University of Medical sciences supported this investigation. The authors thank students' research committee for their support.

Conflict of Interest

The authors report no conflicts of interest.

References

1. Woeber KA. Methimazole-induced hepatotoxicity. *Endocr Pract* 2002;8(3):222-4.

2. Genter MB, Deamer NJ, Blake BL, Wesley DS, Levi PE. Olfactory toxicity of methimazole: dose-response and structure-activity studies and characterization of flavin-containing monooxygenase activity in the Long-Evans rat olfactory mucosa. *Toxicol Pathol* 1995;23(4):477-86.

3. Mizutani T, Murakami M, Shirai M, Tanaka M, Nakanishi K. Metabolism-dependent hepatotoxicity of methimazole in mice depleted of glutathione. *J Appl Toxicol* 1999;19(3):193-8.

4. Bergstrom U, Giovanetti A, Piras E, Brittebo EB. Methimazole-induced damage in the olfactory mucosa: effects on ultrastructure and glutathione levels. *Toxicol Pathol* 2003;31(4):379-87.

5. Xie F, Zhou X, Genter MB, Behr M, Gu J, Ding X. The tissue-specific toxicity of methimazole in the mouse olfactory mucosa is partly mediated through target-tissue metabolic activation by CYP2A5. *Drug Metab Dispos* 2011;39(6):947-51.

6. Heidari R, Babaei H, Eghbal M. Mechanisms of methimazole cytotoxicity in isolated rat hepatocytes. *Drug Chem Toxicol* 2013;36(4):403-11.

7. Bergman U, Brittebo EB. Methimazole toxicity in rodents: covalent binding in the olfactory mucosa and detection of glial fibrillary acidic protein in the olfactory bulb. *Toxicol Appl Pharmacol* 1999;155(2):190-200.

8. Mizutani T, Yoshida K, Murakami M, Shirai M, Kawazoe S. Evidence for the involvement of N-methylthiourea, a ring cleavage metabolite, in the hepatotoxicity of methimazole in glutathione-depleted mice: structure-toxicity and metabolic studies. *Chem Res Toxicol* 2000;13(3):170-6.

9. Huq F. Molecular Modelling Analysis of the Metabolism of Methimazole. *J Pharmacol Toxicol* 2008;3(1):11-9.

10. Sahu S, Rani Sahoo P, Patel S, Mishra BK. Oxidation of thiourea and substituted thioureas: a review. *J Sulfur Chem* 2011;32(2):171-97.

11. Mansuy D, Dansette PM. Sulfenic acids as reactive intermediates in xenobiotic metabolism. *Arch Biochem Biophys* 2011;507(1):174-85.

12. Drew R, Miners JO. The effects of buthionine sulphoximine (BSO) on glutathione depletion and xenobiotic biotransformation. *Biochem Pharmacol* 1984;33(19):2989-94.

13. Valoti M, Fusi F, Frosini M, Pessina F, Tipton KF, Sgaragli GP. Cytochrome P450-dependent N-dealkylation of L-deprenyl in C57BL mouse liver microsomes: effects of in vivo pretreatment with ethanol, phenobarbital, beta-naphthoflavone and L-deprenyl. *Eur J Pharmacol* 2000;391(3):199-206.

14. Moezi L, Heidari R, Amirghofran Z, Nekooeian AA, Monabati A, Dehpour AR. Enhanced anti-ulcer effect of pioglitazone on gastric ulcers in cirrhotic rats: the role of nitric oxide and IL-1beta. *Pharmacol Rep* 2013;65(1):134-43.

15. Sedlak J, Lindsay RH. Estimation of total, protein-bound, and nonprotein sulfhydryl groups in tissue with Ellman's reagent. *Anal Biochem* 1968;25(1):192-205.

16. Mihara M, Uchiyama M. Determination of malonaldehyde precursor in tissues by thiobarbituric acid test. *Anal Biochem* 1978;86(1):271-8.

17. de Oliveira IMV, Fujimori E, Pereira VG, Lima AR. Relationship between liver gamma-glutamyltranspeptidase activity and glutathione content in chronic-malnourished pups of adolescent rats. *Nutr Res* 2000;20(1):103-11.

18. Vogt BL, Richie JP, Jr. Glutathione depletion and recovery after acute ethanol administration in the aging mouse. *Biochem Pharmacol* 2007;73(10):1613-21.

19. Masubuchi Y, Nakayama J, Sadakata Y. Protective effects of exogenous glutathione and related thiol compounds against drug-induced liver injury. *Biol Pharm Bull* 2011;34(3):366-70.

20. Gillissen A, Scharling B, Jaworska M, Bartling A, Rasche K, Schultze-Werninghaus G. Oxidant scavenger function of ambroxol in vitro: a comparison with N-acetylcysteine. *Res Exp Med (Berl)* 1997;196(6):389-98.

21. Heidari R, Babaei H, Eghbal MA. Cytoprotective effects of organosulfur compounds against methimazole-induced toxicity in isolated rat hepatocytes. *Adv Pharm Bull* 2013;3(1):135-42.

22. Erve JC. Chemical toxicology: reactive intermediates and their role in pharmacology and toxicology. *Expert Opin Drug Metab Toxicol* 2006;2(6):923-46.

23. Mehta R, Wong L, O'brien PJ. Cytoprotective mechanisms of carbonyl scavenging drugs in isolated rat hepatocytes. *Chem Biol Interact* 2009;178(1-3):317-23.

24. Iba MM, Fung J, Thomas PE, Park Y. Constitutive and induced expression by pyridine and beta-naphthoflavone of rat CYP1A is sexually dimorphic. *Arch Toxicol* 1999;73(4-5):208-16.

25. Runge D, Kohler C, Kostrubsky VE, Jager D, Lehmann T, Runge DM, et al. Induction of cytochrome P450 (CYP)1A1, CYP1A2, and CYP3A4 but not of CYP2C9, CYP2C19, multidrug resistance (MDR-1) and multidrug resistance associated protein (MRP-1) by prototypical inducers in human hepatocytes. *Biochem Biophys Res Commun* 2000;273(1):333-41.

17

Therapeutic Effects of Myeloid Cell Leukemia-1 siRNA on Human Acute Myeloid Leukemia Cells

Hadi Karami[1,2], Behzad Baradaran[1]*, Ali Esfahani[3], Masoud Sakhinia[4], Ebrahim Sakhinia[5,6]*

[1] Immunology Research Center, Tabriz University of Medical Sciences, Tabriz, Iran.

[2] Department of Biochemistry, Faculty of Medicine, Tabriz University of Medical Sciences, Tabriz, Iran.

[3] Hematology and Oncology Research Center, Shahid Ghazi Hospital, Tabriz University of Medical Sciences, Tabriz, Iran.

[4] Faculty of Medicine, University of Liverpool, Liverpool, United Kingdom.

[5] Department of Genetics, Faculty of Medicine, Tabriz University of Medical Sciences, Tabriz, Iran.

[6] Tuberculosis and Lung Disease Reseach Center, Tabriz University of Medical Sciences, Tabriz, Iran.

ARTICLE INFO

Keywords:
Mcl-1
siRNA
Leukemia
HL-60
Apoptosis
Proliferation

ABSTRACT

Purpose: Up-regulation of Mcl-1, a known anti-apoptotic protein, is associated with the survival and progression of various malignancies including leukemia. The aim of this study was to explore the effect of Mcl-1 small interference RNA (siRNA) on the proliferation and apoptosis of HL-60 acute myeloid leukemia (AML) cells.

Methods: siRNA transfection was performed using Lipofectamine™2000 reagent. Relative mRNA and protein expressions were quantified by quantitative real-time PCR and Western blotting, respectively. Trypan blue assay was performed to assess tumor cell proliferation after siRNA transfection. The cytotoxic effect of Mcl-1 siRNA on leukemic cells was measured using MTT assay. Apoptosis was detected using ELISA cell death assay.

Results: Mcl-1 siRNA clearly lowered both Mcl-1 mRNA and protein levels in a time-dependent manner, leading to marked inhibition of cell survival and proliferation. Furthermore, Mcl-1 down-regulation significantly enhanced the extent of HL-60 apoptotic cells.

Conclusion: Our results suggest that the down-regulation of Mcl-1 by siRNA can effectively trigger apoptosis and inhibit the proliferation of leukemic cells. Therefore, Mcl-1 siRNA may be a potent adjuvant in AML therapy.

Introduction

Acute myeloid leukemia (AML) is a lethal disorder characterized by the accumulation of abnormal myeloid progenitor cells in the bone marrow, which results in hematopoietic failure. Despite various efforts in detection and treatment, many patients with AML continue to die of this cancer.[1-3] Therefore, understanding the cellular mechanisms linked to the AML formation and progression could be beneficial in designing of the new therapeutic strategies for AML.

Myeloid cell leukaemia-1 (Mcl-1) is a highly regulated member of the anti-apoptotic B-cell lymphoma-2 (Bcl-2) family of proteins, was originally isolated from the ML-1 human myeloid leukemia cells during differentiation.[4] This protein was founded in various tissue and tumor cells and has a critical role in the regulation of cell cycle program and apoptosis. Some previous studies have revealed that Mcl-1 is needed for the survival of hematopoietic and tumor cells.[5-7]

Furthermore, other studies have demonstrated that Mcl-1 is overexpressed in different malignances including leukemia, and suppression of this protein by RNA interference (RNAi) or antisense oligonucleotide (ASO) technology triggered apoptosis and inhibited the growth of tumor cells.[8-13]

RNAi or post-transcriptional gene-silencing technology is a potent phenomenon in which a double stranded RNA (called siRNA) is transfered into the cells where it suppresses the expression of a specific gene by cleavage of the homologous mRNA. There have been many confirmed studies that RNAi-mediated gene silencing can successfully induce apoptosis and arrest the proliferation of the malignant cells in vivo and in vitro, and siRNA-based gene therapy has been turned into an effective approach for cancer therapy.[14-16]

In this study, Mcl-1 small interference RNA (siRNA) was transfected into AML cell line HL-60 in vitro, to

*Corresponding author: Behzad Baradaran, Immunology Research Center, Tabriz University of Medical Sciences, Tabriz, Iran. Email: baradaranb@tbzmed.ac.ir; Ebrahim Sakhinia, Department of Genetics, Faculty of Medicine, Tabriz University of Medical Sciences, Tabriz, Iran. Email: esakhinia@yahoo.co.uk.

investigate the impact of Mcl-1 gene suppression on the human AML cell apoptosis and proliferation.

Materials and Methods
Cell culture conditions
The HL-60 AML cell line (Pasteur Institute, Tehran, Iran) was maintained in RPMI-1640 culture medium (Sigma-Aldrich, St. Louis, MO, USA) supplemented with 15% fetal bovine serum (FBS) (Sigma-Aldrich), 2 mM of glutamine, 1% sodium pyruvate and 1% antibiotics (100 IU/ml penicillin, 100 µg/ml streptomycin) (Sigma-Aldrich) at 37 °C in a humidified atmosphere containing 5% CO_2. The cells were sub-cultured 48-72 h later with an initial concentration of 5 $\times$ 10^4 cells/ml and used in the logarithmic growth phase in whole experiments.

siRNA transfection
The Mcl-1 specific and negative control (NC) siGENOME siRNA sequences were ordered from Dharmacon (Lafayette, CO, USA). Just before transfection, the cells were grown in RPMI-1640 medium free of antibiotics and FBS. siRNA transfection (at a final concentration of 50 nM in all experiments) was performed using Lipofectamine™2000 reagent (Invitrogen, Carlsbad, CA, USA) according to the manufacturer's instructions. In brief, siRNAs and lipofectamine (4 µl/ml of transfection medium) were separately diluted in Opti-MEM I Reduced Serum Medium (Invitrogen) and incubated for 10 min at ambient temperature. The diluted solutions were then combined and incubated for 20 min at ambient temperature. Following on, the mixtures were added to each well containing medium and cells. Furthermore, the treated cells with only lipofectamine were considered as a siRNA blank control group. The cells were then incubated for 6 h at 37 °C in a humidified CO_2 incubator. Subsequently, complete cell culture medium (with final FBS concentration of 15%) was added and the cells were incubated under the same mentioned conditions. To monitor the effect of siRNA on gene silencing, transfection (5 $\times$ 10^5 cells/well) were done in 6-well plates for 24-48 h. Down-regulation of Mcl-1 expression was then measured by quantitative real-time PCR (qRT-PCR) and Western blot analysis.

Cytotoxicity assay
The cytotoxic effect of Mcl-1 siRNA on HL-60 was determined using 3-(4, 5 Dimethylthiazol-2-yl)-2, 5-Diphenyltetrazolium Bromide (MTT) assay. The experiment was subdivided into three groups: Mcl-1 siRNA, NC siRNA and blank control. Briefly, leukemic cells were seeded at a density of 15 $\times$ 10^3 cells in 96-well cell culture plates. The cells were then transfected with siRNAs as described previously. After 24 and 48 h of incubation, the cytotoxicities of the treatments were measured using the MTT assay kit (Roche Diagnostics GmbH, Mannheim, Germany)

following the manufacturer's recommendations. The amounts of formazan dyes were quantified by measuring their absorbance (A) at 570 nm with a reference wavelength of 650 nm using an ELISA plate reader (Awareness Technology, Palm City, FL, USA). The cell survival rate (SR) was measured from the following formula:

$$SR\ (\%) = (A_{Experiment}\ /A_{Blank\ control}) \times 100\%.$$

Cell proliferation assay
The antiproliferative effect of Mcl-1 siRNA was evaluated using trypan blue exclusion assay. The cells (5 $\times$ 10^4 cells/well) were transfected with Mcl-1 specific and NC siRNAs in 24-well cell culture plates and then incubated for 24-120 h. At different time points after transfections, the cells were collected and stained with equal volume of 0.4% trypan blue dye (Merck KGaA, Darmstadt, Germany) for 1 min. Following on, the number of viable cells (N, unstained cells) was quantified using a hemocytometer and an inverted microscope (Nikon Instrument Inc., Melville, NY, USA). The percentage of viable cells was then determined from the equation as follows: Cell viability (%) = (N $_{Experiment}$ /N $_{Blank\ control}$) $\times$ 100. The percentage of viable cells in each time was also considered as 100% for blank control group.

qRT-PCR
Following transfections, total RNA was extracted by AccuZol™ reagent (Bioneer, Daedeok-gu, Daejeon, Korea) as described by the manufacturer. Complementary DNA (cDNA) was generated from 1 µg of total RNA by use of oligo-dT primer and MMLV reverse transcriptase (Promega, Madison, WI, USA) according to the manufacturer's recommendations. qRT-PCR was then performed using SYBR Premix Ex Taq (Takara Bio, Otsu, Shiga, Japan) in the Rotor-Gene™ 6000 system (Corbett Life Science, Mortlake, NSW, Australia). The PCR was done in a 20 µl reaction system containing 12 µl of SYBR green reagent, 0.2 µM of each primer, 1 µl of cDNA template and 6 µl of nuclease-free distilled water. The primer sequences were as follows: forward, 5'-TCCCTGGAGAAGAGCTACG-3', reverse, 5'-GTAGTTTCGTGGATGCCACA-3', for β–actin and forward, 5'-TAAGGACAAAACGGGACTGG-3', and reverse, 5'-ACCAGCTCCTACTCCAGCAA-3', for Mcl-1. The initial denaturation step at 95 °C for 10 min was followed by 45 cycles at 95 °C for 20 sec and 60 °C for 1 min. Relative Mcl-1 mRNA expression was calculated with the $2^{-(\Delta\Delta C_T)}$,[17] using β-actin as a reference gene.

Western blot analysis
At indicated time points after transfection, the cells were harvested, washed with cold PBS and resuspended in lysis buffer (1% SDS, 50 mM Tris-HCl, pH 7.4, 150 mM NaCl, 1% Triton X-100 and 1 mM EDTA, pH 8) containing protease inhibitor cocktail

complete (Roche Diagnostics GmbH) for 30 min on ice. Cell suspensions were then centrifuged at 12,000 rpm for 10 min at 4 °C and cellular debrises were removed. Protein concentrations were measured using Bradford reagent (Sigma-Aldrich). Next, 50 µg of each protein sample was separated by 12% SDS-PAGE, transferred to PVDF membrane (GE Healthcare, Amersham, Buckinghamshire, UK), and then blocked with 3% skim milk in PBS/Tween-20 (0.05%, v/v) for 45 min at room temperature. Subsequently, the membrane was probed overnight at 4 °C with primary monoclonal antibodies against β-actin (1:1000, Abcam, Cambridge, MA, UK) and Mcl-1 (1:500, Abcam) diluted in 3% skim milk in PBS. After three 7 min washes with a buffer containing PBS and 0.05% Tween-20, membrane was incubated with appropriate horseradish peroxidase-linked secondary antibody (1:4,000, Abcam) diluted in PBS for 1.5 h at room temperature. Following on, the membrane was washed and protein bands visualized using enhanced chemiluminescence detection Kit (GE Healthcare) and X-ray film (Estman Kodak, Rochester, NY, USA). The protein bands were then analyzed by ImageJ 1.62 software (National Institues of Health, Bethesda, Maryland, USA) and signal intensity of each band was normalized to its corresponding β-actin loading control.

Apoptosis ELISA assay

The HL-60 leukemia cells were seeded at a density of 5 × 10⁴ cells/well in 24-well cell culture plates and then transfected with Mcl-1 specific and NC siRNAs as described above. At 24 and 48 h after transfection of siRNAs, cells were collected and apoptosis was detected using an ELISA cell death detection kit (Roche Diagnostics GmbH) according to the supplier's recommendations. This assay determines the amount of cytosolic mono- and oligonucleosomes produced during apoptosis. In brief, the cells were lysed and centrifuged at 500 rpm for 10 min. Following the addition of 20 µl of the cell supernatant and 80 µl of immunoreagent containing anti-histone-biotin and anti-DNA-peroxidase to each well, streptavidin-coated plate was incubated for 2 h at ambient temperature. Following washing with incubation buffer, 100 µl of 2, 2-azino-bis (3-ethylbenzthiazoline-6-sulfonic acid) (ABTS) solution was transfered to each well. The reactions were stopped and absorbance at 405 nm was quantified with a microplate reader (with a reference wavelength of 490 nm). The fold increase in apoptosis was calculated by dividing the absorbance of the experiment group by the absorbance of the control group.

Statistical analysis

Data in this study were presented as mean ± standard deviation (SD). Analysis of variance (ANOVA) followed by two-tailed unpaired t-test was used to determine the significant differences between groups. Values of P less than 0.05 were considered significant.

All statistical analyses were performed using GraphPad Prism 6.01 software (GraphPad Software Inc., San Diego, CA, USA).

Results

siRNA suppressed Mcl-1 mRNA and protein levels in leukemia cells

First, we explored the effect of siRNA on Mcl-1 gene expression in HL-60 cells by qRT-PCR and Western blotting. Relative Mcl-1 gene expression was calculated in relation to the blank control group, which was considered as 100%. As shown in Figure 1 and 2, Mcl-1 siRNA led to a clear time-dependent reduction of both Mcl-1 mRNA and protein levels (P<0.05; compared with the blank control and NC siRNA groups). At 24, 48 and 72 h posttransfection, the relative Mcl-1 mRNA expression levels were 45.11%, 37.24% and 16.22%, respectively (Figure 1), while the relative Mcl-1 protein expression levels were 60.19%, 39.43% and 20.76%, respectively (Figure 2B) (P<0.05). Notably, transfection with NC siRNA had an insignificant effect on Mcl-1 gene expression compared to the blank control group.

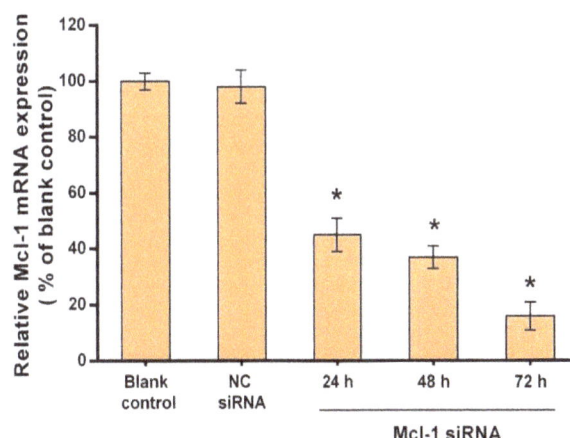

Figure 1. Down-regulation of Mcl-1 mRNA expression by siRNA in HL-60 cells. The cells were transfected with negative control (NC) siRNA or Mcl-1 siRNA for 24, 48 and 72 h. Relative mRNA expression was then measured by qRT-PCR using 2 $^{(-\Delta\Delta Ct)}$ method. The results are expressed as mean ± SD (n = 3); *P<0.05 versus blank control and NC siRNA.

Mcl-1 siRNA decreased the cell survival rate of the leukemic cells

To assess the cytotoxic effect of Mcl-1 down-regulation on HL-60 leukemia cells, the cells were treated with Mcl-1 siRNA for 24 and 48 h and then analyzed in MTT assay. As shown in Figure 3, the cytotoxicity significantly enhanced at 24 and 48 h in the Mcl-1 siRNA transfected cells relative to the blank control and NC siRNA transfected cells. The results showed that Mcl-1 siRNA significantly lowered the cell survival rate to 81.21% (24 h) and 65.15% (48 h) compared with the blank control group (P<0.05). In contrast, transfection with NC siRNA had a minimal cytotoxic effect on the leukemic cells relative to the blank control group (P>0.05; Figure 3).

A)

B)

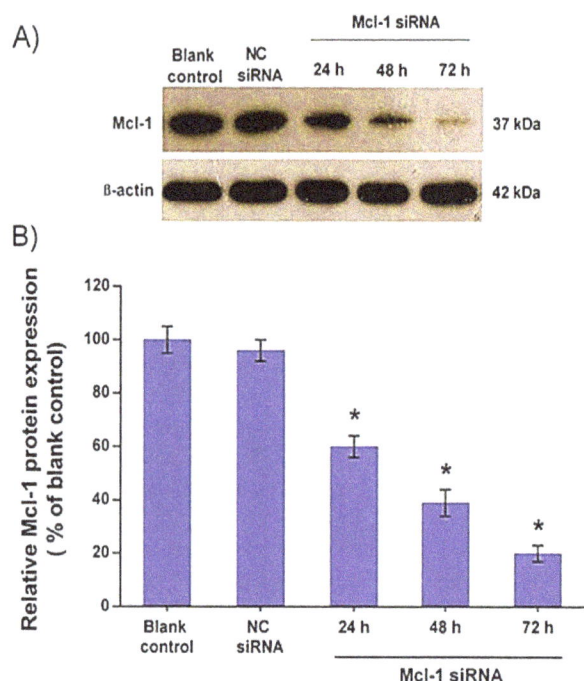

Figure 2. Mcl-1 protein expression levels in HL-60 cells transfected with siRNAs. (A) Representative western blot of β-actin and Mcl-1 proteins from cells transfected with NC siRNA or Mcl-1 siRNA. (B) The expression level of each band was quantified using densitometry and normalized to the respective β-actin. The results are expressed as mean ± SD (n = 3); *P<0.05 versus blank control and NC siRNA.

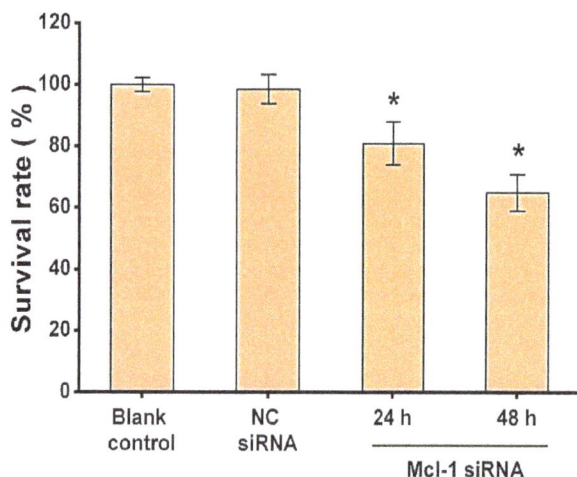

Figure 3. Effect of Mcl-1 siRNA on the survival rate of leukemia cells. The HL-60 cells were transfected with NC siRNA or Mcl-1 siRNA for 24 and 48 h and then the cytotoxicities of the treatments were measured by MTT assay. The results are expressed as mean ± SD (n = 4); *P<0.05 versus blank control and NC siRNA.

Down-regulation of Mcl-1 expression inhibited the proliferation of HL-60 cells

As up-regulation of Mcl-1 is involved in the survival of leukemia cells; we therefore sought to examine whether suppression of this protein could inhibit the proliferation of AML cells. The HL-60 cells were therefore transfected with Mcl-1 specific and NC

siRNAs for 5 days and cell viability was measured every 24 h by trypan blue exclusion assay. Results showed that compared with the blank control or NC siRNA groups, Mcl-1 siRNA significantly inhibited the proliferation of HL-60 cells over a period of 5 days (P<0.05; Figure 4). At 24 h after transfection of Mcl-1 siRNA, the percentage of viable cells dropped to 84.40% and then to a further 53.37% at the end of the experiment (day 5). Meanwhile, no significant differences in cell proliferation was observed between the NC siRNA group and the blank control groups (P>0.05; Figure 4).

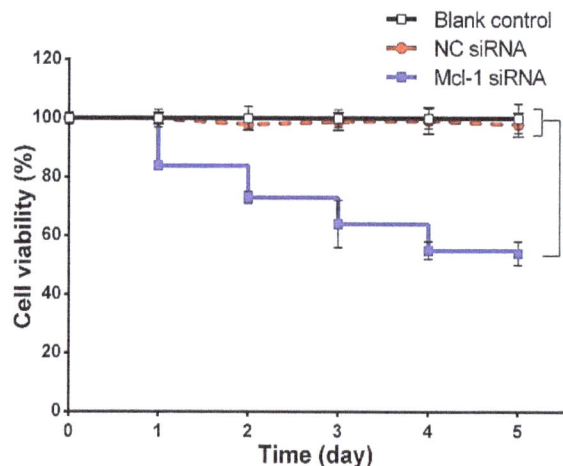

Figure 4. Proliferation inhibition of HL-60 cells transfected with NC siRNA or Mcl-1 siRNA. Cell viability was determined by trypan blue assay over a period of 5 days. The results are expressed as mean ± SD (n = 3); *P<0.05 versus blank control and NC siRNA.

Suppression of survivin expression enhanced apoptotic cell death

To analyze whether the observed cytotoxic effect of Mcl-1 Down-regulation was linked to the enhancement of apoptosis, the effect of Mcl-1 siRNA on apoptosis were examined using an ELISA cell death assay. Results showed that Mcl-1 siRNA significantly enhanced the extent of apoptosis at 24 and 48 h relative to the blank control group and the NC siRNA transfected group (Table 1; P<0.05). However, NC siRNA transfected cells displayed no distinct alteration in the extent of apoptosis relative to the blank control group (P>0.05). These results indicate that the cytotoxic effect of survivin suppression is partially due to the induction of apoptosis.

Table 1. Fold increase in apoptosis of HL-60 cells after transfection of siRNAs.

Groups	Fold increase in apoptosis
Blank control	1
NC siRNA	1.33
Mcl-1 siRNA (24 h)	7.01*
Mcl-1 siRNA (48 h)	11.38*
Results from the ELISA cell death assay showed that Mcl-1 siRNA significantly enhanced the extent of apoptosis at 48 and 72 h after transfection relative to the blank control and the NC siRNA groups. *P <0.05.	

Discussion

Molecular targeted therapy is a new emerging technology for treatment of cancer. Gene therapy is a potent kind of targeted therapy, in which the target is a specific gene overexpressed in tumor cells. The therapeutic agents, including ASO, ribozyme and siRNA are used to interfere with the expression of the target gene. As a result, the formation, growth and metastasis of tumors are inhibited.[14-16] Overexpression of Mcl-1, a member of the anti-apoptotic Bcl-2 family of proteins, is attributed to the tumor formation, development and metastasis.[13] On the contrary, different reports have shown that suppression of Mcl-1 expression can induce apoptosis and inhibit the proliferation of tumor cells.[8,9] Thus, we used a siRNA-based gene therapy strategy to target Mcl-1 and evaluate its antileukemic effects.

Quantitative PCR and Western blotting findings showed that transfection with Mcl-1 siRNA led to steady decrease in the expression levels of both Mcl-1 mRNA and protein over a 3-day period. These data revealed that Mcl-1 siRNA effectively blocked the synthesis of the Mcl-1 protein by cleavage of its corresponding mRNA. The results of cytotoxicity assay exhibited that Mcl-1 siRNA distinctly lowered the cell survival rate. Most notably, the results of the cell proliferation assay demonstrated that the suppression of Mcl-1 expression significantly decreased the viability of HL-60 cells during a 5-day period, suggesting the critical role of Mcl-1 in the proliferation of leukemic cells. In contrast, treatment with NC siRNA or lipofectamine displayed no significant changes in the gene expression and cellular events, demonstrating the specific impact of Mcl-1 siRNA.

To further investigate the cellular role of Mcl-1 in the development of leukemic cells, we examined the effect of Mcl-1 suppression on induction of apoptosis. Results of ELISA cell death assay indicated that siRNA-mediated silencing of Mcl-1 led to a remarkable spontaneous apoptosis. These results are in contrast to the other studies on solid tumors.[18,19] Meanwhile, our observations are in agreement with the results of similar studies on hematological tumors,[11,20] illustrating the important biological role of Mcl-1 in the survival and growth of leukemia cells. The above-mentioned results confirm that the presence of Mcl-1 protein is required for the development and progression of HL-60 cells. Therefore, silencing of Mcl-1 expression could induce spontaneous apoptosis and inhibit the proliferation of AML cells.

Cellular apoptosis can be controlled by two major signaling pathways. The intrinsic pathway responds to toxic intracellular stimuli, resulting in release of cytochrome c from inner mitochondrial membrane space which leads to the activation of caspases-9. The extrinsic pathway triggers by ligands binding to extracellular death receptors and causes caspase-8 activation. Both pathways converge at caspase-3 that activates the other caspases and leading to a proteolytic cascade and the next apoptotic events. Mcl-1 mainly blocks the mitochondrial pathway by the sequestering and neutralization of pro-apoptotic Bcl-2 family members such as Bim, Bax and Bak, thereby preserving mitochondria integrity. This action inhibits the release of cytochrome c that is necessary for caspase-9 activation.[12,13,21]

Moreover, recent studies on melanoma cells have revealed that overexpression of Mcl-1 inhibited the death receptor pathway of apoptosis.[8,22] Our study showed that transfection of Mcl-1 siRNA induced apoptosis in leukemia cells. Therefore, we suggest that suppression of Mcl-1 expression by siRNA may trigger apoptosis through caspase-3-dependent mechanisms. However, the exact roles of Mcl-1 in the regulation of the apoptosis pathways remain unclear.

RNAi-mediated gene silencing is a powerful strategy for the knockdown of a particular gene in which siRNA is introduces to the target cells and suppresses the expression of specific gene by degradation of the corresponding complementary mRNA. Because of its unique characteristics such as specificity, high efficacy and low cytotoxicity, siRNA is extensively used in gene-based medicine investigations.[14-16] Moreover, owing to its advantages such as the greater resistance to cellular nucleases, siRNA is preferred to the ribozyme and ASO technologies.[23,24] On the other hand, transient nature of double-stranded siRNA is one of the major drawbacks of long term siRNA-based therapeutics which can be overcome by use of the siRNA-based vector systems.[14-16]

Conclusion

In summary, we have demonstrated that Mcl-1 has a critical role in the survival and growth of HL-60 cells. Specific knockdown of Mcl-1 by siRNA induced apoptosis and inhibited the proliferation of leukemia cells in vitro. We therefore suggest that the siRNA-mediated silencing of Mcl-1 may be considered as a novel treatment strategy for AML patients in the future. Future studies on animal models could further examine whether Mcl-1 can be efficiently suppressed by siRNA expressed from a vector-based system, such that siRNA can effectively silence Mcl-1 in AML cells in a long term period.

Acknowledgements

This work was supported by a grant from the Immunology Research Center (IRC), Tabriz University of Medical Sciences (No. 9032). We thank staff of the IRC and Biochemistry Department for their technical assistance.

Conflict of Interest

The authors declare that they have no conflict of interest.

References

1. Smits EL, Berneman ZN, Van Tendeloo VF. Immunotherapy of acute myeloid leukemia: current approaches. *Oncologist* 2009;14(3):240-52.

2. Szer J. The prevalent predicament of relapsed acute myeloid leukemia. *Hematology Am Soc Hematol Educ Program* 2012;2012:43-8.

3. Kupsa T, Horacek JM, Jebavy L. The role of cytokines in acute myeloid leukemia: a systematic review. *Biomed Pap Med Fac Univ Palacky Olomouc Czech Repub* 2012;156(4):291-301.

4. Kozopas KM, Yang T, Buchan HL, Zhou P, Craig RW. MCL1, a gene expressed in programmed myeloid cell differentiation, has sequence similarity to BCL2. *Proc Natl Acad Sci U S A* 1993;90(8):3516-20.

5. Derenne S, Monia B, Dean NM, Taylor JK, Rapp MJ, Harousseau JL, et al. Anti sense strategy shows that Mcl-1 rather than Bcl-2 or Bcl-x(L) is an essential survival protein of human myeloma cells. *Blood* 2002;100(1):194-9.

6. Opferman JT, Letai A, Beard C, Sorcinelli MD, Ong CC, Korsmeyer SJ. Development and maintenance of B and T lymphocytes requires antiapoptotic MCL-1. *Nature* 2003;426(6967):671-6.

7. Craig RW. MCL1 provides a window on the role of the BCL2 family in cell proliferation, differentiation and tumorigenesis. *Leukemia* 2002;16(4):444-54.

8. Chetoui N, Sylla K, Gagnon-Houde JV, Alcaide-Loridan C, Charron D, Al-Daccak R, et al. Down-regulation of mcl-1 by small interfering RNA sensitizes resistant melanoma cells to fas-mediated apoptosis. *Mol Cancer Res* 2008;6(1):42-52.

9. Skoda C, Erovic BM, Wachek V, Vormittag L, Wrba F, Martinek H, et al. Down-regulation of Mcl-1 with antisense technology alters the effect of various cytotoxic agents used in treatment of squamous cell carcinoma of the head and neck. *Oncol Rep* 2008;19(6):1499-503.

10. Kaufmann SH, Karp JE, Svingen PA, Krajewski S, Burke PJ, Gore SD, et al. Elevated expression of the apoptotic regulator Mcl-1 at the time of leukemic relapse. *Blood* 1998;91(3):991-1000.

11. Aichberger KJ, Mayerhofer M, Krauth MT, Skvara H, Florian S, Sonneck K, et al. Identification of mcl-1 as a BCR/ABL-dependent target in chronic myeloid leukemia (CML): evidence for cooperative antileukemic effects of imatinib and mcl-1 antisense oligonucleotides. *Blood* 2005;105(8):3303-11.

12. Akagi H, Higuchi H, Sumimoto H, Igarashi T, Kabashima A, Mizuguchi H, et al. Suppression of myeloid cell leukemia-1 (Mcl-1) enhances chemotherapy-associated apoptosis in gastric cancer cells. *Gastric Cancer* 2013;16(1):100-10.

13. Warr MR, Shore GC. Unique biology of Mcl-1: therapeutic opportunities in cancer. *Curr Mol Med* 2008;8(2):138-47.

14. Yang M, Mattes J. Discovery, biology and therapeutic potential of RNA interference, microRNA and antagomirs. *Pharmacol Ther* 2008;117(1):94-104.

15. Shan G. RNA interference as a gene knockdown technique. *Int J Biochem Cell Biol* 2010;42(8):1243-51.

16. Devi GR. siRNA-based approaches in cancer therapy. *Cancer Gene Ther* 2006;13(9):819-29.

17. Livak KJ, Schmittgen TD. Analysis of relative gene expression data using real-time quantitative PCR and the 2(-Delta Delta C(T)) Method. *Methods* 2001;25(4):402-8.

18. Thallinger C, Wolschek MF, Wacheck V, Maierhofer H, Gunsberg P, Polterauer P, et al. Mcl-1 antisense therapy chemosensitizes human melanoma in a SCID mouse xenotransplantation model. *J Invest Dermatol* 2003;120(6):1081-6.

19. Thallinger C, Wolschek MF, Maierhofer H, Skvara H, Pehamberger H, Monia BP, et al. Mcl-1 is a novel therapeutic target for human sarcoma: synergistic inhibition of human sarcoma xenotransplants by a combination of mcl-1 antisense oligonucleotides with low-dose cyclophosphamide. *Clin Cancer Res* 2004;10(12 Pt 1):4185-91.

20. Zhang B, Gojo I, Fenton RG. Myeloid cell factor-1 is a critical survival factor for multiple myeloma. *Blood* 2002;99(6):1885-93.

21. Dai Y, Grant S. Targeting multiple arms of the apoptotic regulatory machinery. *Cancer Res* 2007;67(7):2908-11.

22. Boisvert-Adamo K, Longmate W, Abel EV, Aplin AE. Mcl-1 is required for melanoma cell resistance to anoikis. *Mol Cancer Res* 2009;7(4):549-56.

23. Brantl S. Antisense-RNA regulation and RNA interference. *Biochim Biophys Acta* 2002;1575(1-3):15-25.

24. Aoki Y, Cioca DP, Oidaira H, Kamiya J, Kiyosawa K. RNA interference may be more potent than antisense RNA in human cancer cell lines. *Clin Exp Pharmacol Physiol* 2003;30(1-2):96-102.

18

The Effect of Adenosine A_{2A} and A_{2B} Antagonists on Tracheal Responsiveness, Serum Levels of Cytokines and Lung Inflammation in Guinea Pig Model of Asthma

Laleh Pejman[1], Hasan Omrani[1], Zahra Mirzamohammadi[1], Amir Ali Shahbazfar[2], Majid Khalili[3], Rana Keyhanmanesh[3]*

[1] Department of Physiology, Faculty of Medicine, Tabriz University of Medical Sciences, Tabriz, Iran.

[2] Department of Pathology, Faculty of Veterinary Medicine, Tabriz University, Tabriz, Iran.

[3] Tuberculosis and Lung Research Center, Tabriz University of Medical Sciences, Tabriz, Iran.

ARTICLE INFO

Keywords:
ZM241385
MRS1706
Adenosine A_{2A} and A_{2B} receptor
Asthma
Guinea pig

ABSTRACT

Purpose: Nowadays adenosine is specified as an important factor in the pathophysiology of asthma. For determining the effect of different A_2 receptors, in this investigation the effect of single dose of selective adenosine A_{2A} and A_{2B} antagonists (ZM241385 and MRS1706) on different inflammatory parameters; tracheal responsiveness to methacholine and ovalbumin, total and differential cell count in bronchoalveolar lavage (BAL), blood levels of IL-4 and IFN-γ and lung pathology of guinea pig model of asthma were assessed.

Methods: All mentioned parameters were evaluated in two sensitized groups of guinea pigs pretreated with A_{2A} and A_{2B} antagonists (S+Anta A_{2A}, S+Anta A_{2B}) compared with sensitized (S) and control (C) groups.

Results: The tracheal responsiveness to methacholine and OA, total cell and eosinophil and basophil count in BAL, blood IL-4 level and pathological changes in pre-treated group with MRS1706 (S+Anta A_{2B}) was significantly lower than those of sensitized group ($p<0.01$ to $p<0.05$). In pretreated group with Anta A_{2A}(S+Anta A_{2A}), all the above changes were reversed.

Conclusion: These results showed a preventive effect of A_{2B} antagonist (MRS1706) on tracheal responsiveness to methacholine and OA, total and differential cell count in bronchoalveolar lavage, blood cytokines and pathological changes. Administration of ZM241385, selective A_{2A} antagonist, deteriorated the induction effect of ovalbumin.

Introduction

Asthma is a chronic disease characterized by a variety of features including reversible airways obstruction, airway inflammation and an increased airway responsiveness.[1] Evidence has increasingly implicated adenosine in the pathophysiology of asthma.[2] Adenosin is the breakdown product of ATP via endogenous ecto-ATPases and is also present at cell surface in cultured airway epithelial cells.[3] Adenosine in a signaling nucleoside is eliciting many physiological responses. Elevated levels of adenosine have been found in bronchoalveolar lavage, blood and exhaled breath condensate of patients with asthma. In addition, inhaled adenosine-5'-monophosphate induces bronchoconstriction in asthmatics but not in normal subjects. Studies on animals and humans have shown that bronchoconstriction is most likely due to the release of inflammatory mediators from mast cells. However a number of evidences suggest that adenosine modulates

the function of many other cells involved in airway inflammation such as neutrophils, eosinophils, lymphocytes and macrophages.[4]

It has become clear that biological functions of adenosine are mediated by four distinct subtypes of receptors (A_1, A_{2A}, A_{2B}, and A_3) and that biological responses are determined by the different pattern of receptors distribution in specific cells. Adenosine receptors are ubiquitously expressed throughout the body, with virtually all cells expressing one or more adenosine receptor subtype. With respect to the lung, little is known about the relative expression of adenosine receptor subtypes; however, binding studies in healthy peripheral lung tissue have suggested that A_2 receptor subtypes are much more abundant than the A_1 and A_3 receptor subtypes.[5]

For determining the effect of different A_2 receptors in pathophysiology of asthma, in this investigation the

*Corresponding author: Rana Keyhanmanesh, Tuberculosis and Lung Research Center, Tabriz University of Medical Sciences, Tabriz, Iran.
Email: keyhanmaneshr@tbzmed.ac.ir, rkeyhanmanesh@gmail.com

effect of selective adenosine A_{2A} and A_{2B} antagonists (ZM241385 and MRS1706) on tracheal responsiveness to methacholine and ovalbumin (OA), total and differential cell count in bronchoalveolar lavage, blood levels of IL-4 and IFN-γ and lung pathology of guinea pig model of asthma were assessed.

Materials and Methods
Animal sensitization and animal groups
Forty male adult Dunkin-Hartley guinea pigs (400–700 g) were used throughout the study. They were allowed to acclimatize to the new situation for ten days. The animals were group-housed in individual cages in climate-controlled animal quarters and were given water and food ad libitum, while a12-h on/12-h off light cycle was maintained.

Animals randomly divided to four groups; Control group (C), Sensitized group with ovalbumin (OA, S), sensitized groups pretreated with selective A_{2A} antagonist (ZM241385) and selective A_{2B} antagonist (MRS1706) (S+Anta A_{2A} and S+Anta A_{2B} groups). Each of these antagonists (Tocris bioscience, UK) with 3 mg/kg dose was injected i.p. on day 10 of induction protocol.[6,7]

Sensitization of animals to OA (Grade II Sigma Chemical Ltd., UK) was performed according to our previous study.[8] Briefly, on the first day, 100 mg of OA, dissolved in saline, injected intraperitoneally and other 100 mg of OA subcutaneously. A week later, subsequent 10 mg of OA was injected intraperitoneally. Then from day 14, sensitized animals were exposed to an aerosol of 4% OA for 18 ± 1 days, 4 min daily. The aerosol was administered in a closed chamber with dimensions 30 × 20 × 20 cm. Control animals were treated similarly but saline was used instead of OA solution. The study was approved by the ethical committee of the Tabriz University of Medical Sciences.

Tissue preparation
Guinea pigs were killed by a blow on the neck and the trachea was removed. In each animal, after separation of the trachea from adjacent tissues, one tracheal chain was prepared as follows: The trachea was cut into 10 rings (each containing 2–3 cartilaginous rings) and sutured together to form a tracheal chain. Then all the rings (except terminal rings) were cut open opposite the trachealis muscle to clarify the muscular response. Finally tissue was suspended in a 20-mL organ bath (Schuler organ bath type 809, Germany) containing Krebs-Henseliet solution of the following composition (mM): NaCl; 120, $NaHCO_3$; 25, $MgSO_4$; 0.5, KH_2PO_4; 1.2, KCl; 4.72, $CaCl_2$; 2.5 and dextrose 11. The Krebs solution was maintained at 37 °C and gassed with 95% O_2 and 5% CO_2. Tissue was suspended under isotonic tension of 1 g and allowed to equilibration for at least 1 hour while it was washed with Krebs solution every 15 min.[9]

Responses were measured using an isometric transducer (ADInstruments, spain) with a sensitivity range of 0–25 g. These responses after amplifying with ML/118 quadribridge amplifier (March-Hugstetten, Germany) were recorded on a powerlab (ML-750, 4 channel recorder; March-Hugstetten, Germany).

Assessment of tracheal response to Methacholine
In each experiment, a concentration-response curve of the tracheal chain was obtained. Consecutive concentrations of methacholine hydrochloride (Sigma Chemical Ltd., UK); including 10^{-7} to 10^{-2} M, dissolved in saline; were added every 3 minutes. The contraction due to each concentration was recorded at the end of 3 minutes and the effect reached a plateau in all experiments. Then the percentage of the tracheal smooth muscle contraction due to each concentration of methacholine in proportion to the maximal contraction obtained by its final concentration was plotted against log concentration of methacholine. A concentration-response curve of methacholine was performed in the tracheal chain of each studied animal. The effective concentration of methacholine causing 50% of maximum response (EC50) was measured from the methacholine response curve in each experiment using 50% of the maximum response in the Y axis and measuring the dose of methacholine causing this response in the X axis. The contractility response to 10 μM methacholine as the magnitude of contraction was also measured.

Measurement of tracheal response to Ovalbumin (OA)
The tracheal response of all animals to a 0.1% solution of OA was measured in each studied animal as follows: 0.5 mL of 4% OA solution (dissolved in saline) was added to the 20-mL organ bath and the degree of tracheal chain contraction was recorded after 10 min and was expressed as a proportion (in percentage) to the contraction obtained with 10 μM methacholine.

The measurements of tracheal response to methacholine and OA were performed in random order.

Lung lavage and its white blood cell count
Coincident with preparing the tracheal chain, a cannula was located into the remaining trachea and the lungs were lavaged with 5mL of saline 4 times (total: 20 mL). One mL of lung lavage fluid (LLF) was stained with Turk solution and counted in duplicate in a hemocytometer (in a Burker chamber). The Turk solution consisted of 1mL of glacial acetic acid, 1 mL of gentiac violet solution 1% and 100 mL of distilled water.

The remaining LLF was centrifuged at 2500 × g at 4 °C for 10 min. The supernatant was removed. The smear was prepared from the cells and stained with Wright-Giemsa. According to staining and morphological criteria, differential cell analysis was carried out under a light microscope by counting 100 cells twice and the percentage of each cell type calculated.[10]

Measurement of blood interleukin 4 (IL-4) and interferon-γ (IFN-γ) levels

Ten milliliters of peripheral blood was obtained immediately after sacrificing the animals and placed at room temperature for 1 hour. The samples were then centrifuged at 3500g 4 °C for 10 min. The supernatant was collected and immediately stored in deep freezer at −70°C until analyzed. Finally, blood IL-4 and IFN-γ levels were measured using the sandwich ELISA method.[11]

Pathological evaluation

Guinea pigs were sacrificed by a cervical dislocation, and their lungs and trachea were removed and placed into 10% buffered formalin (37%, Merck, Germany).

Seven days later, the tissues were dried using an Autotechnicon apparatus by passage of the tissues through 70% ethanol and xylol to clear the tissues and then paraffin block the tissues. The specimens were cut into 4-μm slices and stained with hematoxylin and eosin (H&E stain). The tissues were then evaluated under a light microscope. For each specimen, at least 10 airways and vessels were evaluated.[8]

The following pathological changes in the lungs of the sensitized groups were observed: vascular and airway membrane hyperplasia, mucosal plug, local epithelial denudation, eosinophil and lymphocyte infiltration and emphysema. These changes were scored as follows: no pathologic changes = 0, patchy changes =1, local changes =2, scattered changes =3 and severe changes =4.

Statistical analysis

The data of tracheal response to methacholine (EC50), tracheal contractility response, tracheal response to OA, total WBC numbers and differential WBC counts are quoted as mean ± SEM. The data of three sensitized groups were compared with controls using one-way analysis of variance (ANOVA) with Tukey-Kramer post-test. Moreover, the data of the sensitized group were compared with control and treated guinea pigs using one-way analysis of variance (ANOVA) with Tukey-Kramer post-test. The data between groups of animals treated with antagonists using the unpaired t-test. Significance was accepted at p<0.05.

Results

Tracheal response to methacholine

Concentration response curves to methacholine in non incubated tissues showed left ward shift of the curve in group S compared to group C. However, the curve of S+Anta A_{2B} group was shifted to right compared to group S. Pretreatment with Anta A_{2A} caused left ward shift compared to S group (Figure 1).

The mean value of EC_{50} in tracheal chains of group S (1.50±0.36 μM) was significantly lower than in group C (5.31±0.71 μM, p<0.001, Figure 2). The mean value of EC_{50} in tracheal chains in pre-treated group with Anta A_{2A} (1.38±0.24μM) was non significantly lower than sensitized group; but administration of Anta A_{2B}

(3.10±0.54 μM, P<0.01) caused significant improvment compared to the group S (Figure 2). However, the mean value of EC_{50} in tracheal chains of S+Anta A_{2B} group was still significantly lower than in group C (P<0.05, Figure 2).

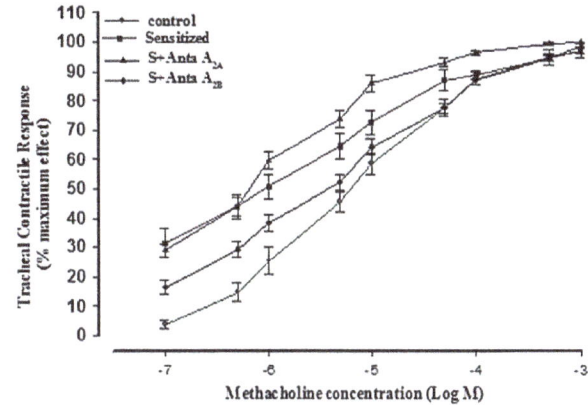

Figure 1. Cumulative log concentration-response curves of methacholine induced contraction of isolated trachea in control (C), sensitized (S), S treated with Anta A2A (S+Anta A2A) and Anta A2B (S+Anta A2B) guinea pigs in the organ bath (for each group, n=7).

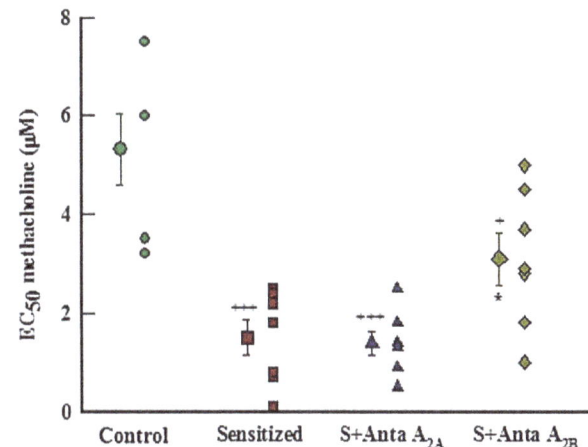

Figure 2. Individual values and mean±SEM (big symbols with bars) of tracheal response to methacholine (EC_{50}) in control (C), sensitized (S), S treated with Anta A_{2A} (S+Anta A_{2A}) and Anta A_{2B} (S+Anta A_{2B}) guinea pigs (for each group, n=6). Statistical differences between control and different groups: +; p<0.05, ++; p<0.01, +++; p<0.001. Statistical differences between sensitized and treated groups: *: p<0.05, **: p<0.01, ***: p<0.001.

Tracheal response to ovalbumin

Tracheal response to OA in tracheal chains of group S (62.889.12%, range 42.80-100%) was significantly higher than in group C (4.853.18%, range 0-23%, p<0.001, Figure 3). Tracheal response to OA in group S+Anta A_{2A} (64.729.01%, range 45-114.45%) was non significantly higher than that of S group but pre-treatment with Anta A_{2B} (45.7810.24%, range 12-78%) was significantly improved compared to sensitized group (p<0.05, Figure 3). However, tracheal response to OA in S+Anta A_{2B} group was still significantly higher than in group C (P<0.01, Figure 3).

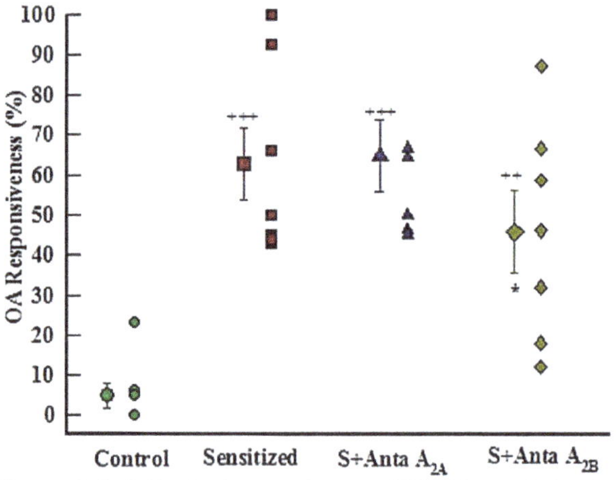

Figure 3. Individual values and mean±SEM (big symbols with bars) of tracheal response to ovalbumin in control (C), sensitized (S), S treated with Anta A_{2A} (S+Anta A_{2A}) and Anta A_{2B} (S+Anta A_{2B}) guinea pigs (for each group, n=6). Statistical differences between control and different groups: +; p<0.05, ++; p<0.01, +++; p<0.001. Statistical differences between sensitized and treated groups: *: p<0.05, **: p<0.01, ***: p<0.001.

Contractility

The contractility response of tracheal chains to methacholine of group S (1.63±0.08 g) was significantly higher than that of group C (0.58±0.04 g, p<0.05). The contractility response in treated group with Anta A_{2B} (1.27±0.05 g) caused significant decrease compared with S group (p<0.01) although this response was still significantly higher than controls (p<0.001). There was no significant difference in the contractility response of S+Anta A_{2A} group (1.84±0.21 g) with group S (Figure 4).

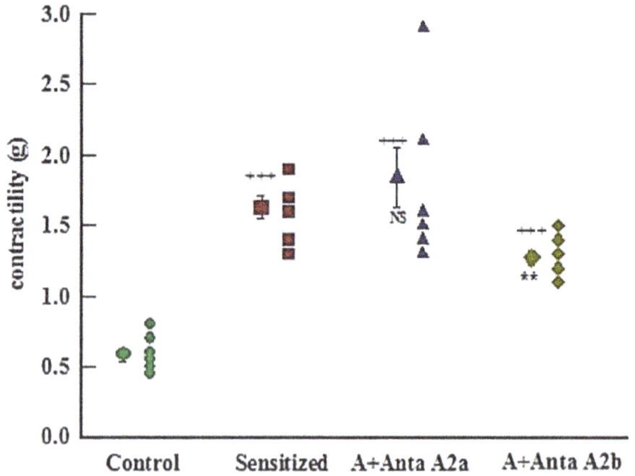

Figure 4. Individual values and mean±SEM (big symbols with bars) of tracheal contractility response to 10 µM methacholine in control (C), sensitized (S), S treated with Anta A_{2A} (S+Anta A_{2A}) and Anta A_{2B} (S+Anta A_{2B}) guinea pigs (for each group, n=6). Statistical differences between control and different groups: +; p<0.05, ++; p<0.01, +++; p<0.001. Statistical differences between sensitized and treated groups: *: p<0.05, **: p<0.01, ***: p<0.001.

Total white blood cell count

The mean value of total white blood cell (WBC) in LLF of group S (9421.43±169.1) was significantly higher than that of group C (2580±180.02, P<0.01)

(Figure 5). The WBC in S+Anta A_{2A} group (9896.43±288.80) was non significantly higher than sensitized animals. The WBC in S+Anta A_{2B} group (5950±1035.7) showed significant improvement compared to that of S group (p<0.05, Figure 5). However, the mean value of WBC in this group was still significantly higher than in group C (p<0.01, Figure 5).

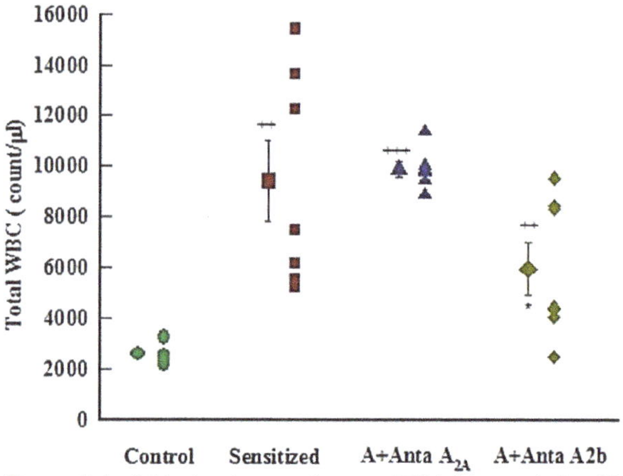

Figure 5. Individual values and mean±SEM (big symbols with bars) of total LLF WBC number in control (C), sensitized (S),S treated with Anta A_{2A} (S+Anta A_{2A}) and Anta A_{2B} (S+Anta A_{2B}) guinea pigs (for each group, n=6). Statistical differences between control and different groups: +; p<0.05, ++; p<0.01, +++; p<0.001. Statistical differences between between sensitized and treated groups: *: p<0.05, **: p<0.01, ***: p<0.001.

Differential count of WBC in Lung Lavage fluid

There was a significant decrease in neutrophil, lymphocyte and monocyte but significant increase of eosinophil and non-significant increase of basophil in LLF of group S compared to those of group C (p<0.001 for all cases, Figure 6a-e). Administration of Anta A_{2A} caused significant decline in lymphocyte (p<0.01) and significant increment in eosinophil count (p<0.05) but the neutrophil, monocyte and basophil counts were not significantly different from S group. However treatment of sensitized animals with Anta A_{2B} caused significant improvement in all LLF different cell counts (p<0.001 for all cases) but there were still significant differences in eosinophil and lymphocyte count of this group in comparison with those of group C (p<0.05 to P<0.001, Figure 6a-e).

Blood IL-4 and IFN-γ levels

The mean value of the blood IL-4 levels in groups S (47.41± 1.98), S + Anta A_{2A} (49.48 ± 2.74) and S + Anta A_{2B} (45.24 ± 2.15) were significantly higher than that of group C (39.78± 2.10, p < 0.05, Figure 7a). However, the mean values of the IL-4 in these pretreated groups were not significantly lower than those of group S (Figure 7a).

The mean value of the blood IFN-γ levels of group S (117.37 ± 2.7) and S + Anta A_{2B} (120.02 ± 2.95) was significantly higher than that of group C (104.97 ± 2.70,

$p < 0.05$, Figure 7b). The mean value of IFN-γ in S+Anta A$_{2A}$ group (101.14±3.24) was significantly lower than in group S ($p<0.01$, Figure 7b).

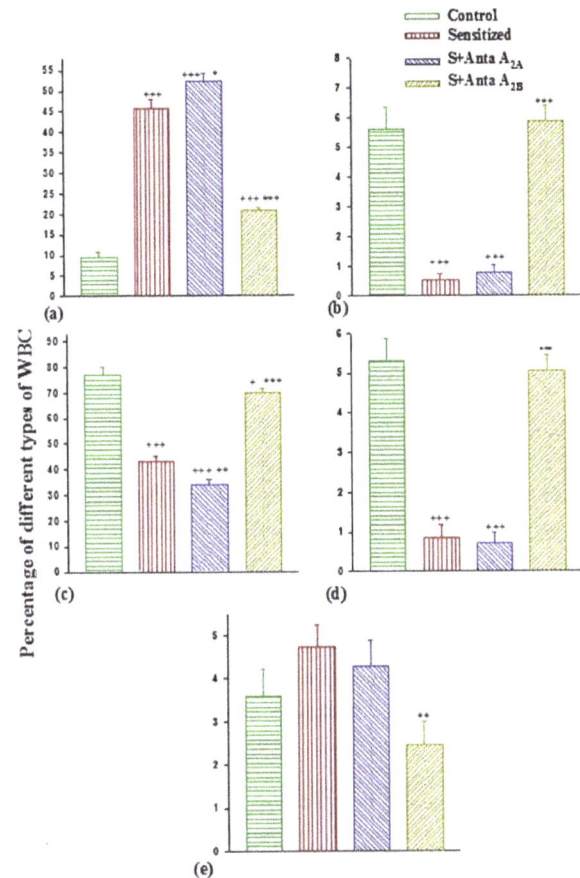

Figure 6. The percentages of eosinophil (a), neutrophil (b), lymphocyte (c), monocyte (d) and basophil (e) of lung lavage fluid in control , sensitized (S), S treated with Anta A$_{2A}$ (S+Anta A$_{2A}$) and Anta A$_{2B}$ (S+Anta A$_{2B}$) guinea pigs (for each group, n=15). Statistical differences between control and different groups: +; $p<0.05$, ++; $p<0.01$, +++; $p<0.001$. Statistical differences between sensitized and treated groups: *: $p<0.05$, **: $p<0.01$, ***: $p<0.001$.

Pathological results

All pathological changes in the S and S+A$_{2A}$ groups, including vascular membrane hyperplasia (3.0±0.3 and 2.90±0.28 respectively), airway membrane hyperplasia (2.54±0.28 and 2.54±0.31 respectively), mucosal plug (2.72±0.14 and 2.27±0.23 respectively), local epithelial denudation (2.18±0.23 and 2.45±0.21 respectively), eosinophil and lymphocyte infiltration (1.55±0.20 and 2.18±0.22 respectively) and emphysema (2.0±0.27 and 2.18±0.23 respectively) were significantly higher than control group (0.33±0.21, 0.17±0.16, 0±0, 0.17±0.16, 0±0 and 0.17±0.16 for vascular and airway membrane hyperplasia, mucosal plug, local epithelial denudation, infiltration and emphysema respectively, $p<0.05$ for all, Figure 8, 9 a-f).
In S+A$_{2B}$ group, some of pathological changes; the mucosal plug (1.14±0.34), local epithelial denudation (0.86±0.26) and emphysema (1.42±0.30) were

significantly higher than controls ($p<0.05$). however, the pathological changes such as vascular membrane hyperplasia (1.42±0.48) and airway membrane hyperplasia (0.86±0.34), the mucosal plug , local epithelial denudation in group S+A$_{2B}$ were significantly lower than S group ($p<0.05$, Figure 8, 9 a-f).

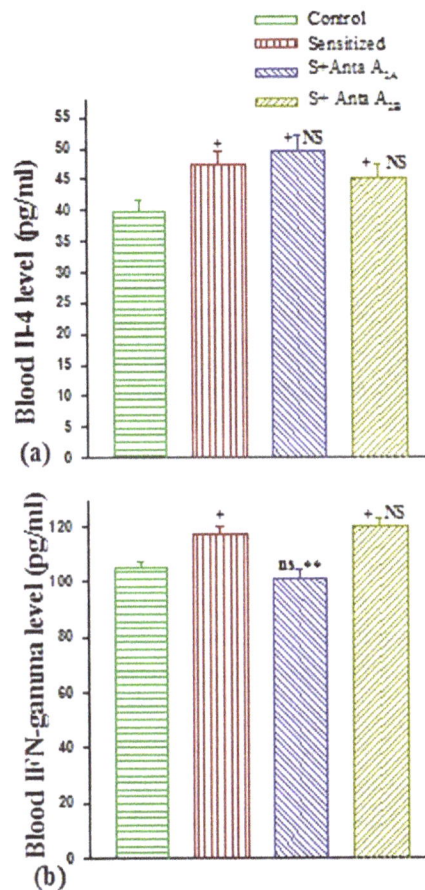

Figure 7. The blood IL-4 (a) and IFN-γ (b) levels (pg/ml) in control, sensitized (S), S treated with Anta A$_{2A}$ (S+Anta A$_{2A}$) and Anta A$_{2B}$ (S+Anta A$_{2B}$) guinea pigs (for each group, n = 8). Statistical differences between the control and the different groups: ns; no significant difference, +; $p < 0.05$. Statistical differences between sensitized and treated groups: NS; no significant difference,** $p < 0.01$.

Discussion

In the present study, the effect of ZM241385 (selective adenosine A$_{2A}$ antagonist) and MRS1706 (selective adenosine A$_{2B}$ antagonists) on tracheal responsiveness to methacholine and OA, total and differential cell count in bronchoalveolar lavage, blood levels of IL-4 and IFN-γ and lung pathology of guinea pig model of asthma were examined. The results showed increased tracheal responsiveness to methacholine and OA, increased contractility response, increment of LLF total WBC count, eosinophil and basophil number (non-significantly), elevated blood IL-4 and IFN-γ and numerous lung tissue pathological changes but decreased neutrophil, lymphocyte and monocyte in sensitized compared to control animal which was similar to the results of our previous studies.[11,12]

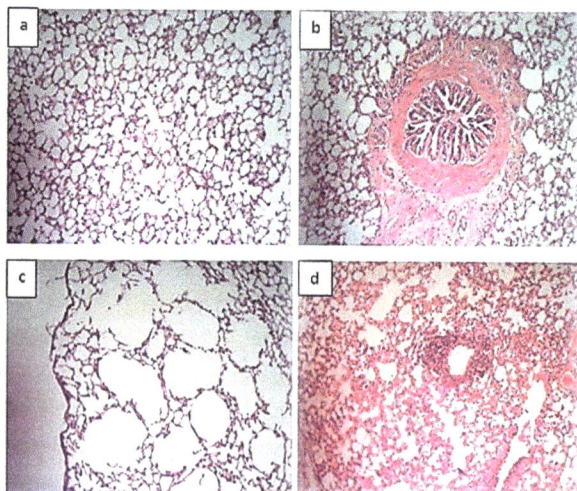

Figure 8. Photographs of a lung specimen in guinea pigs: a- control normal lung tissues (C); b- sensitized (S) with airway membrane hyperplasia and mucosal plug; c- S treated with Anta A_{2A} (S+Anta A_{2A}) with severe emphysema and d- S treated with Anta A_{2B} (S+Anta A_{2B}) with local epithelial denudation (magnification for each group; 10×20).

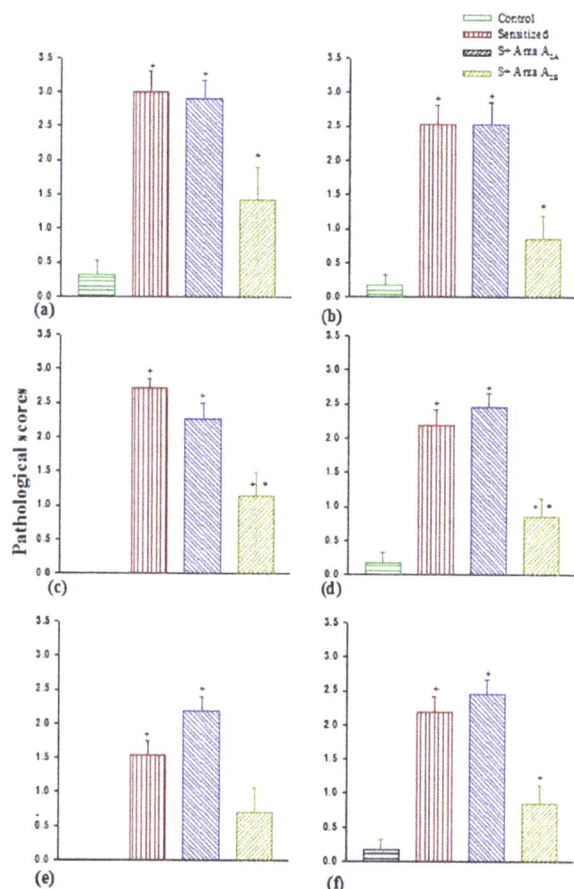

Figure 9. The vascular (a) and airway membrane hyperplasia (b), mucosal plug (c), local epithelial denudation (d), eosinophil and lymphocyte infiltration (e) and emphysema (f) of lungs in control, sensitized (S), S treated with Anta A_{2A} (S+Anta A_{2A}) and Anta A_{2B} (S+Anta A_{2B}) guinea pigs (for each group, n = 8). Statistical differences between the control and the different groups: ns; no significant difference, +; p < 0.05. Statistical differences between sensitized and treated groups: NS; no significant difference,* p < 0.05.

Exogenous and endogenous adenosine; a ubiquitous purine nucleoside, has essential role in the pathogenesis of asthma and other lung inflammatory disorders. This concept is based on the fact that adenosine receptors are present in many cell types involved in airway inflammation.[13] It is now clear that the main mechanism responsible for exogenous adenosine inhalation-induced bronchoconstriction is mediators release from mast cells although there are some evidences for neural pathways activation.[14] In addition to this effect, the increased level of adenosine found in biological fluids, such as bronchoalveolar lavage and exhaled breath condensate of patients with asthma.[15] Although the precise source of adenosine release (mast cells, smooth muscle, epithelial cells) remains uncertain it is likely that adenosine may contribute to the bronchoconstriction induced by other stimuli such as allergens, hypoxia, lung injury and chronic inflammation.[16] However the bio-availability of adenosine is an important determinant of its biological functions, the pattern of expression and distribution of its different receptors (A_1, A_{2A}, A_{2B}, A_3) in the anatomical and structural sites of the respiratory system and in immune or inflammatory cells, are responsible for this matter that adenosine may exert either deleterious or protective roles in the lung. However the inflammatory cytokines can regulate the expression of adenosine receptors, adenosine had a role in the inflammatory environment.[17]

The data strongly suggest that activation of adenosine A_{2A} receptors, which are present in most of the inflammatory cells (such as neutrophils, mast cells, macrophages, eosinophils, platelets and T cells) inhibit inflammatory responses via affecting multiple aspects of the inflammatory process, modulating neutrophils activation and degranulation, oxidative species production, adhesion molecules expression, cytokines release and mast cells degranulation.[5,18-20]

In this study, single dose administration of ZM241385, selective adenosine A_{2A} antagonist, caused increased tracheal responsiveness (decreased EC50 and incremental contractility), tracheal response to OA and total WBC count and eosinophil and basophil number in LLF and pathological changes and decrease in neutrophil, monocyte and lymphocyte count in comparison to controls. These changes were more than those of sensitized group. It showed that this A_{2A} receptor antagonist deteriorated the effect of ovalbumin in inducing asthma in guinea pigs. It has been predicted by exerting inhibitory effects of activation of these receptors on multiple inflammatory cell types mentioned before.

In addition, administration of selective adenosine A_{2A} antagonist, ZM241385, caused increased IL-4 level and decreased IFN-γ in blood. In asthma, the inflammation is regulated by two subsets of CD4+ helper T cells; Th1 and Th2 balance. IFN-γ secretes mostly by Th1 cells whereas IL-4 produces mostly by Th2 cells. In fact, asthma is associated with a shift in immune responses away from a Th1 (IFN-γ) pattern and toward a Th2 (IL-4, IL-5 and IL-13) profile.[21] So one of proposed mechanisms of selective adenosine A_{2A} antagonist could be its effect on regulation of T helper cells subtypes. Also the decreased lymphocyte count in this study can support this suggested mechanism.

Expression of adenosine A_{2B} receptors has been found in bronchial epithelium, cultured human airway smooth muscle, human mast cells, monocytes and fibroblasts.[4] Increasing evidences suggest that in rodents and man activation of adenosine A_{2B} receptors modulates mast cells function. Adenosine signaling through the A_{2B} receptors can stimulate the production of IL-8, IL-4, IL-13 and VEGF from mast cells. This receptors signaling is an important factor of aberrant dendritic cell differentiation and generation of tolerogenic, angiogenic, and pro-inflammatory cells that produce VEGF, IL-8, IL-6, IL-10, COX-2 and TGF-β. In addition, A_{2B} receptors engagement can promote the production of IL-6 and osteopontin from macrophages; IL-6 and MCP-1 from bronchial smooth muscles; increases in IL-6 release from fibroblasts; induces myofibroblasts differentiation; and induces the expression of fibronectin in type II lung epithelial cells. A_{2B} receptor signaling also contributes to the maintenance of airway surface liquid height in airway epithelial cells and vascular barrier function in endothelial cells.[22] It suggests that adenosine, via A_{2B} receptors participates in the remodelling process occurring in chronic inflammatory lung diseases.[23] Taken together these evidences suggest that adenosine A_{2B} receptor are deeply involved in the mechanisms underlying mediators release by mast cells, the major mechanism by which adenosine induces bronchoconstriction and airway inflammation in asthma. Therefore it has been suggested that targeting adenosine receptors might be a possible approach for the development of anti-inflammatory treatments in diseases characterized by chronic airway inflammation such as asthma and COPD. Currently there is an agreement that development of selective adenosine A_{2B} receptor antagonists might be the most appealing approach.[14,24]

Some authors have speculated that the pro- and anti-inflammatory property of adenosine may be dictated by its level in the lung. [14,16] Lung inflammation determines a hypoxic environment in which adenosine is generated. In the initial stage, low levels of adenosine activate high affinity receptors, such as adenosine A_{2A} receptors, and this triggers a protective pathway. However higher levels of adenosine are released when lung inflammation is severe, and these, activating the low affinity adenosine A_{2B} receptors, may trigger deleterious signaling pathways that further exacerbate inflammation.[16]

Single dose administration of MRS1706, selective adenosine A_{2B} antagonist, in this study, improved the changes in tracheal responsiveness, total WBC count and lung pathological changes. This drug ameliorated the variations in differential WBC compared to asthmatic guinea pigs. However it could not prevent completely in comparison to controls. Moreover, this drug caused increase in IFN-γ and decrease in IL-4 level in comparison to sensitized animals although it could not reach those of controls. The lymphocyte count was also higher than sensitized group. These results were in line with previous studies. Mustafa and his colleagues in 2007 showed that other antagonist of adenosine A_{2B} receptors, CVT-6883, inhibited the airway inflammation.[25] These studies confirmed the role of A_{2B} receptors in the pathophysiology of asthma.

Conclusion
In Conclusion, the results showed that administration of single dose of selective adenosine A_{2A} (ZM241385) deteriorated the inflammatory changes of ovalbumin induced asthma and single dose prescription of A_{2B} antagonists (MRS1706) could prevent these changes.

Acknowledgements
This investigation was supported by Tuberculosis and lung research center of Tabriz University of medical sciences as the part of the thesis of Msc student, Miss Pejman.

Conflict of Interest
The authors declare that they have no conflict of interest.

References
1. Keir S, Page C. The rabbit as a model to study asthma and other lung diseases. *Pulm Pharmacol Ther* 2008;21(5):721-30.
2. Rorke S, Holgate ST. Targeting adenosine receptors: novel therapeutic targets in asthma and chronic obstructive pulmonary disease. *Am J Respir Med* 2002;1(2):99-105.
3. Kornerup KN, Page CP, Moffatt JD. Pharmacological characterisation of the adenosine receptor mediating increased ion transport in the mouse isolated trachea and the effect of allergen challenge. *Br J Pharmacol* 2005;144(7):1011-6.
4. Spicuzza L, Di Maria G, Polosa R. Adenosine in the airways: implications and applications. *Eur J Pharmacol* 2006;533(1-3):77-88.
5. Brown RA, Spina D, Page CP. Adenosine receptors and asthma. *Br J Pharmacol* 2008;153 Suppl 1:S446-56.
6. Fozard JR, Mccarthy C. Adenosine receptor ligands as potential therapeutics in asthma. *Curr Opin Investig Drugs* 2002;3(1):69-77.
7. Smith N, Broadley KJ. Adenosine receptor subtypes in the airways responses to 5'-adenosine monophosphate inhalation of sensitized guinea-pigs. *Clin Exp Allergy* 2008;38(9):1536-47.
8. Keyhanmanesh R, Boskabady MH, Khamneh S, Doostar Y. Effect of thymoquinone on the lung pathology and cytokine levels of ovalbumin-

sensitized guinea pigs. *Pharmacol Rep* 2010;62(5):910-6.

9. Keyhanmanesh R, Boskabady MH. Relaxant effects of different fractions from Tymus vulgaris on guinea-pig tracheal chains. *Biol Res* 2012;45(1):67-73.

10. Keyhanmanesh R, Boskabady MH, Eslamizadeh MJ, Khamneh S, Ebrahimi MA. The effect of thymoquinone, the main constituent of Nigella sativa on tracheal responsiveness and white blood cell count in lung lavage of sensitized guinea pigs. *Planta medica* 2010;76(3):218-22.

11. Boskabady MH, Keyhanmanesh R, Khameneh S, Doostdar Y, Khakzad MR. Potential immunomodulation effect of the extract of Nigella sativa on ovalbumin sensitized guinea pigs. *J Zhejiang Univ Sci B* 2011;12(3):201-9.

12. Boskabady MH, Keyhanmanesh R, Khamneh S, Ebrahimi MA. The effect of Nigella sativa extract on tracheal responsiveness and lung inflammation in ovalbumin-sensitized guinea pigs. *Clinics (Sao Paulo)* 2011;66(5):879-87.

13. Spicuzza L, Bonfiglio C, Polosa R. Research applications and implications of adenosine in diseased airways. *Trends Pharmacol Sci* 2003;24(8):409-13.

14. Polosa R, Rorke S, Holgate ST. Evolving concepts on the value of adenosine hyperresponsiveness in asthma and chronic obstructive pulmonary disease. *Thorax* 2002;57(7):649-54.

15. Huszar E, Vass G, Vizi E, Csoma Z, Barat E, Molnar Vilagos G, et al. Adenosine in exhaled breath condensate in healthy volunteers and in patients with asthma. *Eur Respir J* 2002;20(6):1393-8.

16. Blackburn MR. Too much of a good thing: adenosine overload in adenosine-deaminase-deficient mice. *Trends Pharmacol Sci* 2003;24(2):66-70.

17. Khoa ND, Montesinos MC, Reiss AB, Delano D, Awadallah N, Cronstein BN. Inflammatory cytokines regulate function and expression of adenosine A(2A) receptors in human monocytic THP-1 cells. *J Immunol* 2001;167(7):4026-32.

18. Lappas CM, Sullivan GW, Linden J. Adenosine A2A agonists in development for the treatment of inflammation. *Expert Opin Investig Drugs* 2005;14(7):797-806.

19. Thiel M, Chouker A, Ohta A, Jackson E, Caldwell C, Smith P, et al. Oxygenation inhibits the physiological tissue-protecting mechanism and thereby exacerbates acute inflammatory lung injury. *PLoS Biol* 2005;3(6):e174.

20. Constance N, Wilson S, Mustafa J, Abbracchio MP, Heidelberg SD. Adenosine receptors in health and disease. Dordrecht: Springer; 2009.

21. Schmidt-Weber CB, Blaser K. The role of the FOXP3 transcription factor in the immune regulation of allergic asthma. *Curr Allergy Asthma Rep* 2005;5(5):356-61.

22. Zhoua Y, Schneidera DJ, Blackburna MR. Adenosine signaling and the regulation of chronic lung disease. *Pharmacol Ther* 2009;123(1):105-16.

23. Zhong H, Belardinelli L, Maa T, Zeng D. Synergy between A_{2B} adenosine receptors and hypoxia in activating human lung fibroblasts. *Am J Respir Cell Mol Biol* 2005;32(1):2-8.

24. Holgate ST. The Quintiles Prize Lecture 2004. The identification of the adenosine A_{2B} receptor as a novel therapeutic target in asthma. *Br J Pharmacol* 2005;145(8):1009-15.

25. Mustafa SJ, Nadeem A, Fan M, Zhong H, Belardinelli L, Zeng D. Effect of a specific and selective A(2B) adenosine receptor antagonist on adenosine agonist amp and allergen-induced airway responsiveness and cellular influx in a mouse model of asthma. *J Pharmacol Exp Ther* 2007;320(3):1246-51.

19

ABT-737, Synergistically Enhances Daunorubicin-Mediated Apoptosis in Acute Myeloid Leukemia Cell Lines

Hassan Dariushnejad[1], Nosratallah Zarghami[1,2]*, Mohammad Rahmati[1,2], Samaneh Ghasemali[1], Zohreh Sadeghi[1], Zahra Davoodi[1], Hossein Jafari Tekab[3], Masoud Gandomkar Ghalhar[1]

[1] Department of Medical Biotechnology, Faculty of Advance Medical Sciences, Tabriz University of Medical Sciences, Tabriz, Iran.

[2] Department of Clinical Biochemistry, Faculty of Medicine, Tabriz University of Medical Sciences, Tabriz, Iran.

[3] Department of Medical Genetics, Faculty of Medicine, Tabriz University of Medical Sciences, Tabriz, Iran.

ARTICLE INFO

Keywords:
Acute myeloid leukemia
Daunorubicin
ABT-737
Combination
Apoptosis

ABSTRACT

Purpose: Intensive chemotherapy with daunorubicin (DNR) is associated with serious side effects in acute myeloid leukemia (AML) patients. In this study the effect of small-molecule BH3-mimetic, ABT-737, on the sensitivity of HL60 and U937 AML cell lines was investigated.

Methods: The cytotoxic effects of DNR and ABT-737, alone or in combination were assessed using MTT assay and combination index analysis. The effects of treatments on the cell proliferation was determined by trypan blue assay. ELISA cell death assay was used for measurement of apoptosis.

Results: IC50 values of DNR and ABT-737 were 2.52 and 0.59 μM for HL-60 cells line and 1.31 and 0.80 μM for U937 cell line at 24 h, respectively. Surprisingly, combination treatment significantly lowered the IC50 values in a synergic manner in both cell lines. Moreover, treatment with a mixture of two agents had more growth inhibition effect relative to the monotherapy. Results of apoptosis assay showed that the cytotoxic effects are related to the enhancement of apoptosis.

Conclusion: Our study suggests that ABT-737 synergistically enhances the cytotoxic effect of DNR in AML cell lines and therefore may be useful to overcome chemoresistance of leukemia patients.

Introduction

Acute myeloid leukemia (AML) is an aggressive blood disorder that known with the accumulation of immature hematopoietic stem cells in bone marrow.[1] AML is the most common type of leukemia in adults with lowest survival rate of all leukemias.[2,3] AML treatment includes at least one course of induction chemotherapy including daunorubicin (DNR) and cytarabine.[4] More than 50% of patient with AML do not achieve complete remission or show relapse after high-dose induction chemotherapy.[5] In addition, the cardiotoxicity and nephrotoxicity of anthracyclines remain as a major problem in clinical treatment of AML.[6] Studies have shown that the use of biological modifiers in combination with conventional cytotoxic agents is useful to reduce undesirable toxicity.[7]

Mitochondria play a central role in the regulation of apoptosis (programmed cell death).[8] B-cell lymphoma-2 (Bcl-2) family of proteins are regulated the intrinsic pathway of apoptosis by the stabilization of the outer membrane of mitochondria (OMM). The members of this family are divided into three main groups based on function and regions of the Bcl-2 homology (BH) domains: multi-domain anti-apoptotic proteins (Bcl-2, Bcl-x_L, Bcl-w, Mcl-1 and A1) multi-domain pro-apoptotic proteins (Bax and Bak), and BH3-only pro-apoptotic proteins (Bid, PUMA, Bim and NOXA). Studies have showed that BH1, BH2 and BH3 domains of anti-apoptotic proteins interact with the α-helixes formed by BH3 domains of pro-apoptotic members. When the cells received the apoptosis signals, BH3-only pockets of anti-apoptotic proteins bind to the hydrophobic cleft formed by anti-apoptotic proteins resulting in release of Bax and Bak. Oligomerized Bax and Bak permeabilize OMM that cause release of cytochrome c and thereby execution of apoptosis.[9-11]

It is shown that the overexpression of anti-apoptotic Bcl-2 family of proteins have been correlated with survival and therapeutic resistance of tumor cells including leukemia.[12,13] Moreover,

*Corresponding author: Nosratallah Zarghami, Department of Medical Biotechnology, Faculty of Advanced Medical Sciences, Tabriz University of Medical Sciences, Golgasht Street, 51664, Tabriz, Iran, Email: zarghamin@yahoo.com

others have demonstrated that targeting of anti-apoptotic Bcl-2 family members can induce apoptosis and reverse multi-drug resistance of cancer cells.[14] Since, the BH3 binding pockets of anti-apoptotic proteins are essential for their functions, it is hypothesized that the small molecules that bind to these pockets may be able to block the hetero-dimerization of anti-apoptotic and pro-apoptotic proteins and trigger apoptosis.[15]

ABT-737 is a potent small molecule inhibitor of the Bcl-2, Bcl-xL and Bcl-w proteins, developed by Abbott laboratories. This compound, like BH3-only proteins, binds to anti-apoptotic Bcl-2 family members and antagonizes their effects, thereby diminishing their ability to inhibit apoptosis.[16] Furthermore, ABT-737 was found to exhibit chemosensitization effect, and single anti-cancer activity was observed in lymphoma and small-cell lung carcinoma (SCLC) tumor cells with low toxicity.[17]

The aims of this study were to investigate the anti-tumor effect of anthracycline DNR on AML cells and to determine whether this effect can be enhanced by ABT-737. To this end, we have examined the effects of either agent, alone and in combination, in HL-60 and U937 cell lines.

Materials and Methods
Cell lines and culture
HL-60 (acute promyelocytic leukemia) and U937 (human leukemic monocyte leukemia) cell lines were purchased from Pasteur Institute Cell Bank of Iran. RPMI-1640 medium (Sigma, USA) supplemented with 10% heat inactivated fetal bovine serum (FBS) (Gibco, Invitrogen, USA), 2 mg/ml sodium bicarbonate, 0.05 mg/ml penicillin G (Serva co, Germany) and 100 µg/ml streptomycin (Gibco) was used for cell culture. The cell lines were cultured in 25 cm2 flasks and maintained in a humidified incubator containing 5% CO_2 at 37 °C.

In vitro cytotoxicity
The cytotoxicity of treatments was determined by MTT assay. This test detects the reduction of yellow MTT [3-(4, 5-dimethylthiazolyl)-2, 5-diphenyl-tetrazolium bromide] into purple formazan crystals by mitochondrial dehydrogenases, which reflects the normal function of mitochondria. Just before treatments, leukemia cell lines were cultured in complete medium at a density of 3×10^4 cells/well in 96-well U-shape bottom tissue culture plates (Nunc, Denmark) and incubated overnight at 37 °C. The next day, the culture medium was replaced with 200 µl of fresh complete medium and then the cells were treated with different concentrations (0.001, 0.01, 0.1, 0.5, 1 and 2 µM) of either ABT-737 (Active Biocheminals, HongKong) or DNR (Sigma, Germany) alone. Moreover, a combination treatment with equal concentrations of two agents was performed. Treatments with 1% DMSO (solvent of ABT-737) and

RPMI (solvent of DNR) without drugs were also considered as a blank control. After 24 h of incubation, the culture medium was removed and the cells were incubated with MTT solution (Sigma) (0.2 mg/ml, 200 µl) for 4 h at 37 °C in a humidified atmosphere. The cell culture plates were centrifuged at 1500 g for 5 min and the supernatants were discarded. Subsequently, 200 µl of DMSO and 25 µl of Sorenson's glycine buffer were added to the wells to dissolve the formazan crystals. Finally, the amount of soluble formazan was determined by quantification of the absorbance at 570 nm (with a reference wavelength of 650 nm) using EL × 800 ELISA plate reader (Bio Tech Instruments, USA). After correction of the background absorbance, the percentage of cell viability was determined using the following formula:

Cell viability (%) = $Absorbance_{Test}$ / $Absorbance_{Control}$ × 100.

The IC_{50} values (concentrations that induced 50% cytotoxicity) were calculated using GraphPad Prism 6.01 software (GraphPad Software Inc., USA).

Combination index analysis
To investigate the interaction effect between ABT-737 and DNR, combination index analysis, based on Chou and Talalay method was performed.[18] The combination index (CI) was calculated using the following equation: CI = (A/B) + (A/C), which A, B and C are the IC_{50} values of the combination treatment, ABT-737 and DNR, respectively. The values of CI less than 1, equal to 1 and bigger than 1, indicate synergistic, additive and antagonist effects respectively.

Cell proliferation assay
Trypan blue exclusion assay was used to determine anti-proliferative effects of treatments. In brief, the cells (5×10^4 cells/well) were treated with the IC_{50} doses of either ABT-737 or DNR and their combination in 24-well tissue culture plate (Nunc). Following treatments, the cells were incubated in appropriate culture conditions for 24-96 h. At the end of each day, the cells were stained with 0.4% trypan blue dye (Merck KGaA, Germany) and then the number of viable cells was counted using neubauer chamber under an Olympus inverted microscope.

Apoptosis assay
HL-60 and U937 cells were seeded at a density of 5×10^4 cells/well in 96-well plates and treated with drugs as described in the cytotoxicity assay section. Following the treatments, apoptosis was detected using an apoptosis ELISA assay kit (Roche Diagnostics GmbH, Germany) according to the manufacturer's protocol. This test is based on the identification of mono and oligonucleosomes in the cytoplasmic fraction of apoptotic cell lysates. In brief, 24 h after treatments, the cells were centrifuged and lysed. Then, 20 µl of supernatants and 80 µl of immunoreagent containing monoclonal antibodies directed against DNA and histones were transfered to each wells of ELISA

microplate. After 2 h of incubation, the wells were washed and 100 µl of ABTS solution was added. The resulting colors were quantified using a plate reader at 405 nm (with reference wavelength in 490 nm).

Statistical analysis
Statistical analyses were performed with GraphPad Prism 6.01 software. Results were expressed as the mean ± standard deviation (SD). Statistical differences were assessed by unpaired student t-test; and a value of P less than 0.05 was considered significant.

Results
ABT-737, synergistically enhanced the cytotoxic effects of DNR in leukemia cells
To analyze the effect of ABT-737 on sensitivity of leukemic cells to DNR, a combination treatment of two agents was investigated. HL-60 and U937 leukemia cells were exposed to the various concentrations of drugs (0.001-2 µM), alone or in combination, and cytotoxicity was measured by MTT assay after 24 h. As shown in Figure 1a and b, monotherapy with BAT-737 or DNR markedly decreased the viability of the two cell lines in a dose-dependent manner. Results of MTT assay showed that, compare with the single agent treatment, the combination therapy further decreased the percentage of viable cells (P<0.05, Figure 1a and b). Moreover, combination of two agents resulted in significant decrease in the IC_{50} values relative to the monotreatment (Table 1). Results of combination index analyses indicated that the interaction effect between drug combinations was synergistic with CI values of 0.93 and 0.80 in HL-60 and U937 cell lines, respectively.

Table 1. The IC_{50} values determined by MTT assay

	IC₅₀ (µM)	
-	**HL-60**	**U937**
ABT-737	0.59	0.80
DNR	2.52	1.31
Combination	0.45*	0.41*
* P<0.05 relative to single agent reatments		

ABT-737 enhanced the growth inhibitory effect of DNR
We investigated whether treatment with DNR, ABT-737 or the combination of them affects cell proliferation. Cell proliferation was assessed by trypan blue exclusion assay at 24-96 h after treatments. The cell growth curves of HL-60 and U937 cells showed that the treatment with DNR or ABT-737 alone, significantly suppressed cell growth over a period of 5 days (relative to the blank control) (Figure 2a and b). Moreover, two treatments with DNR or ABT-737 further inhibited the growth of two cell lines (P<0.05).

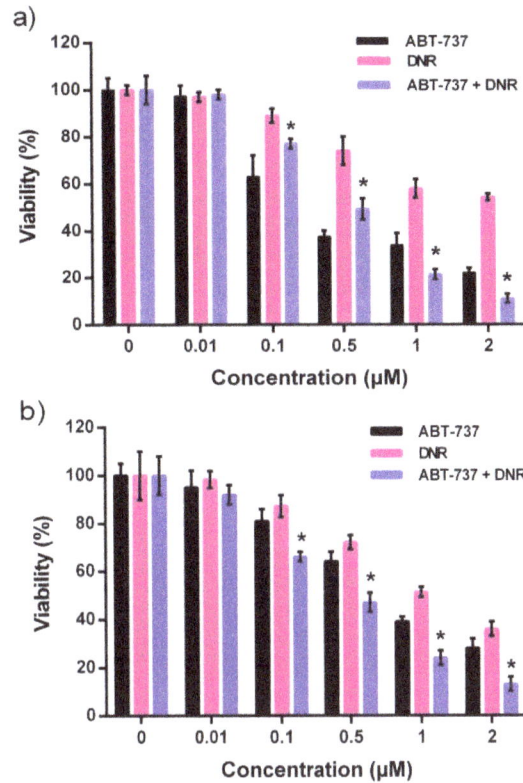

Figure 1. The cytotoxic effects of ABT-737, DNR and their combination on HL-60 (a) and U937 (b) cells were determined by MTT assay. Results expressed as the mean ± SD (n=3), *p<0.05 versus DNR or ABT-737 alone.

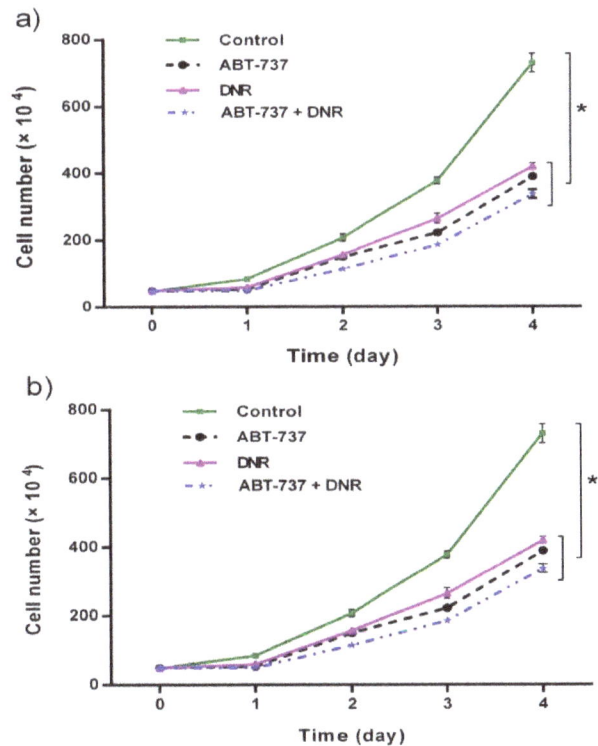

Figure 2. Effects of ABT-737, DNR and their combination on the proliferation of HL-60 (a) and U937 (b) cell lines. The growth curves of leukemic cells were constructed from the results of trypan blue dye exclusion assay. Results expressed as the mean ± SD (n=3), *p<0.05 versus control.

ABT-737 increased the sensitivity of leukemia cells to DNR-mediated apoptosis

To investigate whether the cytotoxic effects of treatments are linked to the enhancement of apoptosis, an apoptosis ELISA assay was performed. HL-60 and U937 tumor cells were treated with both IC_{50} dose of ABT-737 or DNR alone and IC_{50} dose of combination for 24 h, and then validated for apoptosis. Results showed that, Compare with the blank control, treatment with ABT-737 resulted in 5.56 and 7.25 fold increase in apoptosis in HL-60 and U937 cells, respectively (P<0.05, Figure 3). In addition, exposure of HL-60 and U937 cells with DNR significantly enhanced the extent of apoptosis to 4.42 and 5.39 fold, respectively. Moreover, with the combination treatment of two agents, fold increases in apoptosis were 5 for HL-60 cells and 7.59 for U937 Cells.

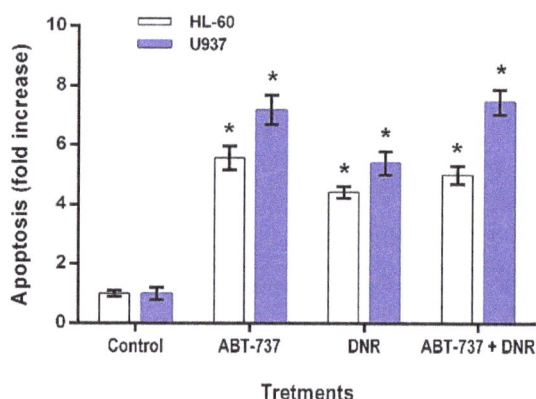

Figure 3. ABT-737 enhanced the sensitivity of leukemia cells to DNR-mediated apoptosis. HL-60 and U937 cells were treated with the drugs and apoptosis was measured by ELISA cell death assay. Results expressed as the fold increase in apoptosis compare with the blank control. Data are the mean ± SD of independent experiments (n=3), *p<0.05 versus blank control.

Discussion

The use of anthracyclines (daunorubicin or idarubicin) in combination with cytarabine is one of the effective induction treatments for AML patients.[19] Since, intensive chemotherapy with DNR is associated with undesirable side effects such as cardiotoxicity; the use of lower doses of daunorubicin is one of great clinical interests.[6] Overexpression of anti-apoptotic proteins plays a critical role in the inherent resistance of tumor cells to cytotoxic agents.[12] Studies have indicated that the suppression of these mediators of apoptosis pathway by various strategies could induce apoptosis and overcome drug resistance of cancer cells.[13,14] In this study, the effect of, BH3-memetic ABT-737, on the apoptosis and sensitivity of HL-60 and U937 AML cells to DNR investigated.

Our data demonstrated that the treatment with ABT-737 or DNR alone causes significant cytotoxic and growth inhibitory effects in leukemic cells. MTT assay and combination index analysis showed that ABT-737 synergistically enhances the cytotoxic effect of DNR in two cell lines. Moreover, apoptosis assay findings

revealed that the chemosensitization effect of ABT-737 is contribute to the induction of apoptosis. These results were in agreement with the other reports describing the important role of mitochondrial anti-apoptotic proteins in drug resistance of tumor cells.[12-14]

Apoptosis can be triggered via two distinct pathways: the intrinsic and the extrinsic pathways. Anti-apoptotic Bcl-2 family of proteins commonly inhibit the intrinsic pathway of apoptosis by interaction with the BH3-only pro-apoptotic proteins (Bid, PUMA, Bim and NOXA), thereby release multi-domain pro-apoptotic proteins (Bax and Bak) to cytoplasm. Oligomerization of Bax and Bak proteins in OMM causes release of cytochrome c from the inner mitochondrial membrane space that lead to caspases activation and the next apoptosis events.[8-11] Our study shows that treatment of leukemic cells with either DNR or ABT-737 triggers marked apoptotic cell death. Furthermore, ABT-737 enhances the apoptosis effect caused by DNR. Thus, it is conceivable that BH3-memetic ABT-737 that interacts with anti-apoptotic proteins, triggers apoptosis through the intrinsic pathway. Chemotherapeutic drug, DNR, is a DNA intercalating agent that induces apoptosis by the inhibition of DNA and RNA synthesis.[4] However, the exact cellular mechanisms of DNR-mediated apoptosis and chemosensitization effect of ABT-737 remain unclear. Further investigations are needed.

Small-molecule BH3-mimetic, ABT-737, strongly inhibits Bcl-2, Bcl-xL, and Bcl-w pro-apoptotic proteins (K_i < 1 nM), but not Mcl-1(K_i > 1 μM).[9,17] ABT-737 has shown promise for treatment of follicular B-cell lymphoma and small-cell lung cancer with low levels of Mcl-1 expression.[20] In addition, it was confirmed that the cells with high levels of Mcl-1 are more resistance to ABT-737, indicates the correlation between the cellular levels of Mcl-1 and response to the compound.[21-24] Our study demonstrated that HL-60 cells are more sensitive to ABT-737 relative to U937 cells (Table 1) that have higher levels of Mcl-1 expression.[25] Our findings support the above-mentioned reports and further confirm the cytoprotective role of Mcl-1 against ABT-737.

Conclusion

In conclusion, the present study has demonstrated that targeted down-regulation of anti-apoptotic proteins by ABT-737 results in a significant single-agent activity against leukemic cells. Furthermore, combination of DNR with ABT-737 exhibited synergistic anti-tumor effect. These findings highlight anti-apoptotic Bcl-2 family of proteins as a relevant target and drug resistance factor in AML patients. Our findings underline the potential of ABT-737 to induce tumor cell apoptosis and reduce the serious side effects caused by high dose chemotherapy. We suggest that the specific suppression of Mcl-1 may further enhance the chemosensitization effect of ABT-737.

Acknowledgments
This study was supported by a grant from Hematology and Oncology Research Center, Tabriz University of Medical Sciences. We acknowledge Dr. Hadi Karami, Molecular Medicine Research Center, Arak University of Medical Sciences, Arak, Iran, for technical assistance and critical review of the manuscript.

Conflict of Interest
The authors declare that they have no conflict of interest.

References
1. Lowenberg B, Downing JR, Burnett A. Acute myeloid leukemia. *N Engl J Med* 1999;341(14):1051-62.
2. Kupsa T, Horacek JM, Jebavy L. The role of cytokines in acute myeloid leukemia: a systematic review. *Biomed Pap Med Fac Univ Palacky Olomouc Czech Repub* 2012;156(4):291-301.
3. Kersemans V, Cornelissen B, Minden MD, Brandwein J, Reilly RM. Drug-resistant AML cells and primary AML specimens are killed by 111In-anti-CD33 monoclonal antibodies modified with nuclear localizing peptide sequences. *J Nucl Med* 2008;49(9):1546-54.
4. Rabbani A, Finn RM, Ausio J. The anthracycline antibiotics: antitumor drugs that alter chromatin structure. *Bioessays* 2005;27(1):50-6.
5. Robak T, Wierzbowska A. Current and emerging therapies for acute myeloid leukemia. *Clin Ther* 2009;31 Pt 2:2349-70.
6. Bardi E, Bobok I, A VO, Kappelmayer J, Kiss C. Anthracycline antibiotics induce acute renal tubular toxicity in children with cancer. *Pathol Oncol Res* 2007;13(3):249-53.
7. Gu C, Ye T, Wells RA. Synergistic effects of troglitazone in combination with cytotoxic agents in acute myelogenous leukaemia cells. *Leuk Res* 2006;30(11):1447-51.
8. Bras M, Queenan B, Susin SA. Programmed cell death via mitochondria: different modes of dying. *Biochemistry (Mosc)* 2005;70(2):231-9.
9. Cheng EH, Levine B, Boise LH, Thompson CB, Hardwick JM. Bax-independent inhibition of apoptosis by Bcl-XL. *Nature* 1996;379(6565):554-6.
10. Lutz RJ. Role of the BH3 (Bcl-2 homology 3) domain in the regulation of apoptosis and Bcl-2-related proteins. *Biochem Soc Trans* 2000;28(2):51-6.
11. Oltersdorf T, Elmore SW, Shoemaker AR, Armstrong RC, Augeri DJ, Belli BA, et al. An inhibitor of Bcl-2 family proteins induces regression of solid tumours. *Nature* 2005;435(7042):677-81.
12. Varin E, Denoyelle C, Brotin E, Meryet-Figuiere M, Giffard F, Abeilard E, et al. Downregulation of Bcl-xL and Mcl-1 is sufficient to induce cell death in mesothelioma cells highly refractory to conventional chemotherapy. *Carcinogenesis* 2010;31(6):984-93.
13. Akagi H, Higuchi H, Sumimoto H, Igarashi T, Kabashima A, Mizuguchi H, et al. Suppression of myeloid cell leukemia-1 (Mcl-1) enhances chemotherapy-associated apoptosis in gastric cancer cells. *Gastric Cancer* 2013;16(1):100-10.
14. Kang MH, Reynolds CP. Bcl-2 inhibitors: targeting mitochondrial apoptotic pathways in cancer therapy. *Clin Cancer Res* 2009;15(4):1126-32.
15. Pommier Y, Sordet O, Antony S, Hayward RL, Kohn KW. Apoptosis defects and chemotherapy resistance: molecular interaction maps and networks. *Oncogene* 2004;23(16):2934-49.
16. Witham J, Valenti MR, De-Haven-Brandon AK, Vidot S, Eccles SA, Kaye SB, et al. The Bcl-2/Bcl-XL family inhibitor ABT-737 sensitizes ovarian cancer cells to carboplatin. *Clin Cancer Res* 2007;13(23):7191-8.
17. Warr MR, Shore GC. Unique biology of Mcl-1: therapeutic opportunities in cancer. *Curr Mol Med* 2008;8(2):138-47.
18. Chou TC, Talalay P. Quantitative analysis of dose-effect relationships: the combined effects of multiple drugs or enzyme inhibitors. *Adv Enzyme Regul* 1984;22:27-55.
19. Tallman MS, Gilliland DG, Rowe JM. Drug therapy for acute myeloid leukemia. *Blood* 2005;106(4):1154-63.
20. Lucas KM, Mohana-Kumaran N, Lau D, Zhang XD, Hersey P, Huang DC, et al. Modulation of NOXA and MCL-1 as a strategy for sensitizing melanoma cells to the BH3-mimetic ABT-737. *Clin Cancer Res* 2012;18(3):783-95.
21. Chen S, Dai Y, Harada H, Dent P, Grant S. Mcl-1 down-regulation potentiates ABT-737 lethality by cooperatively inducing Bak activation and Bax translocation. *Cancer Res* 2007;67(2):782-91.
22. Lin X, Morgan-Lappe S, Huang X, Li L, Zakula DM, Vernetti LA, et al. 'Seed' analysis of off-target siRNAs reveals an essential role of Mcl-1 in resistance to the small-molecule Bcl-2/Bcl-XL inhibitor ABT-737. *Oncogene* 2007;26(27):3972-9.
23. Tahir SK, Yang X, Anderson MG, Morgan-Lappe SE, Sarthy AV, Chen J, et al. Influence of Bcl-2 family members on the cellular response of small-cell lung cancer cell lines to ABT-737. *Cancer Res* 2007;67(3):1176-83.
24. Van Delft MF, Wei AH, Mason KD, Vandenberg CJ, Chen L, Czabotar PE, et al. The BH3 mimetic ABT-737 targets selective Bcl-2 proteins and efficiently induces apoptosis via Bak/Bax if Mcl-1 is neutralized. *Cancer Cell* 2006;10(5):389-99.
25. Ugarenko M, Nudelman A, Rephaeli A, Kimura K, Phillips DR, Cutts SM. ABT-737 overcomes Bcl-2 mediated resistance to doxorubicin-DNA adducts. *Biochem Pharmacol* 2010;79(3):339-49.

20

Reduced ABCB1 Expression and Activity in the Presence of Acrylic Copolymers

Ramin Mohammadzadeh[1,2]**, Behzad Baradaran**[3]**, Hadi Valizadeh**[1]**, Bahman Yousefi**[3]**, Parvin Zakeri-Milani**[4]*

[1] *Drug Applied Research Center and Faculty of Pharmacy, Tabriz University of Medical Sciences, Tabriz, Iran.*

[2] *Students Research Committee, Tabriz University of Medical Sciences, Tabriz, Iran.*

[3] *Immunology Research Center and School of Medicine, Tabriz University of Medical Sciences, Tabriz, Iran.*

[4] *Liver and Gastrointestinal Diseases Research Center and Faculty of Pharmacy, Tabriz University of Medical Sciences, Tabriz, Iran.*

A R T I C L E I N F O

Keywords:
ABCB1
P-glycoprotein
Intestinal efflux pump
Rhodamine
Eudragit

A B S T R A C T

Purpose: P-glycoprotein (P-gp; ABCB1), an integral membrane protein in the apical surface of human intestinal epithelial cells, plays a crucial role in the intestinal transport and efflux leading to changes in the bioavailability of oral pharmaceutical compounds. This study was set to examine the potential effects of three Eudragits RL100, S100 and L100 on the intestinal epithelial membrane transport of rhodammine-123 (Rho-123), a substrate of P-gp using a monolayer of human colon cancer cell line (Caco-2).

Methods: The least non-cytotoxic concentrations of the excipients were assessed in Caco-2 cells by the MTT assay. Then the transepithelial transport of Rho-123 across Caco-2 monolayers was determined with a fluorescence spectrophotometer. Besides, the expression of the P-gp in cells exposed to the polymers was demonstrated using Western-blotting analysis.

Results: Treatment of cells with Eudragit RL100 and L100 led to a very slight change while Eudragit S100 showed 61% increase in Rho-123 accumulation (P<0.001) and also reduced transporter expression.

Conclusion: Our studies suggest that using proper concentrations of the Eudragit S100 in drug formulation would improve intestinal permeability and absorption of p-gp substrate drugs.

Introduction

Although oral route for drug administration is the most convenient and favored choice for patients, most hydrophilic drugs and some high molecular weight hydrophobic drugs show poor intestinal permeability and absorption which is a key factor that determines the pharmacokinetics of oral drug compounds and alters their both bioavailability and pharmaceutical effects.[1-4] P-gp, also known as ABCB1, is a plasma-membrane associated efflux pump in humans with an energy dependent function which plays a crucial role in the intestinal transport and is known to be responsible for the occurrence of drug resistances.[5-7] This effect of P-gp, which is encoded by MDR1 gene, is considered to be one defense against toxic agents where it can reduce the bioavailability of a wide range of pharmaceutical compounds as well.[8-10] Caco-2 cells which are human colonic adenocarcinoma cell line and expressing P-gp appear to be used widely for in vitro permeability studies.[11] Previous studies have revealed that some drugs and commonly used substances in drug formulations can alter the ability of P-gp in pumping its

substrates.[12,13] That means excipients, substances other than the pharmacologically active drugs, are not considered to be inert components and may have an important effect on drug metabolism and efflux.[11,14] Polyacrylate polymers have been used widely to achieve the desired drug release profile with the drug being released at the right place and time or, if necessary, over a desired period of time. Other important uses are taste and odor masking to increase patient compliance and also protection from external influences like moisture. Eudragit® polymers are copolymers derived from esters of acrylic and methacrylic acid, whose physicochemical properties are determined by functional groups. Eudragit S100 is an anionic polymer showing a pH-dependent solubility and has been utilized for oral drug delivery because of its solubility and consequently drug release at pH above 7. Also Eudragit L100, which is an enteric anionic copolymer, is based on methacrylic acid and methyl methacrylate. On the other hand Eudragit RL100 is a positively charged acrylate polymer which is

Corresponding author: Parvin Zakeri-Milani, Department of Pharmaceutics, Faculty of Pharmacy, Tabriz University of Medical Sciences, Tabriz, Iran. 51664. E-mail: pzakeri@tbzmed.ac.ir

extensively used in pharmaceutical sciences i.e. sustained release film coating, etc.[15-22] This study has been conducted in order to test the ability of the named excipients, whose influence on the expression of P-gp has not been reported until now, in down regulating the P-gp efflux transporter which would probably lead to enhancement in drug bioavailability.

Materials and Methods
Materials
Human carcinoma colorectal (Caco-2) cell line was purchased from National cell bank of Iran, Pastur institute, Iran. All cell culture disposable equipments were obtained from Orange, Belgium. RPMI 1640 – Powdered Cell Culture Medium was from PAA Co, Austria. Fetal Bovine Serum (FBS) was aquired from Gibco, Invitrogen, USA. Dimethylsulfoxide (DMSO) was from Merck, Germany. Penicillin and streptomycin were obtained from Sigma, Germany. MTT reagent (3-(4,5-dimetylthiazol-2-yl)-2,5-diphenyltetrazolium bromide was purchased from Roche Diagnostics GmbH, Germany. Trypsin was provided from Gibco, Invitrogen, USA.

Cell culture
All operations were performed via standard sterile conditions under a laminar flow cabinet. The cabinets were habitually sterilized overnight by exposure to ultra-violet radial ion and then washed in 70% alcohol before use. Cells were grown in RPMI 1640 medium supplemented with 10% fetal bovine serum (FBS), 100 µg/ml streptomycin and 100 U/ml penicillin. Cells were incubated in a humidified incubator having 5% CO_2 at 37 °C. Then cells were subcultured into 96-well plates and 6-well plates during various steps of the study.[23]

MTT assay
Cytotoxicity of the excipients were measured in Caco-2 cells via the MTT reagent (3-(4,5-dimetylthiazol-2-yl)-2,5-diphenyltetrazolium bromide according to the manufacturer's procedure. This method is based on the ability of viable cells to metabolize yellow tetrazolium salt MTT to purple formazan crystals by mitochondrial dehydrogenases. The cells were seeded in 96-well plates with a density of 10^4 cells/well and incubated for 24 h at 37°C and 5% CO_2. The cells were treated with various concentrations of solvent extracts (10, 20, 50, 100, 150, 200, 300, 400 µg/ml) and 0.2 % (v/v) DMSO as a negative control. After 12, 24 and 48 h treatment 10 µl of MTT labeling reagent was added to all wells. The plates were incubated at 37°C and 5% CO2 for 4 hours. Then, 100µl of the solubilization solution was added to each well and followed by incubation overnight at 37°C to dissolve formazan crystals. Finally, absorbance was read using an ELISA plate reader (Bio Teck, Germany) at a wavelength of 570 nm. The percentage of cytotoxicity and cell viability were estimated using following equation[24]:

% Cytotoxicity = 1- [mean absorbance of treated cells/ mean absorbance of negative control]
% Viability = 100 - % Cytotoxicity.

Assessing Uptake of Rhodamine-123
For the uptake studies Caco-2 cells were seeded into 24-well plates; and left for 24 hours. On the other day old medium was removed and cells were washed by PBS. Then new culture media containing different concentrations of excipients and 0.3 mM verapamil, as P-gp inhibitor, were added and left for another 24 hours. On day 3 of experiment, the old medium was removed and cells were washed three times with PBS and Rho-123 solution (RPMI containing 10 mM HEPES (pH=7.4) and 5 µM Rho-123) were added and incubated in 37 °C for 3 hours. After incubation period, Rho-123 solution was removed and cells were washed three times with ice-cold PBS. Cells were lysed in 1% Triton X-100 and centrifuged in 1000 rpm for 5 minutes. Supernatant was used to measure the fluorescence and total protein content. Quantity of Rho-123 was calculated using the obtained calibration curve (R^2=1). Then cellular Rho-123 accumulation was normalized to total protein content determined by protein assay kit.[25]

Western Blotting
Cells were moved to 6-well plate in density of 10^6 cells per well and treated with excipients for 24 hours. Solutions were removed and cells were washed by PBS then incubated in 37°C for 5 minutes with Trypsin/EDTA 0.25%. Supernatant was removed and cell sediment was washed twice with PBS. Lysis buffer was added and cell suspension was centrifuged in 15000 rpm for 5 minutes. The proteins were separated by electrophoresis through SDS-polyacrylamide gel on 12.5% running gel and 4% stacking gel at 80 V for 120 min. The gel was electro blotted to Polyvinylidene difluoride (PVDF) membrane using semi-dry western blotting. 3% non-fat dry milk was used to block the membrane for 1 hour at room temperature and membrane was washed 3 times with PBS-Tween 20 0.1% and then incubated overnight with primary monoclonal antibody (Anti-β-actin), diluted 1/1000 in PBS containing 0.1% tween 20. After washing with PBS-Tween 20 0.1%, the membrane was incubated with horseradish peroxidase-conjugated Rabbit anti-mouse secondary antibody for two hours. Membrane was washed and solution A and B of Enhanced chemiluminescence (ECL) kit was added, then membrane was exposed to X-ray film. Membrane was washed twice and was incubated with MDR1 Antibody (C219) overnight. After washing, membrane was put into horseradish peroxidase-conjugated Rabbit anti-mouse secondary antibody for two hours. Membrane was washed and then solution A and B of ECL kit was added, then membrane was exposed to X-ray film.[26,27]

Results

Cytotoxicity of excipients on cells was estimated via MTT test assay. MTT test assay of excipients specified the proper concentration of excipient which should be used in western blotting and Rho-123 uptake experiment. Optical density (OD) value obtained from ELISA reader was divided to that of control and cell viability was calculated for each excipient after 24 hours exposure to different polymer concentrations. Two maximum nontoxic concentrations were selected for

western blotting and Rho-123 uptake test. According to the results, Eudragit RL100 in concentrations more than 0.5% was toxic for Caco-2 cells (P<0.001). Therefore we used its lower concentrations (0.25% and 0.1% (w/v)) for the subsequent studies. Eudragit S100 and L100 caused significant decrease in cell viability in concentrations more than 0.1% (w/v) and 0.25% (w/v), respectively. Thus lower concentrations were selected for uptake study and also western blotting. The MTT assay results are shown in Figure 1.

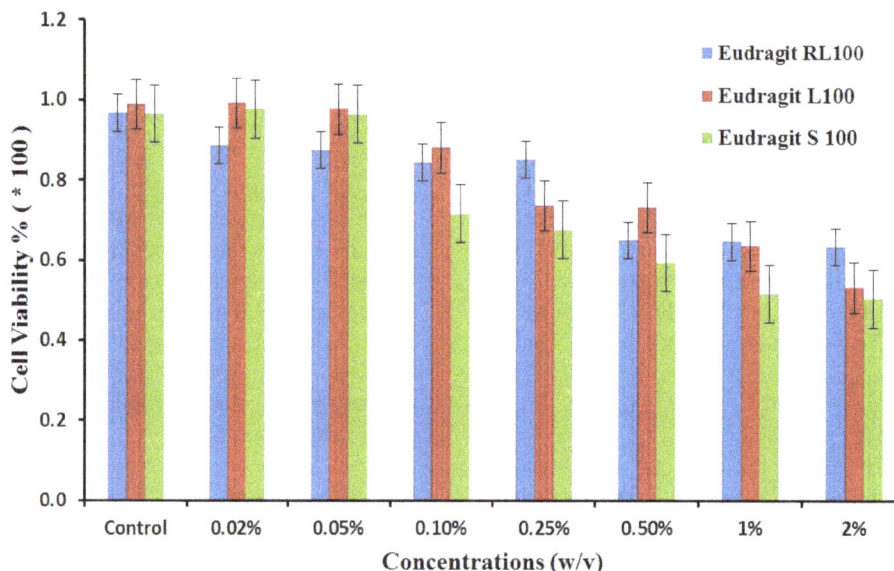

Figure 1. Effects of Eudragit RL100, L100 and S100 on cell viability in Caco-2 cells. Data are expressed as the mean of percent cell viability compared to control after exposure for 24 hours ± standard deviation (n=3).

In order to investigate the functional activity of P-gp, Caco-2 cells were incubated in 48-well plates with different concentrations of the excipients for 24 hours. Afterwards cells were washed with PBS and then exposed to Rho-123 (5 μM) for 3 hours. Cells were lysed and accumulated Rho-123 in cells was measured (excitation at

485 nm and emission measured at 530 nm) for each sample. The protein content of the aliquots was measured by protein assay and cellular Rho-123 accumulation was normalized with respect to the total protein in each well. Eudragit S100 enhanced Rho-123 uptake significantly into Caco-2 cells as shown in the Figure 2.

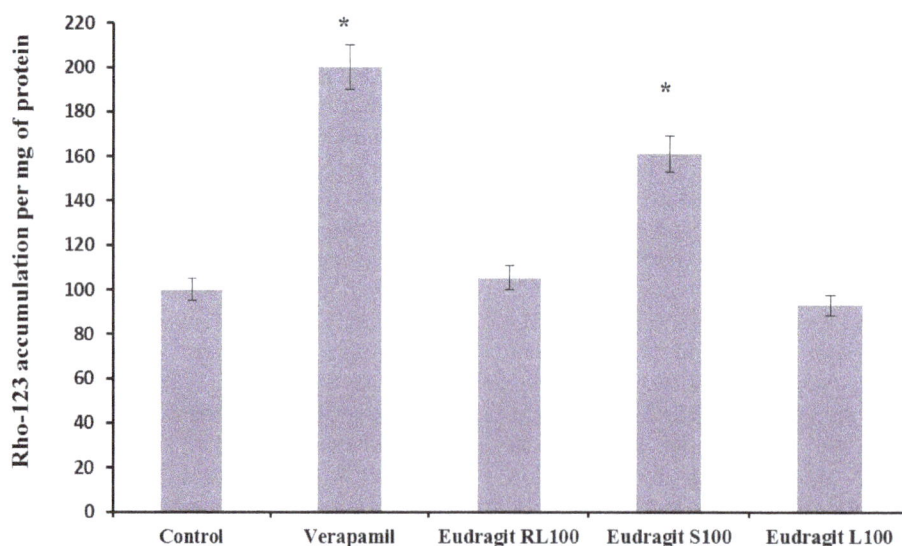

Figure 2. Effect of Eudragit RL100, Eudragit L100 and Eudragit S100 on Rho-123 uptake in Caco-2 cells. Data are expressed by the ratio of quantity of Rho-123 (mg×10⁶/mL) to total protein (mg/mL) in each well. Values are versus control as compared with control group using one way ANOVA with Student-Newman-Keuls post hoc test (*P<0.001).

P-glycoprotein expression was measured in Caco-2 cells which had been treated for 24 hours with excipients and compared to that of control. The protein was separated by electrophoresis on 12.5% running gel and 4% stacking gel. Electrophoretic transfer of separated proteins in gel was transferred to a PVDF membrane using semi-dry blotting. The membrane was blocked in PBS containing 0.1% tween-20 and 3% dried skim milk at room temperature for 1 h and washed three times for 15 min in PBS containing 0.1% tween-20. Encountering with primary and secondary antibody, the bands were visualized using ECL Western Blotting Detection Reagents and exposed to an X-ray film. As shown in the Figure 3 Eudragit S100 had inhibited the P-gp expression which leads to the inhibition of the efflux pump. Other excipients used in the current work had a similar effect as the control group.

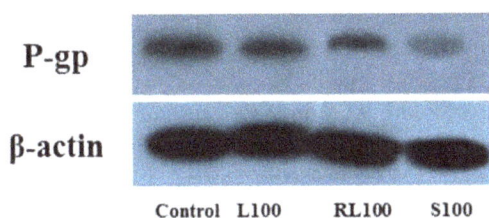

Figure 3. P-gp protein expression after 24 hours exposure to the excipients. Expression in treatment groups were compared with P-gp expression in untreated control cells. 20 μg of total protein were separated by SDS polyacrylamide gel electrophoresis and immunoblotted with monoclonal antibody C219 for P-gp and I-19 for actin.

Discussion

The results of this study showed that there are excipients which could down regulate MDR1 gene and P-gp protein expressions which can lead to enhancement in drug bioavailability. The present study characterizes the effects of the polyacrylate excipients on P-gp expression and activity in Caco-2 monolayer. Sub-toxic concentrations of excipients were prepared using MTT test assay and in the accumulation studies a known P-gp substrate, Rho-123, uptake was tested. Furthermore western blotting confirmed Rho-123 uptake data. Eudragit S100 that was able to increase Rho-123 accumulation decreased P-gp expression either. This study aimed to access a rational drug formulation development strategy for oral dosage forms based on Caco-2 monolayer as an in vitro screening model.

The oral delivery of drugs is generally the most suitable route to administer drugs, as it is painless and easy to use, and therefore it is followed by high patient compliance.[28,29] On the other hand, MDR proteins belonging to ABC transporters are a part of membrane transport proteins that detoxify cells from external substrates. These proteins are identified to limit absorption through biological membranes such as intestinal, brain and cancer cells.[30-32] Several papers have reported data on the effects of different agents and excipients other than Eudragits on the P-gp. For instance a report states that tween 80 can decrease the percentage of serosal-mucosal transport to mucosal-serosal transport of Rho-123 across rat jejunal membrane in vitro and caco-2 cell monolayer, suggestive of p-gp inhibition.[33] In addition, the in vitro absorption of digoxin across an everted rat gut sac (a p-gp substrate) showed a deep increase after treating with 0.5% (w/v) tween 20 and tween 80.[34] Also, digoxin given with tween showed an increase in AUC and C_{max} in rats. Another study has claimed that cremophor EL (0.1%, w/v) only partially inhibits P-gp activity in Caco-2 cells.[35] Lipid excipients Peceol and Gelucire 44/14 decrease P-glycoprotein mediated efflux of rhodamine 123 partially due to modifying P-glycoprotein protein expression within Caco-2 cells.[25] On the other hand there are many other reports on the effects of inhibition of P-gp by co administered drugs on intestinal permeability of drugs.[36,37] Granting these findings, there was no direct study to be conducted on the changes of the expression of MDR1 gene or P-gp induced by Eudragits. In this study, concentrations of 0.1% and 0.25% (w/v) for Eudragit RL100 had no toxic effect on Caco-2 cells so used in the Rho-123 uptake assay. When compared to control group (Intracellular Rho = 2612 pg/mL; total protein = 26 mg/mL), Eudragit RL100 led to a very slight increase in the accumulation of Rho in cells which was not significant (Intracellular Rho = 2754 pg/mL; total protein =96 mg/mL). Moreover from the results of MTT test, Eudragit L100 at 0.25% (w/v) and 0.5% (w/v) concentrations and Eudragit S100 at 1% (w/v) and 2% (w/v) were found to be non-toxic to Caco-2 cells and were subjected to Rho-123 uptake assay and western blotting analysis. Treatment of cells with the Eudragit L100 caused to 7%, decrease in Rho-123 accumulation. (Intracellular Rho = 2429 pg/mL; total protein =93 mg/mL). Eudragit S100 showed significant increase in Rho-123 accumulation in cells. This increase was 61%. (Intracellular Rho = 4205 pg/mL; total protein =89 mg/mL). According to the obtained results, the present study demonstrated the efficacy of Eudragit S100 as an excipient in decreasing the P-glycoprotein expression and consequently its possible role as an inhibitory factor in the efflux process in different absorption regions. Using this polymer as an efflux pump inhibitor would be novel and it apparently will improve the bioavailability and help both substrate drug intestinal permeability and its absorption. Although the study is fulfilled in vitro, the data leave no doubt that Eudragit S100 has beneficial effects in inhibiting P-gp efflux activity.

Conclusion

Taken together, this paper suggests that using proper concentrations of the Eudragit S100 excipient would probably advance the bioavailability and help drug intestinal permeability and absorption which can plausibly have a significant impact on both drug efflux process and metabolism. Of course some other factors including P-gp structure, P-gp environment and substrate partitioning into the tissues have to be understood fully to decide on the ability of these commonly used excipients to inhibit P-gp activity in vitro and to further describe the effect of them on both activity and expression of P-gp. Therefore further tests for example, gut perfusion or pharmacokinetic studies in animals or more specific assays which target specific binding sites on P-glycoprotein should be carried out, later.

Acknowledgements
The authors would like to thank the authorities of Drug Applied Research Center, Tabriz University of Medical Sciences, for their financial support. This article is based on a thesis submitted for PharmD degree (No. 3664) in Faculty of Pharmacy, Tabriz University of Medical Sciences, Tabriz, Iran.

Conflict of Interest
The Authors report no conflict of interests in the present study.

References
1. Sugihara N, Toyama K, Michihara A, Akasaki K, Tsuji H, Furuno K. Effect of benzo[a]pyrene on P-glycoprotein-mediated transport in Caco-2 cell monolayer. *Toxicol* 2006;223(1-2):156-65.

2. Rekha MR, Sharma CP. Oral delivery of therapeutic protein/peptide for diabetes--future perspectives. *Int J Pharm* 2013;440(1):48-62.

3. Jiang L, Long X, Meng Q. Rhamnolipids enhance epithelial permeability in Caco-2 monolayers. *Int J Pharm* 2013;446(1-2):130-5.

4. Amin ML. P-glycoprotein inhibition for optimal drug delivery. *Drug Target Insights* 2013;7:27-34.

5. Arora A, Seth K, Kalra N, Shukla T. Modulation of p-glycoprotein-mediated multidrug resistance in k562 leukemic cells by indole-3-carbinol. *Toxicol Appl Pharmacol* 2005;202(3):237-43.

6. Giacomini KM, Huang SM, Tweedie DJ, Benet LZ, Brouwer KL, et al. Membrane transporters in drug development. *Nat Rev Drug Discov* 2010;9(3):215-36.

7. Xie Z, Cao L, Zhang J. miR-21 modulates paclitaxel sensitivity and hypoxia-inducible factor-1alpha expression in human ovarian cancer cells. *Oncol Lett* 2013;6(3):795-800.

8. Bodo A, Bakos E, Szeri F, Varadi A, Sarkadi B. The role of multidrug transporters in drug availability, metabolism and toxicity. *Toxicol Lett* 2003;140-141:133-43.

9. Schwab M, Eichelbaum M, Fromm MF. Genetic polymorphisms of the human MDR1 drug transporter. *Annu Rev Pharmacol Toxicol* 2003;43:285-307.

10. Sugano K, Kansy M, Artursson P, Avdeef A, Bendels S, Di L, et al. Coexistence of passive and carrier-mediated processes in drug transport. *Nat Rev Drug Discov* 2010;9(8):597-614.

11. Johnson BM, Charman WN, Porter CJ. An in vitro examination of the impact of polyethylene glycol 400, Pluronic P85, and vitamin E d-alpha-tocopheryl polyethylene glycol 1000 succinate on P-glycoprotein efflux and enterocyte-based metabolism in excised rat intestine. *AAPS pharmSci* 2002;4(4):E40.

12. Shen Q, Lin Y, Handa T, Doi M, Sugie M, Wakayama K, et al. Modulation of intestinal P-glycoprotein function by polyethylene glycols and their derivatives by in vitro transport and in situ absorption studies. *Int J Pharm* 2006;313(1-2):49-56.

13. Wempe MF, Wright C, Little JL, Lightner JW, Large SE, Caflisch GB, et al. Inhibiting efflux with novel non-ionic surfactants: Rational design based on vitamin E TPGS. *Int J Pharm* 2009;370(1-2):93-102.

14. Ursino MG, Poluzzi E, Caramella C, De Ponti F. Excipients in medicinal products used in gastroenterology as a possible cause of side effects. *Regul Toxicol Pharmacol* 2011;60(1):93-105.

15. Akhgari A, Abbaspour MR, Pirmoradi S. Preparation and evaluation of pellets using acacia and tragacanth by extrusion-spheronization. *Daru* 2011;19(6):417-23.

16. Aigner D, Ungerbock B, Mayr T, Saf R, Klimant I, Borisov SM. Fluorescent materials for ph sensing and imaging based on novel 1,4-diketopyrrolo-[3,4-c]pyrrole dyes. *J Mater Chem C Mater Opt Electron Devices* 2013;1(36):5685–93.

17. Roy H, Brahma CK, Nandi S, Parida KR. Formulation and design of sustained release matrix tablets of metformin hydrochloride: Influence of hypromellose and polyacrylate polymers. *Int J Appl Basic Med Res* 2013;3(1):55-63.

18. Tsai SW, Yu DS, Tsao SW, Hsu FY. Hyaluronan-cisplatin conjugate nanoparticles embedded in Eudragit S100-coated pectin/alginate microbeads for colon drug delivery. *Int J Nanomedicine* 2013;8:2399-407.

19. Thakral NK, Ray AR, Majumdar DK. Eudragit S-100 entrapped chitosan microspheres of valdecoxib for colon cancer. *J Mater Sci Mater Med* 2010;21(9):2691-9.

20. Thakral NK, Ray AR, Bar-Shalom D, Eriksson AH, Majumdar DK. The quest for targeted delivery in colon cancer: Mucoadhesive valdecoxib microspheres. *Int J Nanomedicine* 2011;6:1057-68.

21. Thakral S, Thakral NK, Majumdar DK. Eudragit: A technology evaluation. *Expert Opin Drug Deliv* 2013;10(1):131-49.

22. Verma P, Gupta RN, Jha AK, Pandey R. Development, in vitro and in vivo characterization of Eudragit RL 100 nanoparticles for improved ocular bioavailability of acetazolamide. *Drug Deliv* 2013;20(7):269-76.

23. Valiyari S, Baradaran B, Delazar A, Pasdaran A, Zare F. Dichloromethane and Methanol Extracts of Scrophularia oxysepala Induces Apoptosis in MCF-7 Human Breast Cancer Cells. *Adv Pharm Bull* 2012;2(2):223-31.

24. Berridge MV, Herst PM, Tan AS. Tetrazolium dyes as tools in cell biology: New insights into their cellular reduction. *Biotechnol Annu Rev* 2005;11:127-52.

25. Sachs-Barrable K, Thamboo A, Lee SD, Wasan KM. Lipid excipients Peceol and Gelucire 44/14 decrease P-glycoprotein mediated efflux of rhodamine 123 partially due to modifying P-glycoprotein protein expression within Caco-2 cells. *J Pharm Pharm Sci* 2007;10(3):319-31.

26. Zibaei M, Firoozeh F, Bahrami P, Sadjjadi SM. Investigation of anti-Toxocara antibodies in epileptic patients and comparison of two methods: ELISA and Western blotting. *Epilepsy Res Treat* 2013;2013:156815.

27. Ferroglio E, Zanet S, Mignone W, Poggi M, Trisciuoglio A, Bianciardi P. Evaluation of a rapid device for serological diagnosis of Leishmania infantum infection in dogs as an alternative to immunofluorescence assay and Western blotting. *Clin Vaccine Immunol* 2013;20(5):657-9.

28. Gradauer K, Dunnhaupt S, Vonach C, Szollosi H, Pali-Scholl I, Mangge H, et al. Thiomer-coated liposomes harbor permeation enhancing and efflux pump inhibitory properties. *J Control Release* 2013;165(3):207-15.

29. Lee CK, Choi JS, Bang JS. Effects of Fluvastatin on the Pharmacokinetics of Repaglinide: Possible Role of CYP3A4 and P-glycoprotein Inhibition by Fluvastatin. *Korean J Physiol Pharmacol* 2013;17(3):245-51.

30. Schinkel AH, Jonker JW. Mammalian drug efflux transporters of the ATP binding cassette (ABC) family: an overview. *Adv Drug Deliv Rev* 2003;55(1):3-29.

31. Sharma M, Prasad R. The quorum-sensing molecule farnesol is a modulator of drug efflux mediated by ABC multidrug transporters and synergizes with drugs in Candida albicans. *Antimicrob Agents Chemother* 2011;55(10):4834-43.

32. Shaikh SA, Li J, Enkavi G, Wen PC, Huang Z, Tajkhorshid E. Visualizing functional motions of membrane transporters with molecular dynamics simulations. *Biochemistry* 2013;52(4):569-87.

33. Rege BD, Kao JP, Polli JE. Effects of nonionic surfactants on membrane transporters in Caco-2 cell monolayers. *Eur J Pharm Sci* 2002;16(4-5):237-46.

34. Cornaire G, Woodley J, Hermann P, Cloarec A, Arellano C, Houin G. Impact of excipients on the absorption of P-glycoprotein substrates in vitro and in vivo. *Int J Pharm* 2004;278(1):119-31.

35. Huang J, Si L, Jiang L, Fan Z, Qiu J, Li G. Effect of pluronic F68 block copolymer on P-glycoprotein transport and CYP3A4 metabolism. *Int J Pharm* 2008;356(1-2):351-3.

36. Zakeri-Milani P, Valizadeh H, Islambulchilar Z, Damani S, Mehtari M. Investigation of the intestinal permeability of ciclosporin using the in situ technique in rats and the relevance of P-glycoprotein. *Arzneimittelforschung* 2008;58(4):188-92.

37. Zakeri-Milani P, Mehtari M, Valizadeh H. Evidence for the enhanced intestinal absorption of digoxin by p-glycoprotein inhibitors. *Trop J Pharm Res* 2012;12(6):939-45.

21

The Anti-Inflammatory Effect of Erythropoietin and Melatonin on Renal Ischemia Reperfusion Injury in Male Rats

Nasser Ahmadiasl[1], Shokofeh Banaei[2]*, Alireza Alihemmati[3], Behzad Baradaran[4], Ehsan Azimian[5]

[1] Drug Applied Research Center, Tabriz University of Medical Sciences, Tabriz, Iran.

[2] Department of Physiology, Tabriz University of Medical Sciences, Tabriz, Iran.

[3] Department of Histology & Embryology, Tabriz University of Medical Sciences, Tabriz, Iran.

[4] Immunology Research Center, Tabriz University of Medical Sciences, Tabriz, Iran.

[5] Department of Linguistics and Foreign Languages, Payame Noor University, Tehran, Iran.

ARTICLE INFO

Keywords:
Erythropoietin
Inflammation
Melatonin
Renal ischemia reperfusion

ABSTRACT

Purpose: Renal ischemia reperfusion (IR) is an important cause of renal dysfunction. It contributes to the development of acute renal failure (ARF). The purpose of this study was to investigate the anti-inflammatory effect of erythropoietin (EPO) and melatonin (MEL), which are known anti-inflammatory and antioxidant agents, in IR-induced renal injury in rats.

Methods: Male Wistar Albino rats were unilaterally nephrectomized and subjected to 45 min of renal pedicle occlusion followed by 24 h reperfusion. MEL (10mg/kg, i.p) and EPO (5000U/kg, i.p) were administered prior to ischemia. After 24 h reperfusion, blood samples were collected for the determination of total antioxidant capacity (TAC), malondialdehyde (MDA) and serum creatinine levels. Also, renal samples were taken for Immunohistochemical evaluation of Bcl2 and TNF-α (tumor necrosis factor-α) expression.

Results: Ischemia reperfusion increased creatinine, TAC, MDA levels and TNF-α expression, also, IR decreased Bcl2 expression. Treatment with EPO or MEL decreased creatinine, MDA levels, and increased TAC level. Also, MEL up-regulated Bcl2 expression and down-regulated TNF-α expression compared with EPO.

Conclusion: Treatment with EPO and MEL had a curative effect on renal IR injury. These results may indicate that MEL protects against inflammation and apoptosis better than EPO in renal IR injury.

Introduction

Renal ischemia reperfusion injury (IRI), which occurs during kidney transplantation, partial nephrectomy, and elective urological operations, is a common cause of acute renal failure (ARF). Ischemia insult, during renal transplantation, is responsible for primary graft dysfunction.[1] Reperfusion (re-establishing blood flow) of ischemic renal tissue is highly damaging and initiates a series of cellular events that lead to necrotic and apoptotic cell death. Several mechanisms contribute to the pathophysiology of ischemia reperfusion injury, such as reactive oxygen species (ROS), ATP depletion and increased neutrophil infiltration.[2] Therefore, increased generation of inflammatory cytokines and ROS in the reperfusion phase is believed to play a pivotal role. The excessive production of reactive oxygen and nitrogen species (RNS) after reperfusion results in the expression of genes for pro-inflammatory mediators, the lipid peroxidation of the cellular membranes and oxidative DNA damage, with the subsequent generation of toxic metabolites causing apoptotic cell death.[3]

Lipid peroxidation is related to IR injury-induced tissue damage and malondialdehyde (MDA) is an indicator of the rate of lipid peroxidation.[4] Several anti-inflammatory and antioxidant agents have been explored to be effective in reducing renal ischemia-reperfusion injury.[5,6]

Erythropoietin (EPO) is a hypoxia-inducible hematopoietic factor, a key protein in red blood cell production, which is predominantly expressed in the kidney. EPO has multiple protective effects, including antioxidant, anti-inflammatory, angiogenic, and anti-apoptotic effects.[7] The biological effects of erythropoietin are mediated by binding to its specific cell surface receptor (EPOR), and the presence of functional EPOR in renal mesangial and tubular epithelial cells has pointed to a potential role for erythropoietin in the kidney.[8] One important effect of erythropoietin is the reduction in apoptosis and oxidative stress.[9] It is also revealed that renal EPO level lowered after renal ischemia reperfusion.[10]

Melatonin (N-acetyl-5-methoxytryptamine) is the major product of the pineal gland that functions as a regulator of sleep, circadian rhythm, and immune function.[11] Melatonin (MEL) and its metabolites have potent antioxidant/anti-inflammatory properties and have been proved to be highly effective in a variety of disorders linked to inflammation and oxidative stress.[12] MEL not only neutralizes RNS and ROS species, but also acts through stimulation of several anti-oxidative systems and stabilizing cell membranes.[13] It modulates the gene expression of several protective enzymes and reduces apoptosis and lipid peroxidation.[14]

Therefore, ROS and inflammation have been shown to contribute to the cellular damage induced by ischemia-reperfusion. The aim of the present study was to examine the potential effects of EPO and MEL on renal IR injury. For this purpose, we measured the plasma levels of MDA, total antioxidant capacity (TAC), creatinine (Cr), and using immunohistochemistry (IHC), expression of anti-apoptotic Bcl2 and inflammatory mediator TNF-α were assessed in renal sections after ischemia reperfusion (IR) in rats subjected to renal IR injury.

Materials and Methods
Animals
In this study, 40 male Wistar- Albino rats (weighing 200 - 300g) were obtained from the experimental animal research center, Medical Faculty, Tabriz University, Iran. The animals were housed in a room temperature (21±2 °C) and humidity (60±5%) controlled room in which a 12-12 h light-dark cycle was maintained. They had free access to standard water and food. The study was approved by the University Ethics Committee.

Surgery and Experimental protocol
Rats were anaesthetized with 75 mg/kg ketamine hydrochloride and 8 mg/kg xylazine, intraperitoneal injection. Right nephrectomy was performed and then, the left renal pedicle (artery and vein) was occluded by placing a microvascular clamp for 45 min to induce ischemia and then subjected to reperfusion for 24h.

The animals were divided into four groups of 10 animals each (n=10).
1. The sham group of animals underwent only nephrectomy without occlusion.
2. IR group (ischemic control)
3. MEL + IR group
4. EPO + IR group

MEL (10 mg/kg; i.p) or vehicle (1% alcohol in saline) was administered 10 min prior to ischemia. MEL (Sigma, St. Louis, MO, USA) was dissolved in absolute ethanol and then diluted in saline to give a final alcohol concentration of 1% ethanol. EPO (Neorecormon, Roche, Mannheim, Germany) was administered as a 5000 U/kg single dose, intraperitoneally 10 min before ischemia.

Biochemical analysis
The blood samples and left kidney tissues of the rats were obtained after 24 h reperfusion in each group for determination of plasma levels of TAC, MDA and creatinine. The blood samples were centrifuged at approximately 4000g for 10 min at 4°C. The Cr level in the serum was determined to assess the renal function, using the Autoanalyser (Alcyon 300 USA).

Malondialdehyde assessment
Plasma MDA levels were measured using the thiobarbituric acid reactive substances (TBARS) method.[15]

Total antioxidant capacity assessment
Plasma TAC was determined using Randox total antioxidant status kit in which ABTS (2, 2-Azino-di [3-ethylbenzthiazolin sulphanatel]) is incubated with a peroxidase and hydrogen peroxide to produce the radical cation ABTS$^+$. This has a stable blue green color, which is determined at 600 nm. Antioxidants in the added sample cause suppression of this color production to a degree which is proportional to their concentration.[16]

Immunohistochemistry
Tissue samples preserved in 10% buffered formalin were dehydrated, embedded in paraffin and sectioned at 5 μm. Sections were mounted on slides and deparaffinized in xylene (3 × 10 min) and ethanol (100% ethanol, 2 × 5 min; 96%, 5 min; 70%, 5 min), then boiled with 10 mM citrate buffer in the microwave for 10 min, cooled down in citrate buffer for 20 min and rinsed with deionized water and PBS (phosphate buffered saline). To quench the endogenous activity, sections were incubated for 30 min in 0.1% H_2O_2 in methanol. They were then washed in PBS for 5 min and incubated with diluted normal rabbit serum (Abcam, Cambridge, UK) for 20 min. After blotting excess serum, the sections were incubated with the primary antibody in the dilution of 1/2000 for TNF-α (rabbit polyclonal to TNF-α, Abcam), the dilution of 1/100 for Bcl-2 (rabbit polyclonal to Bcl-2, Abcam). For negative control, slides were incubated with diluted normal rabbit serum (Abcam) for 1 hr in room temperature. After the sections were rinsed in PBS, a supersensitive biotinylated secondary antibody (Goat polyclonal to Rabbit IgG - H&L (HRP); Vector Laboratories Inc., Burlingame, CA, USA) was applied for 30 min. Slides were then rinsed in PBS again and incubated for 30 min with Vectastain ABC Reagent (Vector Laboratories Inc.), washed in PBS and incubated in peroxidase substrate solution (Vektor DAB Peroxide Substrate; Vector Laboratories Inc.)

until desired stain intensity develops. Under microscope, a color reaction (brown) can be seen and the reaction can then be stopped with water.

Immunohistochemical staining for TNF-α and Bcl-2 was examined using light microscopy by an investigator blinded with respect to the animal group at a magnification of ×40. In each group, 8 representative kidney sections were investigated, 20 view fields were counted per kidney section. To assess tubular staining for TNF-α and Bcl-2 expression, the following scoring system was used: grade 0: no expression; grade 1: minimal expression, grade 2: mild expression; grade 3: moderate expression; grade 4: severe expression.[17]

Statistical analysis

All the data are presented as mean ± standard deviation (M±SD). Significance testing between groups was performed using one-way analysis of variance (ANOVA) with SPSS Version 19 and multiple comparison post hoc test to determine significant differences between groups. A P-value of less than 0.05 was considered statistically significant.

Results

The effect of EPO and MEL on renal ischemia reperfusion injury was investigated in 45 minute of renal ischemia followed by 24 hour reperfusion. Biochemical analysis results are outlined in Table 1, and using immunohistochemistry (IHC), expression of anti-apoptotic Bcl2 and inflammatory mediator TNF-α were assessed in renal sections after IR.

Table 1. Biochemical measurements after 24 h of reperfusion

Groups	Sham group	IR group	MEL+IR group	EPO+IR group
Cr (mg/dl)	0.74±0.13	1.32±0.88[a]	1.14±0.20	0.93±0.21
MDA(nmol/ml)	2.19±0.69	2.64±1.35	2.01±0.61	2.46±0.55
TAC (mmol/l)	0.78±0.08	0.87±0.23	1.15±0.25[b]	1.28±0.21[b]

[a] Significantly increased when compared with sham group, P<0.05.

[b] Significantly increased when compared with IR group, P<0.05.

Cr, creatinine; MDA, malondialdehyde; TAC, total antioxidant capacity; EPO, erythropoietin; MEL, melatonin; IR, ischemia reperfusion.

Effects of ischemia reperfusion

Serum creatinine level was significantly higher in the animals from IR group compared with those from sham group (P<0.05). The levels of MDA and TAC in the IR group were higher than those in the sham group, but the difference was not statistically significant (P > 0.05). In the sham group, there was prominent augmentation of Bcl2 expression and absence of TNF-α expression (Figure 1 a, b). Renal IR caused an absence of Bcl2 expression and great increase in TNF-α expression compared with the sham group (Figure 1 c, d).

Effects of melatonin on renal ischemia reperfusion

MDA and serum creatinine levels in the MEL + IR group were lower than those in IR group, but the difference was not statistically significant (P>0.05).

The TAC level in the MEL + IR group was significantly higher than that in the IR group (P=0.01). MEL administration resulted in severe increase of Bcl2 expression and marked reduction of TNF-α expression compared with IR group (Figure 1 e, f).

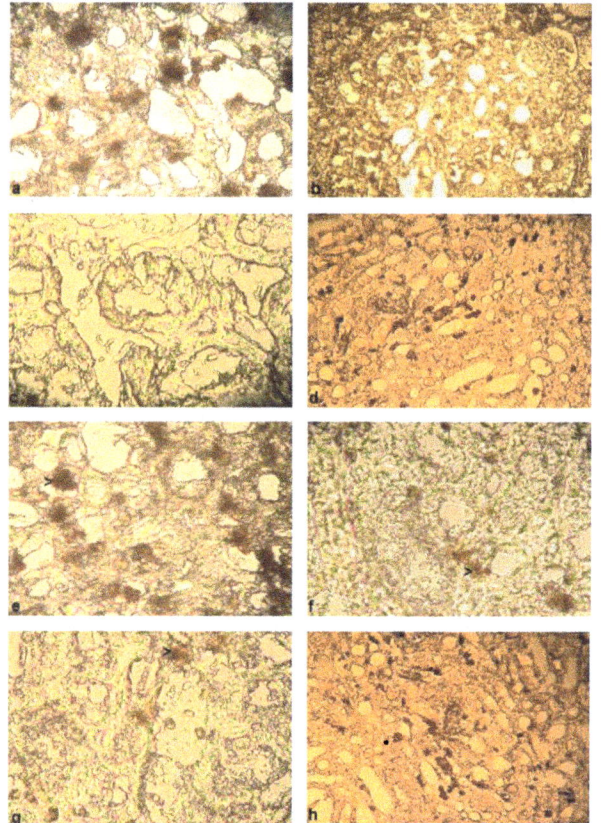

Figure 1. (a, b) Bcl2 and TNF-α expression in renal tubules of the sham group. (c) Expression of Bcl2 after renal IR. The lesser degree of Bcl2 expression in tubular epithelial cells of IR group. Magnification × 40. (d) Expression of TNF-α after renal IR. Increased TNF-α expression in tubular epithelial cells of IR group. Magnification ×20. (e) Expression of Bcl2 after MEL administration. Increased Bcl2 expression in tubular epithelial cells of MEL group compared to IR group. Magnification × 40. (f) Expression of TNF-α after MEL administration. Decreased TNF-α expression in tubular epithelial cells of MEL group compared to IR group. Magnification ×40. (g) Expression of Bcl2 after EPO administration. Minimal increased Bcl2 expression in tubular epithelial cells of EPO group compared to IR group. Magnification × 40. (h) Expression of TNF-α after EPO administration. Lesser decreased TNF-α expression in tubular epithelial cells of EPO group compared to IR group. Magnification ×20.

Effects of erythropoietin on renal ischemia reperfusion

MDA and serum creatinine levels in the EPO + IR group were lower than those in the IR group, but the difference was not statistically significant (P > 0.05).The TAC level in the EPO + IR group was significantly higher than that in the IR group (P=0.000).

EPO administration resulted in minimal Bcl2 expression and moderate TNF-α expression, nearly at the same level of IR group (Figure 1 g, h).

Discussion

Renal IR is a common result of clinical procedures such as organ procurement, vascular surgery, or renal transplantation. Furthermore, renal IR injury is a leading cause of ARF, which is associated with high mortality rates. ARF is characterized by increased vascular resistance in the kidney, a low rate of filtration through the glomeruli, and tubular necrosis. These deleterious effects have been attributed to ROS generation during renal reperfusion.[18] ROS contributes to lethal cell damage. IR injury has been attributed to ROS-mediated lipid peroxidation.[19]

We found that renal IR insignificantly increased the plasma level of TAC. Increased total antioxidant capacity indicates a cellular defensive response to overproduction of ROS after renal IR. ROS generation within cells is countered by sophisticated extracellular and intracellular antioxidant defense systems. These can be divided into enzymatic and non-enzymatic antioxidant systems, which effectively combine different antioxidant activities such as those that prevent ROS formation and distribution, maintain antioxidant enzyme levels and activities, scavenge ROS, and repair ROS –mediated cellular injury.[20]

Our results demonstrated that EPO and MEL significantly increased the level of TAC. This effect of EPO and MEL may be due to their antioxidant properties. Consistent with our finding, Kurcer et al.[21] found that MEL ameliorated the functional and structural alterations in renal IR rats, decreased the total oxidative stress and increased the TAC. On the other hand, Dimitrijevic et al.[22] demonstrated that increase in TAC accompanied increasing durations of EPO treatment and higher levels of TAC were also verified in the group with the longest duration of EPO treatment in hemodialysis patients.

Lipid peroxidation, as a free radical generating system, has been proposed to be closely related to IR induced tissue injury, and MDA is a good indicator of the degree of lipid peroxidation. In the present experiment, the level of MDA is increased by IR, which reflects increased lipid peroxidation due to increased oxidative stress. Erythropoietin decreased the level of MDA, which shows that it decreased the amount of oxidative stress and subsequently lipid peroxidation. Consistent with our findings, Ates et al.[23] demonstrated that EPO decreased the level of MDA after right nephrectomy, clamping of the left renal pedicle, and reperfusion in rats. Our results show that melatonin causes a reduction in MDA production, indicating a reduction in lipid peroxidation and cellular damage. This protective effect of MEL may be in part by scavenging the very reactive ONOO- and OH.[24]

IR injury of the kidney results in both glomerular and tubular dysfunctions.[25] In our study, IR significantly increased creatinine level, suggesting an impaired glomerular function which was greatly reduced after EPO and MEL treatment. It is shown that the administration of EPO before ischemia attenuated the deterioration in renal function as a result of IR injury.[23] Also, it is shown that the administration of MEL retards deterioration of renal function and structure.[26]

In the present study, Immunohistochemical assessment showed that IR caused increase in pro-inflammatory cytokine such as TNF-α. It has been reported that renal IR causes synthesis of pro-inflammatory cytokines such as TNF-α, IL-1, and IL-6.[27,28] EPO treatment did not obviously modify the TNF-α expression in kidney tubules when compared with the IR group. Sølling et al.[29] reported that EPO did not modify the inflammatory response in a porcine model of endotoxemia. MEL severely attenuated the TNF-α expression, this effect of MEL may be due to its anti-inflammatory properties. Consistent with this finding, kireev et al.[30] indicated that MEL administration lowered the expression of TNF-α and IL-1β in hepatic ischemia/reperfusion. In our study, renal IR resulted in decreased expression of Bcl2 protein at 24h reperfusion, indicating that down-regulation of Bcl2 protein could contribute in apoptotic cell death in renal IR. Previous studies conducted in similar animal models of renal IR injury have shown that ischemia leads to an increase in the Bax/Bcl2 ratio suggesting that the fine balance between the activity of pro-apoptotic and anti-apoptotic Bcl2 family members can determine cell survival and modulate the induction of apoptosis.[31] MEL severely increased Bcl2 expression in renal tissue. This effect of MEL may be due to its powerful anti-apoptotic properties. Tunon et al.[32] reported that some anti-apoptotic effects of MEL were related to a reduced expression of Bax and also to the diminished cytochrome C release to the cytosol, to the increased expression of Bcl2 and Bcl-xL, and to the inhibition of caspase-9 activity in an animal model of fulminant hepatic failure. In the EPO group, the Bcl2 expression did not show obvious changes in kidney when compared with IR group. Consistent with this finding, Johnson et al.[33] showed that there was no apparent effect in the model of ischemia ARF on promotion of the anti-apoptotic proteins Bcl2 and Bcl-xL by EPO and darbepoetin.

Conclusion

In conclusion, ROS are considered to be principal components involved in the pathophysiological tissue alterations observed during renal IR. Antioxidant defense systems or TAC activities prevent ROS formation and scavenge ROS. The administration of EPO and MEL, which are potent anti-inflammatory and antioxidant agents, appears to have beneficial effects on IR-induced renal injury as indicated by higher levels of TAC activity, and lower degree of renal dysfunction. However, MEL pretreatment exerted more nephroprotective effect than EPO pretreatment. As MEL administration resulted in severe increase of Bcl2 expression and marked reduction of TNF-α expression compared with EPO group, MEL was probably effective to reverse renal IR by its potent anti-inflammatory and anti-apoptotic effects. These results may indicate that MEL protects against inflammation and apoptosis better than EPO in renal IR injury. However, further investigations are required to explore that the combination treatment of EPO and MEL has a synergistic effect of protection against IR-induced renal injury.

Acknowledgments

This study was financially supported by Drug Applied Research Center of Tabriz University of Medical Sciences. The paper was derived from Ph.D. thesis of Shokofeh Banaei entitled "Effect of erythropoietin and melatonin on renal ischemia-reperfusion injury in rats".

Conflict of Interest

The authors declare that they have no conflict of interest.

References

1. Ploeg RJ, Van Bockel JH, Langendijk PT, Groenewegen M, Van Der Woude FJ, Persijn GG, et al. Effect of preservation solution on results of cadaveric kidney transplantation. The European Multicentre Study Group. *Lancet* 1992;340(8812):129-37.
2. Edelstein CL, Ling H, Schrier RW. The nature of renal cell injury. *Kidney Int* 1997;51(5):1341-51.
3. Lemasters JJ, Thurman RG. Reperfusion injury after liver preservation for transplantation. *Annu Rev Pharmacol Toxicol* 1997;37:327-38.
4. Kacmaz A, Polat A, User Y, Tilki M, Ozkan S, Sener G. Octreotide improves reperfusion-induced oxidative injury in acute abdominal hypertension in rats. *J Gastrointest Surg* 2004;8(1):113-9.
5. Cau J, Favreau F, Zhang K, Febrer G, De La Motte GR, Ricco JB, et al. FR167653 improves renal recovery and decreases inflammation and fibrosis after renal ischemia reperfusion injury. *J Vasc Surg* 2009;49(3):728-40.
6. Korkmaz A, Kolankaya D. The protective effects of ascorbic acid against renal ischemia-reperfusion injury in male rats. *Ren Fail* 2009;31(1):36-43.
7. Ebert BL, Bunn HF. Regulation of the erythropoietin gene. *Blood* 1999;94(6):1864-77.
8. Westenfelder C, Biddle DL, Baranowski RL. Human, rat, and mouse kidney cells express functional erythropoietin receptors. *Kidney Int* 1999;55(3):808-20.
9. Calo LA, Bertipaglia L, Pagnin E. Antioxidants, carnitine and erythropoietin. *G Ital Nefrol* 2006;23 Suppl 34:S47-50.
10. Plotnikov EY, Chupyrkina AA, Jankauskas SS, Pevzner IB, Silachev DN, Skulachev VP, et al. Mechanisms of nephroprotective effect of mitochondria-targeted antioxidants under rhabdomyolysis and ischemia/reperfusion. *Biochim Biophys Acta* 2011;1812(1):77-86.
11. Poeggeler B, Saarela S, Reiter RJ, Tan DX, Chen LD, Manchester LC, et al. Melatonin--a highly potent endogenous radical scavenger and electron donor: new aspects of the oxidation chemistry of this indole accessed in vitro. *Ann N Y Acad Sci* 1994;738:419-20.
12. Mayo JC, Sainz RM, Tan DX, Hardeland R, Leon J, Rodriguez C, et al. Anti-inflammatory actions of melatonin and its metabolites, N1-acetyl-N2-formyl-5-methoxykynuramine (AFMK) and N1-acetyl-5-methoxykynuramine (AMK), in macrophages. *J Neuroimmunol* 2005;165(1-2):139-49.
13. Rodriguez C, Mayo JC, Sainz RM, Antolin I, Herrera F, Martin V, et al. Regulation of antioxidant enzymes: a significant role for melatonin. *J Pineal Res* 2004;36(1):1-9.
14. Reiter RJ, Guerrero JM, Garcia JJ, Acuna-Castroviejo D. Reactive oxygen intermediates, molecular damage, and aging. Relation to melatonin. *Ann N Y Acad Sci* 1998;854:410-24.
15. Yagi K. Assay for blood plasma or serum. *Methods Enzymol* 1984;105:328-31.
16. Miller NJ, Rice-Evans C, Davies MJ, Gopinathan V, Milner A. A novel method for measuring antioxidant capacity and its application to monitoring the antioxidant status in premature neonates. *Clin Sci (Lond)* 1993;84(4):407-12.
17. Bennett WM. The failed renal transplant: in or out? *Seminars in dialysis* 2005;18(3):188-9.
18. Carden DL, Granger DN. Pathophysiology of ischemia reperfusion injury. *J Pathol* 2000;190(3):255-66.
19. McCord JM. The evaluation of free radicals and oxidative stress. *Am J Med* 2000;108:652-9.
20. Evans P, Halliwell B. Micronutrients: oxidant/antioxidant status. *Br J Nutr* 2001;85 Suppl 2:S67-74.
21. Kurcer Z, Oguz E, Ozbilge H, Baba F, Aksoy N, Celik H, et al. Melatonin protects from ischemia/reperfusion-induced renal injury in rats: this effect is not mediated by proinflammatory cytokines. *J Pineal Res* 2007;43(2):172-8.
22. Dimitrijevic ZM, Cvetkovic TP, Djordjevic VM, Pavlovic DD, Stefanovic NZ, Stojanovic IR, et al. How the duration period of erythropoietin treatment influences the oxidative status of hemodialysis patients. *Int J Med Sci* 2012;9(9):808-15.
23. Ates E, Yalcin AU, Yilmaz S, Koken T, Tokyol C. Protective effect of erythropoietin on renal ischemia and reperfusion injury. *ANZ J Surg* 2005;75(12):1100-5.
24. Reiter RJ, Oh CS, Fujimori O. Melatonin Its intracellular and genomic actions. *Trends Endocrinol Metab* 1996;7(1):22-7.
25. Paller MS. Pathophysiologic mechanisms of acute renal failure. In: Goldstein RS, editor. Mechanisms of Injury in Renal Disease and Toxicity. Ann Arbor: CRC Press; 1994. p. 3-13.

26. Quiroz Y, Ferrebuz A, Romero F, Vaziri ND, Rodriguez-Iturbe B. Melatonin ameliorates oxidative stress, inflammation, proteinuria, and progression of renal damage in rats with renal mass reduction. *Am J Physiol Renal Physiol* 2008;294(2):F336-44.

27. Donnahoo KK, Meng X, Ayala A, Cain MP, Harken AH, Meldrum DR. Early kidney TNF-alpha expression mediates neutrophil infiltration and injury after renal ischemia-reperfusion. *Am J Physiol* 1999;277(3 Pt 2):R922-9.

28. Burne-Taney MJ, Kofler J, Yokota N, Weisfeldt M, Traystman RJ, Rabb H. Acute renal failure after whole body ischemia is characterized by inflammation and T cell-mediated injury. *Am J Physiol Renal Physiol* 2003;285(1):F87-94.

29. Sølling C, Christensen AT, Nygaard U, Krag S, Frøkiaer J, Wogensen L, et al. Erythropoietin does not attenuate renal dysfunction or inflammation in a porcine model of endotoxemia. *Acta Anaesthesiol Scand* 2011; 55(4):411-21.

30. Kireev RA, Cuesta S, Ibarrola C, Bela T, Moreno Gonzalez E, Vara E, et al. Age-related differences in hepatic ischemia/reperfusion: gene activation, liver injury, and protective effect of melatonin. *J Surg Res* 2012;178(2):922-34.

31. Gobe G, Zhang XJ, Willgoss DA, Schoch E, Hogg NA, Endre ZH. Relationship between expression of Bcl-2 genes and growth factors in ischemic acute renal failure in the rat. *J Am Soc Nephrol* 2000;11(3):454-67.

32. Tunon MJ, San Miguel B, Crespo I, Jorquera F, Santamaria E, Alvarez M, et al. Melatonin attenuates apoptotic liver damage in fulminant hepatic failure induced by the rabbit hemorrhagic disease virus. *J Pineal Res* 2011;50(1):38-45.

33. Johnson DW, Pat B, Vesey DA, Guan Z, Endre Z, Gobe GC. Delayed administration of darbepoetin or erythropoietin protects against ischemic acute renal injury and failure. *Kidney Int* 2006;69(10):1806-13.

22

Protective Effects of N-acetylcysteine Against the Statins Cytotoxicity in Freshly Isolated Rat Hepatocytes

Narges Abdoli[1,2,3,4], Yadollah Azarmi[2,3], Mohammad Ali Eghbal[2,3]*

[1] *Biotechnology Research Center, Tabriz University of Medical Sciences, Tabriz, Iran.*

[2] *Drug Applied Research Center, Tabriz University of Medical Sciences, Tabriz, Iran.*

[3] *Pharmacology and Toxicology Department, School of pharmacy, Tabriz University of Medical Sciences, Tabriz, Iran.*

[4] *Students' Research Committee, Tabriz University of Medical Sciences, Tabriz, Iran.*

ARTICLE INFO

Keywords:
Statins
Hepatotoxicity
Reactive oxygen species
Mitochondrial membrane potential
N-acetylcysteine

ABSTRACT

Purpose: Hepatotoxicity is one of the most important side effects of the statins therapy as lipid-lowering agents. However, the mechanism(s) of hepatotoxicity induced by these drugs is not clearly understood yet, and no hepatoprotective agent has been developed against this complication.

Methods: The protective effect of N-acetylcysteine (NAC) against statins-induced cytotoxicity was evaluated by using freshly isolated rat hepatocytes. Hepatocytes were prepared by the method of collagenase enzyme perfusion via portal vein. This technique is based on liver perfusion with collagenase after removal of calcium ion (Ca2+) with a chelator (ethylene glycol tetra acetic acid (EGTA) 0.5 mM). The level of parameters such as cell death, ROS formation, lipid peroxidation, mitochondrial membrane potential (MMP) in the statins-treated hepatocytes were determined. Additionally, the mentioned markers were assessed in presence of NAC.

Results: Incubation of hepatocytes by the statins resulted in cytotoxicity characterized by an elevation in cell death, increasing ROS generation and consequently lipid peroxidation and impairment of mitochondrial function. Administration of NAC caused reduction in amount of ROS formation, lipid peroxidation and finally, cell viability and mitochondrial membrane potential (MMP) were improved.

Conclusion: This study confirms that oxidative stress and consequently mitochondrial dysfunction is one of the mechanisms underlying the statins-induced liver injury and treating hepatocytes by NAC (200 μM) attenuates cytotoxicity.

Introduction

Statins (3-hydroxy-3-methylglutaryl co-enzyme A reductase inhibitors) are the most prescribed agents for cholesterol lowering and consequently prevention of obstructive cardiovascular events in the world.[1,2] These pharmaceuticals block the mevalonic acid pathway by inhibition of the rate limiting step in the hepatic *de novo* cholesterol biosynthesis.[3] Severe adverse effects of the statins involving myopathy and hepatotoxicity sometimes limit their usage as lipid lowering agents. Hepatotoxicity characterized by elevation of plasma transaminases is most common and the frequency of elevation is 0.5-5% and dose dependent.[4,5] However the precise molecular mechanisms underlying statins cause hepatotoxicity are not understood.[2] statins are metabolized by cytochrome P450 (3A4) enzymes.[1] The dose- and time-dependent impairment of mitochondrial function caused by statins has been observed in different in vitro models.[6,7]

Different antioxidants administration has been shown to be useful in reducing oxidative stress and cell death in hepatocytes. Efficacy of N-acetylcysteine (NAC) administration as a free radical scavenger in multiple models of oxidative stress induction has been studied.[8]

In the present study, isolated rat hepatocytes were exploited to gain insight into statins hepatotoxicity and to investigate the role of supplementation with NAC in reducing toxicity. Markers like reactive oxygen species (ROS), lipid peroxidation, mitochondrial membrane potential and cell death in the statins-treated freshly isolated rat hepatocytes were assessed and the results were compared to those in NAC-treated hepatocytes. The hepatoprotective properties of NAC(200 μM) supplementation against the statins-induced hepatotoxicity were related to the reduction of ROS generation, lipid peroxidation and maintenance of mitochondrial membrane potential.

---

*Corresponding author: Mohammad Ali Eghbal, Tabriz University of Medical sciences, Pharmacology and Toxicology Department, School of Pharmacy, Tabriz, Iran. Email: m.eghbal@utoronto.ca

Material and Methods
Chemicals
Atorvastatin, Simvastatin and Lovastatin were purchased from sigma-aldrich. NAC was provided from Acros (New Jersey, USA). 2-vinyl pyridine, Triethanolamineand (4-(2-hydroxyethyl) 1-piperazine-ethanessulfonic acid (HEPES) were obtained from Acros (New Jersey, USA). Albumine bovine type was purchased from Roche diagnostic corporation (Indianapolis USA). Rhodamine 123, 5,5'-dithio-bis(2-nitro-benzoicacid)(DTNB), 2,7-Dichlorofluorescin diacetate (DCFDA) and clostridium histolyticum extracted Collagenase (Type II), were obtained from Sigma Aldrich (St. Louis, USA). Trichloroacetic acid (TCA), Ethyleneglycol-bis (ρ-aminoethylether)-N,N,N',N'-tetra acetic acid (EGTA), and Trypan blue were obtained from Merck (Darmstadt, Germany). Thiobarbituric acid (TBA) was obtained from SERVA (Heidenberg, New York). All salts used for preparing buffer solutions were of analytical grade and obtained from Merck (Darmstadt, Germany).

Animals
Male Sprague–Dawley rats (weight range: 250-300g) were provided from Tabriz University of Medical Sciences, Tabriz, Iran, The animals were housed in an animal house unit (temperature 21-23°C and 50-60% relative humidity, fed a standard chow diet and water *ad libitum* were used. The animals were handled and used according to the animal handling protocol of Tabriz University of Medical Sciences, Tabriz, Iran which was approved by a local ethic committee.

Hepatocytes isolation
Hepatocytes were isolated from male Sprague–Dawley rats by a two-step collagenase perfusion as described previously.[9] Approximately 85–90% of hepatocytes excluded Trypan blue (0.1%, w/v) at the time of isolation. The cells were suspended (1×10^6 cell/ml) in Krebs–Henseleit buffer containing 12.5 mM HEPES and incubated under a stream of 95% O_2 and 5% CO_2 in continuously rotating round-bottomed 50 ml flasks at 37°C water bath. Hepatocytes were kept under the relevant atmosphere for 30 minute to achieve equilibrium between gas and liquid phases before the addition of chemicals.

Cell viability
After hepatocyte isolation process, cell viability was assessed by the extent of plasma membrane intactness as determined by Trypan blue exclusion test.[10] Viability was determined immediately after isolation and after one, two and three hours after statins incubation. In experiments NAC (200 µM) and statins were added contemporarily (There were no significant difference between before and co-adding of chemicals).

Reactive oxygen species (ROS) formation
To assess the rate of hepatocytes ROS formation during statins metabolism, 2, 7-dichlorofluorescein diacetate (DCF-DA) 1.6 µM was added to the hepatocyte incubate. DCFH-DA became hydrolyzed to non-fluorescent dichlorofluorescein (DCFH) in hepatocytes. Dichlorofluorescin then reacted with reactive oxygen species to form the highly fluorescent dichlorofluorescein. One ml (10^6 cells) of hepatocytes was taken and the fluorescence intensity was measured using a Jasco® FP-750 spectrofluorometer with excitation and emission wavelengths of 500 and 520 nm, respectively.[11]

Lipid peroxidation
Hepatocyte lipid peroxidation was determined by measuring the amount of thiobarbituric acid-reactive substances (TBARS) such as malondialdehyde (MDA), formed during the decomposition of lipid hydroperoxides by following the absorbance at 532 nm in a Pharmacia Biotech Ultrospec 2000 spectrophotometer after treating a 1.0 ml aliquot of hepatocyte suspension (10^6 cells/ml) with trichloroacetic acid (70%, w/v) and boiling the supernatant with thiobarbituric acid (0.8%, w/v) for 20 min.[12]

Mitochondrial membrane potential assay
Mitochondrial membrane potential (MMP) in hepatocytes was assessed by monitoring the uptake of rhodamine 123, a cationic dye, as described.[13,14] Isolated cells were extracted, and then resuspended in original media containing 1.5µM rhodamine 123. After 10 min of incubation, the cells were centrifuged and the supernatant was measured with a Jasco FP-750 spectrofluorimeter. The amount of dye remaining in the supernatant was inversely proportional to the membrane potential of the cells. The results are reported as the difference in fluorescence intensity between control and treated cells and expressed as percentage of control.

Statistical analysis
The results are shown as mean ±SD, measured at least for 3 different batches of hepatocytes. The differences among the control and experimental groups were determined by one way ANOVA followed by Tukey's post hoc analysis and a $p<0.05$ was considered significant.

Results
By adding different concentrations of atorvastatin, simvastatin and lovastatin to isolated rat hepatocytes and by use of trypan blue exclusion test, the LC_{50}s of statins (the statin concentration that caused 50% death after 120 minutes) were found as 450µM for atorvastatin, simvastatin 200µM and lovastatin 200µM (data not shown). As shown in Table 1, simvastatin 200µM is the most cytotoxic statin, because the amount of dead cell in third hour is more noticeable. Additionally, an optimum effective dose for NAC that provided an appropriate protection was found as 200µM. Hepatocytes were treated

with NAC at the same time that statins were added. It was found that NAC (200μM) effectively prevented cell death induced by the statins (Table 1). Markers such as ROS formation, lipid peroxidation, and mitochondrial membrane potential were assessed to investigate the mechanism by which NAC protects hepatocytes against statins-induced toxicity and elucidate the cause of cell death induced by statins. A significant amount of reactive oxygen species were formed when hepatocytes were treated with atorvastatin (Figure 1), simvastatin (Figure 2) and/or lovastatin (Figure 3) and supplementation with NAC (200μM) significantly reduced the statins-induced ROS generation (Figure 1-3).

Table 1. Prevention of statins cytotoxicity by NAC.

Cytotoxicity (% Trypan blue uptake)			
Addition Incubation time (min)	60	120	180
Control (only hepatocytes)	18±1	22±2	24±1
+NAC(N-acetylcysteine) 200 μM	15±1	17±1	21±1
+Atorvastatin 450 μM	36±1[a]	52±2[a]	68±1[a]
+NAC200 μM	23±1[b]	29±1[b]	38±2[b]
+Simvastatin 200 μM	38±2[a]	54±2[a]	88±2[a]
+ NAC200 μM	25±1[b]	33±2[b]	47±2[b]
+Lovastatin 200 μM	39±2[a]	52±2[a]	74±3[a]
+ NAC200 μM	28±2[b]	38±2[b]	45±4[b]

Statin doses are LD_{50} (The statins concentration caused 50% death after 120 minutes).

NAC (200 μM) was added at the time of statins addition.

Data represent Mean±SE for three independent experiments.

[a]: Significantly different from control group (P<0.05).

[b]: Significantly different from statins-treated group (P<0.05).

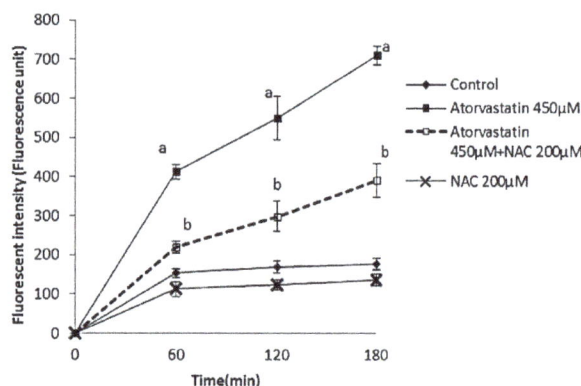

Figure 1. Atorvastatin- induced ROS formation in isolated rat hepatocytes and the protective effect of NAC.
NAC (200 μM) was added at the time of Atorvastatin(450 μM) addition.
Data are shown as Mean±SE for three independent experiments.
[a]: significant *VS* control group(p<0.05).
[b]: significant *VS* Atorvastatin treated group(p<0.05).

It has been shown that ROS formation is usually followed by lipid peroxidation.[15] Lipid peroxidation was determined after 120 and 180 minutes after the statins treatment and it was found that NAC (200μM) significantly prevented lipid peroxidation in the statins-treated hepatocytes (Figure 4-6).
The effect of statins on mitochondria as an essential organelle in energy production was assessed. It was found that statins caused mitochondrial membrane potential (MMP)depression (Figure 7-9). NAC

supplementation showed a significant elevation of mitochondrial membrane potential.

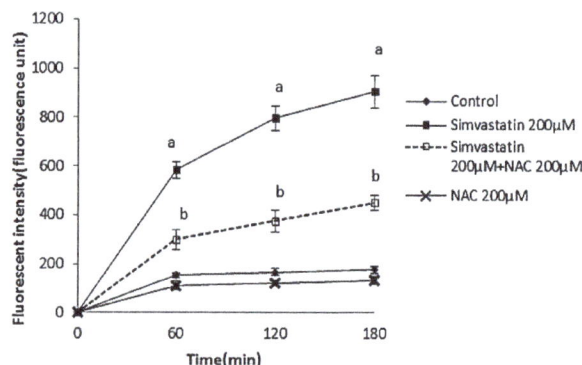

Figure 2. Simvastatin- induced ROS formation in isolated rat hepatocytes and the protective effect of NAC.
NAC (200 μM) was added at the time of Simvastatin (200 μM) addition.
Data are shown as Mean±SE for three independent experiments.
a: significant *VS* control group(p<0.05).
b: significant *VS* Simvastatin - treated group(p<0.05).

Discussion

The results of our study showed the beneficial protective effects of NAC against statin-induced hepatotoxicity. Inhibition of the respiratory chain (complex I and III), depolarization of mitochondrial membrane[7] and releasing of Ca^{2+}, are known as the results of statins exposure.[16] The statins are metabolized by liver cytochrome P450 (CYP 3A4) enzymes.[1] The cytochrome P450 include a superfamily of monooxygenases whose members function critically in xenobiotics catabolism.[17] The major metabolic reactions include oxidation of aliphatic carbons, alkenyl groups and aromatic rings. After oxidation, subsequent reactions involve N-dealkylations, dehydration to form C=C double bonds, dehydrogenation of primary alcohols to an aldehyde and then a carboxylic acid, and finally glutathione conjugation of epoxides.[18] Mitochondria or cytochrome P450-dependent metabolism act as ROS production systems and participate in cell death processes.[19] Our data showed that treating hepatocytes with the statins produces a significant amount of ROS, induces lipid peroxidation, reduces mitochondrial membrane potential and promotes cytotoxicity as compared to the control group and these effect are dose- and time-dependent (different doses of the statins were assessed but data are not shown). Our results are in accordance with the previous study.[7] The amount of ROS formation by Simvastatin was more than that with the others. The intracellular ROS generation is accompanied with cell death in cultured hepatocytes.[20] The efficacy of N-acetylcysteine (NAC) administration as a free radical scavenger in multiple models of oxidative stress induction has been studied.[8,12] The administration of N-acetylcysteine (NAC), as an excellent source of intracellular cysteine and free radical scavenger, has been shown to have clinical applications in conditions such as HIV infection, cancer, heart disease, as well as in smoking, kidney and liver diseases.[21] Adding NAC to the cells incubated with the statins resulted in prevention of ROS formation, lipid peroxidation, mitochondrial dysfunction, and finally improving the cells survival. Therefore, reactive oxygen species formed during the statins metabolism are scavenged by NAC and this may have a role in its protective effects in statins cytotoxicity.

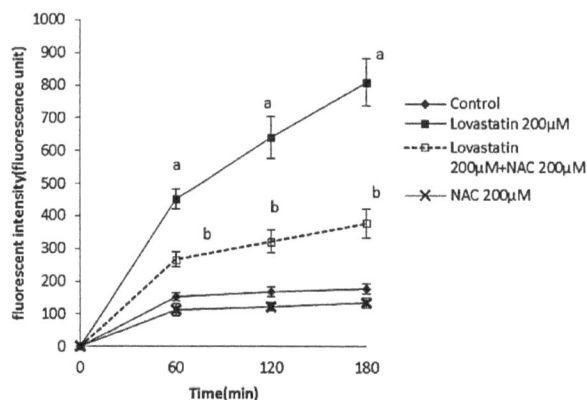

Figure 4. Atorvastatin-induced lipid peroxidation and the protective effect of NAC.
NAC (200 µM) was added at the time of Atorvastatin(450 µM) addition.
Data are shown as Mean±SE for three independent experiments.
a : significant *VS* control group(p<0.05).
b : significant *VS* Atorvastatin treated group(p<0.05).

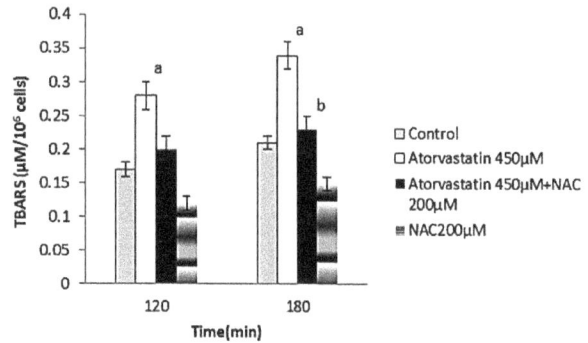

Figure 5. Simvastatin- induced lipid peroxidation and the protective effect of NAC.
NAC (200 µM) was added at the time of Simvastatin(200 µM) addition.
Data are shown as Mean±SE for three independent experiments.
[a] : significant *VS* control group(p<0.05).
[b] : significant *VS* Simvastatin - treated group(p<0.05).

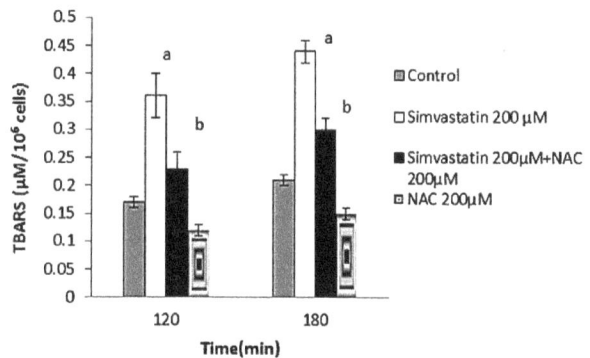

Figure 3. Lovastatin- induced ROS formation in isolated rat hepatocytes and the protective effect of NAC.
NAC(200 µM) was added at the time of Lovastatin(200 µM) addition.
Data are shown as Mean±SE for three independent experiments.
a : significant *VS* control group(p<0.05).
b: significant *VS* Lovastatin - treated group(p<0.05).

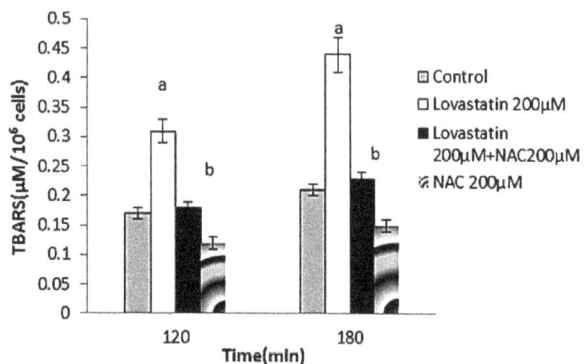

Figure 6. Lovastatin- induced lipid peroxidation and the protective effect of NAC.
NAC (200 µM) was added at the time of Lovastatin (200 µM) addition.
Data are shown as Mean±SE for three independent experiments.
a : significant *VS* control group(p<0.05).
b :significant *VS* Lovastatin - treated group(p<0.05).

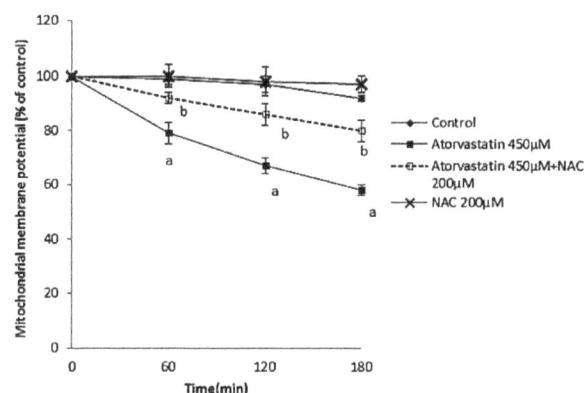

Figure 7. Effect of Atorvastatin on mitochondrial membrane potential and the protective role of NAC.
NAC (200 μM) was added at the time of Atorvastatin (450 μM) addition.
Data are shown as Mean±SE for three independent experiments.
a : significant VS control group(p<0.05).
b: significant VS Atorvastatin -treated group(p<0.05).

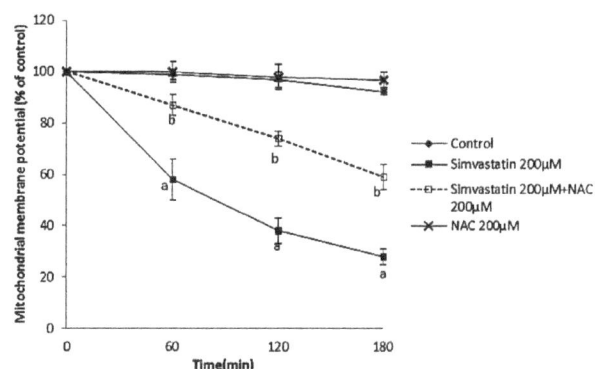

Figure 8. Effect of simvastatin on mitochondrial membrane potential and the protective role of NAC.
NAC (200 μM) was added at the time of Simvastatin(200 μM) addition.
Data are shown as Mean±SE for three independent experiments.
a : significant VS control group(p<0.05).
b:significant VS Simvastatin -treated group(p<0.05).

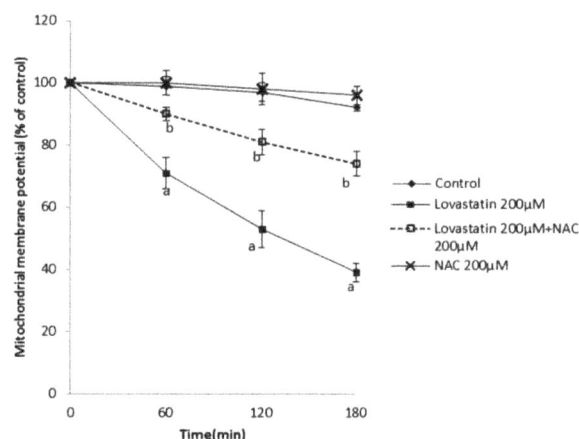

Figure 9. Effect of lovastatin on mitochondrial membrane potential and the protective role of NAC.
NAC (200 μM) was added at the time of lovastatin (200 μM) addition.
Data are shown as Mean±SE for three independent experiments.
a : significant VS control group(p<0.05).
b: significant VS lovastatin -treated group(p<0.05).

Conclusion

In summary, in accordance with a previous study[7], we have shown that, statins act as the inducers of oxidative stress that severely inhibits mitochondria respiration and decreases mitochondrial membrane potential in rat hepatocytes. They also promote peroxidation of lipids and subsequently induce cytotoxicity and cell death. The treatment of hepatocytes with NAC protected cells from the statins-induced ROS production, lipid peroxidation, mitochondrial impairment and cell death. Hence, supplementation with NAC may be an effective therapeutic strategy for the prevention and treatment of clinical conditions caused by statins.

Acknowledgements

The authors thank Biotechnology and Drug Applied Research Centers of Tabriz University of Medical Sciences, Tabriz-Iran, for providing facilities to carry out this study. This research was a part of Narges Abdoli's PhD thesis that was supported by students' research committee. The authors are thankful to the students' research committee of Tabriz University of Medical Sciences, Tabriz-Iran, for providing supports to the study.

Conflict of Interest

The authors declare that they have no conflict of interest.

References

1. Ellesat KS, Tollefsen KE, Asberg A, Thomas KV, Hylland K. Cytotoxicity of atorvastatin and simvastatin on primary rainbow trout (Oncorhynchus mykiss) hepatocytes. *Toxicol In Vitro* 2010;24(6):1610-8.

2. Kubota T, Fujisaki K, Itoh Y, Yano T, Sendo T, Oishi R. Apoptotic injury in cultured human hepatocytes induced by HMG-CoA reductase inhibitors. *Biochem Pharmacol* 2004;67(12):2175-86.

3. Guzman M, Cortes JP, Castro J. Effects of lovastatin on hepatic fatty acid metabolism. *Lipids* 1993;28(12):1087-93.

4. Kromer A, Moosmann B. Statin-induced liver injury involves cross-talk between cholesterol and selenoprotein biosynthetic pathways. *Mol Pharmacol* 2009;75(6):1421-9.

5. Hsu I, Spinler SA, Johnson NE. Comparative evaluation of the safety and efficacy of HMG-CoA reductase inhibitor monotherapy in the treatment of primary hypercholesterolemia. *Ann Pharmacother* 1995;29(7-8):743-59.

6. Callegari S, Mckinnon RA, Andrews S, De Barros Lopes MA. Atorvastatin-induced cell toxicity in yeast is linked to disruption of protein isoprenylation. *FEMS Yeast Res* 2010;10(2):188-98.

7. Abdoli N, Heidari R, Azarmi Y, Eghbal MA. Mechanisms of the statins cytotoxicity in freshly

isolated rat hepatocytes. *J Biochem Mol Toxicol* 2013;27(6):287-94.

8. Gonzalez R, Ferrin G, Hidalgo AB, Ranchal I, Lopez-Cillero P, Santos-Gonzalez M, et al. N-acetylcysteine, coenzyme Q10 and superoxide dismutase mimetic prevent mitochondrial cell dysfunction and cell death induced by d-galactosamine in primary culture of human hepatocytes. *Chem Biol Interact* 2009;181(1):95-106.

9. Heidari R, Babaei H, Eghbal M. Mechanisms of methimazole cytotoxicity in isolated rat hepatocytes. *Drug Chem Toxicol* 2013;36(4):403-11.

10. Heidari R, Babaei H, Eghbal MA. Ameliorative effects of taurine against methimazole-induced cytotoxicity in isolated rat hepatocytes. *Sci Pharm* 2012;80(4):987-99.

11. Heidari R, Babaei H, Eghbal MA. Cytoprotective effects of taurine against toxicity induced by isoniazid and hydrazine in isolated rat hepatocytes. *Arh Hig Rada Toksikol* 2013;64(2):15-24.

12. Heidari R, Babaei H, Roshangar L, Eghbal MA. Effects of enzyme induction and/or glutathione depletion on methimazole-induced hepatotoxicity in mice and the protective role of N-acetylcysteine. *Adv Pharm Bull* 2014;4(1):21-8.

13. Heidari R, Babaei H, Eghbal MA. Cytoprotective Effects of Organosulfur Compounds against Methimazole Induced Toxicity in Isolated Rat Hepatocytes. *Adv Pharm Bull* 2013;3(1):135-42.

14. Heidari R, Babaei H, Eghbal MA. Amodiaquine-induced toxicity in isolated rat hepatocytes and the cytoprotective effects of taurine and/or N-acetyl cysteine. *Res Pharm Sci* 2014;9(2):97-105.

15. Benzie IF. Lipid peroxidation: a review of causes, consequences, measurement and dietary influences. *Int J Food Sci Nutr* 1996;47(3):233-61.

16. Liantonio A, Giannuzzi V, Cippone V, Camerino GM, Pierno S, Camerino DC. Fluvastatin and atorvastatin affect calcium homeostasis of rat skeletal muscle fibers in vivo and in vitro by impairing the sarcoplasmic reticulum/mitochondria Ca2+-release system. *J Pharmacol Exp Ther* 2007;321(2):626-34.

17. Tafazoli S, O'brien PJ. Peroxidases: a role in the metabolism and side effects of drugs. *Drug Discov Today* 2005;10(9):617-25.

18. Caron G, Ermondi G, Testa B. Predicting the oxidative metabolism of statins: an application of the MetaSite algorithm. *Pharm Res* 2007;24(3):480-501.

19. Orrenius S, Gogvadze V, Zhivotovsky B. Mitochondrial oxidative stress: implications for cell death. *Annu Rev Pharmacol Toxicol* 2007;47:143-83.

20. Gonzalez-Aragon D, Ariza J, Villalba JM. Dicoumarol impairs mitochondrial electron transport and pyrimidine biosynthesis in human myeloid leukemia HL-60 cells. *Biochem Pharmacol* 2007;73(3):427-39.

21. Kelly GS. Clinical applications of N-acetylcysteine. *Altern Med Rev* 1998;3(2):114-27.

23

The Prelude on Novel Receptor and Ligand Targets Involved in the Treatment of Diabetes Mellitus

Venu Gopal Jonnalagadda[1]*, Allam Venkata Sita Ram Raju[2], Srinivas Pittala[3], Afsar shaik[4], Nilakash Annaji Selkar[5]

[1] Shree Dhootapapeshwar Ayurvedic Research Foundation (SDARF), Panvel, Navi Mumbai-410206, Maharastra, India.

[2] National Institute of Pharmaceutical Education and Research, Bala Nagar, Hyderabad, Andhra Pradhesh-500037, India.

[3] CSIR-Institute of Genomics and Integrative Biology, Near Jubilee Hall, Mall Road, Delhi-110 007, India.

[4] Gokula Krishna college of Pharmacy, Sullurpet - 524121, Nellore dist, A.P, India.

[5] National Institute for Research in Reproductive Health, Parel, Mumbai-400012, Maharastra, India.

ARTICLE INFO

Keywords:
Diabetes Mellitus
Ligands
Receptors
Signalling

ABSTRACT

Metabolic disorders are a group of disorders, due to the disruption of the normal metabolic process at a cellular level. Diabetes Mellitus and Tyrosinaemia are the majorly reported metabolic disorders. Among them, Diabetes Mellitus is a one of the leading metabolic syndrome, affecting 5 to 7 % of the population worldwide and mainly characterised by elevated levels of glucose and is associated with two types of physiological event disturbances such as impaired insulin secretion and insulin resistance. Up to now, various treatment strategies are like insulin, alphaglucosidase inhibitors, biguanides, incretins were being followed. Concurrently, various novel therapeutic strategies are required to advance the therapy of Diabetes mellitus. For the last few decades, there has been an extensive research in understanding the metabolic pathways involved in Diabetes Mellitus at the cellular level and having the profound knowledge on cell-growth, cell-cycle, and apoptosis at a molecular level provides new targets for the treatment of Diabetes Mellitus. Receptor signalling has been involved in these mechanisms, to translate the information coming from outside. To understand the various receptors involved in these pathways, we must have a sound knowledge on receptors and ligands involved in it. This review mainly summarises the receptors and ligands which are involved the Diabetes Mellitus. Finally, researchers have to develop the alternative chemical moieties that retain their affinity to receptors and efficacy. Diabetes Mellitus being a metabolic disorder due to the glucose surfeit, demands the need for regular exercise along with dietary changes.

Introduction

The human body has eleven systems, namely central nervous, cardiovascular, endocrine system etc. Among all, the endocrine system works in a distinct fashion i.e. away from the synthesis area. To function normally in every aspect of cellular pathway, there is a need for the cells to be in a harmonised state. Every cellular part has different sensors, namely receptors. Receptors are dynamic protein structures, in inactive mode at the cell surface or in the cytoplasm or in nucleus, activated by ligands to receive the chemical signals from outside. Ligands are the binding molecules that mediate their action through their receptors. Ligands are mainly of two types i.e. agonists and antagonists. The cellular response depends on the type of molecule which binds to the receptor. In the present days, vast research being carried out on the cellular pathways involves the reaction between the receptor and the ligand. This, in turn provides new pathways to discover more selective therapeutic drugs.

Diabetes Mellitus (DM) is a chronic multifactorial metabolic disorder resulted due to the altered homeostasis between glucose production and its metabolism.[1] DM is mainly characterised by hyperglycaemia, altered lipid metabolism ascribed due to the unsubstantial amount of insulin production by the β-cells, secretion or both and insulin resistance, oxidative stress, and inflammation.[2] DM is a 5th leading cause for mortality, prevalence of DM in adults was 285 million (6.4%) in 2010, and this value is predicted to reach around 439 million (7.7%) by 2030. DM is

---

Corresponding author: Venu Gopal Jonnalagadda, Shree Dhootapapeshwar Ayurvedic Research Foundation (SDARF), Panvel, Navi Mumbai, Maharastra-410206, India. Email: venu.gopal@teamsdl.in

mainly of two types i.e., Type-1 or Insulin dependent DM (IDDM) and Type 2 or non-insulin dependent DM (NIDDM).[3] Type 2 DM is accounts for at least 90% of cases and it is the predominant form.[4] Up to now, various types of treatments are used in the management of DM based on different types of pharmacological actions, but these drugs aren't able to mitigate the disease progress, although the insulin resistance is an unravel mechanism for scientists. Moreover, DM is associated with various microvascular (retinopathy, nephropathy, and neuropathy) and macrovascular (coronary, cerebral, and peripheral) complications, which necessitated further extensive multidisciplinary research aimed to treat the DM.

The main pathological event in the DM is insulin resistance (IR). Generally IR is defined as decreased insulin action to activate downstream signalling at a cellular level to normalize the glucose surfeit.[5] The major proposed mechanism for the negative insulin signalling was phosphorylation of serine residues like IRS-1, which includes ser636, ser312, and ser1101. In the phosphorylated state, IRS-1 impedes interaction with insulin receptor signalling and ultimately results in insulin resistance.[6]

In this review, we have summarised, a detail description of receptors and ligands of the DM which includes glucose-transporters, calcium-sensing receptors (CaR), epidermal-growth factor(EGF), estrogen-receptor(ER), farnesoid-X-receptor(FXR), gastrin-releasing peptide(GRP), lyso-phosphatidic acid, muscarinic-receptor, neurotensin, peroxisome-proliferator activated receptor (PPAR), insulin receptor, adiponectin receptor, adenosine receptor, cholecystokinin(CCK), cannabinoid receptor(CB), Insulin-like growth factor(IGF), neuropeptide Y(NPY),toll-like receptor(TLR), and protein-tyrosine phosphatase (PTPs)-1B inhibitors.

In this review we underscore the quick glance over the receptors and ligands involved in the DM, and their interaction in physiological, pathological events in the DM.

Glucose transporters (GLUT)

Glucose is a major metabolic fuel for all living mammalian cells, which is required for their normal physiological functions. Generally, glucose was transported across the cell-membrane by the two different mechanisms i.e sodium-independent (facilitated diffusion, GLUT transporters) and sodium-dependent (secondary active transport, SGLT transporters) with varied kinetic properties. Glucose transporters (GLUT) are available in 12 different isomeric forms belonging to SLC2A hexose transport family, and six different SGLT are available belonging to SLC5A co-transport family. Among them all $GLUT_4$ is mainly involved in glucose transport across cell-membrane of brown and white adipose tissue, muscle (skeletal), heart (myocardium)[7], owing to which, a mutation in $GLUT_4$ causes the DM.[8] Almost, 90% of

the filtered glucose was reabsorbed by the sodium-glucose cotransporter-2, at the S1 segment of the proximal tubule, remaining is absorbed by the $SGLT_1$ at the S3 segment.[9] The maximum level of reabsorption was observed in the Type-1 Diabetic patients, implying one of the cause of diabetic condition. The increased levels of $SGLT_2$ was observed in alloxan-induced diabetic rats,[10] and $GLUT_2$ levels were increased in streptozotocin diabetic rats.[11] The inhibition of SGLT transporters improves diabetic conditions in streptozotocin induced diabetic rats.[12] By inhibiting the $SGLT_2$ receptors, the levels of plasma glucose were reduced significantly.[13] Indeed, $SGLT_2$ receptor antagonists are the promising approach to treat DM.

Calcium Sensing Receptors (CaR)

Calcium sensing receptors plays a major role in regulation of pancreatic β-cells' insulin secretion to maintain the glucose homeostasis, and also involve in β-cell development, and growth. Levels of calcium sensing receptors are variable qualitatively or quantitatively in diabetic animal models. Extracellular calcium is involved in insulin secretion, followed by concentration dependent, reversible inhibition of secretion. The mechanism involved in that is increase in cyclic AMP levels, through the phospholipase C–IP$_3$ pathway. CaR are mainly stimulated by the cations like Ca^{2+}, Mg^{2+} and amino acids like L-Phe in HEK-293 cell lines. Apart from that, these are activated by the calcimimetic agents like phenylalkylamines, NPS R-467 and NPS R-568.[14] Elizabeth Gray et al. observed that calcimimetic R-568 agonist activates the concentration of extracellular Ca^{2+} and subsequently activates CaR receptors and induces the insulin release from human islets and MIN6 cells. The mechanism involved in CaR mediated activation is associated with p42/44 mitogen-activated protein kinases (MAPK), and its activation is inhibited by the p42/44 inhibitors. Moreover, CaR mediated insulin secretion is decreased by inhibitors of Phospholiase c, calcium-calmodulin dependent kinase inhibitors and also there is involvement of protein-kinase C inhibitors. Thus, Calcium is involved in exocytosis of insulin secretion.[15] Thus, calcium sensing becomes effective in the treatment of DM.[16]

Epidermal Growth Factor (EGF)

Development and progression of DM is associated with the EGF-receptor ligand system. EGF receptor is an 1186 amino acid glycoprotein, single transmembrane tyrosine-kinase type of receptor, mainly involved in the development of microvessel myogenic tone nature and cell processes like proliferation, survival, and differentiation during development, tissue homeostasis. Leptin level in DM increases the EGFR tyrosine kinase phosphorylation, leading to activation of ERK1/2 MAP-kinase. However, increasing the activity of EGFR phosphorylation leads to increase in glucose levels.[17,18] And, EGFR ligand like betacellulin is associated with the increase in β-cell proliferation and its neogenesis and increase in the activity of gut hormone like GLP-1.[19] This provides new direction to discover the new molecular targets in DM.

Estrogen Receptor(ER)

Estrogen is having the effect on vascular system and DM.[20] The prevalence of DM is more in men, when compared to women,[21] explains the role of steroid hormone estrogen in the protective ability against the disease progress. ER receptors are of two types namely ERα and ERβ. Estrogen is mainly involved in the regulation of glucose homeostasis. ERβ agonists also helpful in DM.[22] ERα may interfere with the one of the inflammatory pathway i.e cytokine-driven iNOS pathway in DM hyperglycaemic rats.[23] This warrants, selective ER agonists are useful in DM along with further extensive research in this area.

Farnesoid X Receptor (FxR)

Farnesoid X receptor (FXR) is a nuclear receptor involved in hepatic glucose and lipid metabolism is mainly found in the intestine, kidneys, and adrenal glands. It is widely expressed in the gastro-intestinal tract. In the last few years the Farnesoid receptor activity has been reviewed.[24] Bile acids (BA) play an important role in Farnesoid receptor activation through gluconeogenesis.[25] FxR activates the induction of the glucose regulated transcription factor KLF11, and FxR receptor activation in beta TC6 cells increases the AkT phosphorylation subsequently causing translocation of GLUT2 transporters at cellular membrane. In another, experiment in non obese diabetic (NOD) mice activation of FxR receptor delay the development of signs and symptoms of hyperglycaemia, diabetes, and glycosuria.[26] In another experiment FxR activation led to the reduced expression of glucogenic enzymes like G6Pase (glucose-6-phosphatase), PEPCK (phosphoenol pyruvate kinase), and FBP1 (fructose-1,6-bisphosphatase).[27,28] FxR receptor activation by the synthetic agonist like GW4064 in insulin-resistant ob/ob mice reduced hyperinsulinemia and improved glucose tolerance.[29] These results suggest that FxR agonists are helpful in the treatment of DM in future.

Gastrin releasing peptide (GRP) Receptor

Gastrin releasing peptide (GRP) is a 27 amino acid, neuropeptide strongly present in the gastro-intestinal tract mainly involved in the digestion, and metabolism. GRP primarily activates the insulin secretion in-vitro and in-vivo by both direct activation of islet cells and indirect activation of ganglionic neurons through gastrin releasing peptide receptor (GRPR).[30] GRP stimulation in L cells of intestine activates the mitogen activated protein kinase (MAPKK) and subsequent phosphorylation of p44/42 mitogen activated protein kinase (MAPK). In another, GRP mediated stimulation activates the cholecystokinin through protein kinase C (PKC).[31] Inactivation of PKCs by the phorbol myristate

prevents the insulin secretion from β-cells which is mediated by the GRPs.[32]

Lyso-phosphatidic acid (LPA)

Lysophosphatidic acid (LPA) is a potent arbitatory agent that mediates mainly smooth muscle contraction, platelet aggregation, anti apoptosis, cell rounding, and cell proliferation regulation.[33] LPA mainly present in the blood, which is produced by lysophospholipase D (Lyso PLD) enzyme.[34] LPA was found to enhance the glucose uptake in 3T3-L1 adipocytes and GLUT4myc myotubes by triggering GLUT4 translocation to the plasma membrane. Although, if the effect of LPA on glucose uptake was inhibited by the LPA antagonists like Ki16425 and G$_i$ inhibitor pertussis toxin, LPA showed the blood glucose lowering effect in streptozotocin induced DM.[35] So, LPA acts as a potent modulator of glucose homeostasis in adipose and muscle tissues.

Muscarinic receptors

Muscarinic receptors are G-protein coupled receptors (GPCR) involves in calcium mobilisation, phospholipase-c and protein kinase-c activation. In human beings, the known endogenous cholinergic agonists are acetylcholine (Ach), and conjugated secondary bile acids (BAs).[36] CHRM3 are located in many places in the body, e.g. smooth muscle, the endocrine glands, exocrine glands, pancreas. Elevated levels of CHRM3 mainly expressed in pancreatic B-cells, and muscarinic receptors activate the GLP-1 peptide secretion by the indirect mechanism involving vagus nerve and from the from the proximal intestine L cells.[37]

Muscarinic receptor signalling in Insulin secretion

Muscarinic receptor ligands, such as secondary BAs and Ach stimulate the extracellular muscarinic receptors. The main mechanism involved in insulin release is through G-protein coupled receptor signalling to the calcium and PKC pathways. The activation of M3 receptor induces the hydrolysis of membrane component phospholipid phosphatidyl inositol- 4,5-biphosphate (PIP2), catalyzed by phospholipase C (PLC). This reaction generates the formation of two secondary messengers i.e. inositol-1,4,5- triphosphate (IP3) and diacylglycerol (DAG). IP3 in turn drives the calcium release from the IP3 sensitive stores, simultaneously DAG activates PKC.[38]

However, G-protein-independent pathway is also involved in the insulin secretion through the protein-kinase D1(PKD1). The principle involved is, phosphorylated form of M3 activates the G-protein-independent pathway through β-arrestin dependent process resulting in secretory releasing.[39] In addition, it activates the sodium channel designated as NALCN, a non-selective sodium-leak channel which plays an important role in insulin release. M3R has showed to activate this channel in the model of MIN-6, pancreatic β cell line via the Src family of tyrosine kinases (SFKs).[40] In particular, there is a need of extensive research studies on this mechanism to develop better therapeutic drugs.

Neurotensin (NT)

Neurotensin (NT) is a peptide neurohormone or neuromodulator in the central nervous system and peripheral nervous system.[41] Neurotensin receptors are present throughout the gut, to express their activity. Neurotensin is involved in different variety of functions including stimulation of pancreatic secretions, stimulation of colonic motility and biliary secretions.[42] Neurotensin receptors are G-protein coupled type of receptors, i.e NTSR1, NTSR2, NTSR3. NTSR2/NTSR3 involved in the pancreatic β-receptor signalling to mediate the insulin secretion. The mechanism involved in this secretion is that the NT binds to the NTSR2/NTSR3 complex leading to the activation of downstream signalling mechanism and causes activation of phospholipase C which enhances the release of calcium, responsible for insulin secretion. NTSR2 selective agonist, levocabastine, causes a transient increase in intracellular calcium levels in Ins1-E cell line.[43] This suggests that refinement of NT can serve as a better novel therapeutic approach for further investigation.

Peroxisome proliferator-activated receptor (PPAR)

PPARs come under the members of nuclear hormone receptor super family and ligand-activated transcription factors. PPARs comprise of mainly three different isoforms: PPARα, PPARβ/γ and PPARγ.[44] Activation of PPARα possesses an anti-diabetic effect. PPARγ agonists were used as therapeutic agents for treatment of DM. PPARγ directly activates the GLUT-2 and B-glucokinase in liver.[45] Till now, the different well known mechanisms have been reported in the antidiabetic activity of PPARγ agonists, like thiazolidines (TZD), they increase the expression of insulin receptor substrate (IRS)-1,[46] IRS-2,[47] the cbl-associated protein,[48] and the p85 subunit of phosphatidyl inositol.[49]

Insulin Receptor (IR)

Insulin receptor is a tyrosine-kinase mediated heterotetrameric membrane glycoprotein receptor comprising of two α and two β subunits linked by disulphide linkage involved in pleiotropic actions of insulin. The mechanism involved in the insulin receptor signalling is, insulin binds to the extra cellular subunit, bringing the two α subunits to come together. By this conformational change ATP binds to the β subunit intracellularly and causes autophosphorylation and enables its kinase activity, leading to IRS/PK-I3 pathway and starts the PIP3 dependent kinases.[50,51] Along with this, another pathway involved in this is exchange factors SOS and growth factor receptor binding protein 2 (GRB2) for stimulation of insulin

mediated actions on growth and proliferation.[52] Insulin Receptor substrates are insulin, IGF-1,and other cytokine receptors that phosphorylate the specific Y-x-x-M motifs.[53] This explains the potential diversity of insulin action.

Adiponectin Receptors

Adipose tissue produces different types of small bioactive molecules, i.e adipocytokines[54] also called adipocyte complement-related protein of 30 kDa (Acrp30).[55] Obesity is a principal cause of cardiovascular disease, and DM. Adiponectin receptors are found to be available in two isomeric forms viz. Adiponectin Receptor R1 (Adipo R1) and Adiponectin Receptor R2 (Adipo R1 is abundantly expressed in muscle, and Adipo R2 is mainly present in liver). Adiponectin mediates its action through these receptors via intracellular signalling pathway by using AMP-activated protein Kinase (AMPK), Peroxisome-proliferated activated receptor-α (PPAR-α), fatty-acid oxidation and glucose uptake in liver. Adiponectin levels were measured by the Enzyme-linked immunosorbent Assay (ELISA), to correlate the adiponectin and DM.[56] Adiponectin levels were decreased in DM type-2 i.e inversely related to glucose levels. But, excitingly the levels of adiponectin were increased in type-1 DM i.e positively correlated with insulin sensitivity.[57] In-case of anti-diabetic drugs increased serum adiponectin levels in insulin resistant cases,[58] and increased levels of adiponectin decrease the risk for DM.[59] Further more extensive research work needs to elucidate the detailed information.

Adenosine Receptor

Adenosine is a purine metabolic product, one of the potent endogenous autocrine immunosuppressive and anti-inflammatory molecules, released into the extracellular space at the time of tissue injury and inflammation. Adenosine receptors are different types like A_1, A_{2A}, A_{2B}, and A_3 belongs to G-protein coupled receptors.[60] All four receptors are involved in adaptive immunity response by adenosine receptor activation. Moreover, single cup of tea or coffee suffices for the blockade of A_1, A_{2A}, A_{2B} receptors, mainly, A2B adenosine receptor (A2bAR) involved in regulation of inflammation. A2B receptor modulated activity in DM was performed by Hillary Johnston-Cox. Up-regulation of A2BAR receptor in control mice along with A2AR knock-out mice, the hallmarks of DM were observed in knock-out mice. Mechanism involved in that A2bAR regulation of SREBP-1 expression, a repressor of insulin-receptor signalling-2(IRS-2), and also A2BAR ligand was observed for 28 days after the high fat, high cholesterol diet (HFD) restored the IRS-2 levels and subsequently abrogated the development of T2D. A1AR receptors were expressed in adipose tissue, principally involved in the dyslipidaemia, insulin resistance, and diabetes. Selective A2AR agonists are helpful in DM by inhibiting the cAMP through G-protein coupled adenylyl cyclase using N[6]-cyclopentyladenosine.[61] However, there is a need for the discovery of adenosine receptor agonists.

Cholecystokinin (CCK)

Cholecystokinin (CCK)[62] and its analogue cerulean[63] leads to the pancreatic cell growth. CCK_A receptors were involved in regulation of pancreatic cell growth and to stimulate the secretion of the digestive enzyme pancreatic lipase, this response was blocked by simultaneous administration of CCK_A receptor antagonists[64] or CCK_A deficient mice.[65] Cholecystokinin acts through the G-protein coupled mechanism, like G_q along with phosphoinositide-specific phospholipase C (PLC-β) and thereby elevates intracellular calcium. And also, CCK activates the NFAT pathway through the calcineurin pathway, in a dose-dependent manner this effect was blocked by inhibitors of this phosphatase, cyclosporine A and immune suppressants FK506.[66]

Cannabinoid Receptor (CB)

Cannabinoid receptors are of two types, i.e. 7 transmembrane CB1 and CB2, belong to Vanilloid-type-1 receptors.CB1 receptors are mainly expressed in the central nervous system, where as CB2 receptors are available in haempoietic system and immune system, mainly regulating the immunological activities.[67] Cannabinoid receptors are partly responsible for the activities of natural constituents of *Cannabis sativa*. CB respond functionally and biochemically to two natural cannabidiol and Δ^9 tetrahydrocannabivarin. Oxidative stress is involved in different pathological events ranging from pain, cancer, obesity, inflammation, and metabolic disorders especially diabetes and its vascular complications.[68] Most of the diabetic complications are due to reactive oxygen species or reactive nitrogen species. Activation of CB1 receptors causes increased insulin secretion. Cannabinoids also activates one of the nuclear receptors peroxisome-proliferated activated receptor-α (PPAR-α). Endocannabinoids like virodhamine, anandamide, and noladin activate the PPAR-α.[69] But, conversely CB1 receptor antagonist rimonabant, showed insulin resistance, C-reactive protein and reduced the glycated haemoglobin (Hb1c) levels in insulin treated diabetic patients, in drug naïve and metformin and sulphonylurea treated type 2 diabetic patients.[70] CB receptors having the modulatory activity in the DM warrants further extensive research in this area.

Insulin like growth factor (IGF) Receptor

Insulin like growth factor (IGF) has two types of ligands, namely IGF-1 and IGF-2. IGF-1 receptor is a tyrosine-kinase membrane associated receptor, existed as a heterotetramer with two- α and two-β subunits linked through the disulphide linkage. Binding of IGF molecules promotes the intramolecular autophosphorylation and phosphorylation of its critical targets. Moreover, it also activates several other signalling pathways such as P13k/AKT pathway and Ras/MAPK.[71] IGF receptors are abundantly present in skeletal muscle, where as adipose, hepatic tissues have fewer. IGF-1 is structurally related to insulin. IGF-1 showed the positive effects like β-cell growth, survival, and insulin secretion.[72] Along with these effects, it also produces increased glucose transport in skeletal, adipose tissue, increased glycogenesis, lipogenesis, and decreased lipolysis. It also decreases the blood glucose, free fatty acids levels similar to insulin.[73] Thus, targeting the IGF pathway provides an efficient strategy to treat the DM.

Neuro Peptide (NP)Y Receptor

Peptide YY and NPY belonging the family of pancreatic polypeptide hormones, comprise a chain of length 36 amino acids, secreted from the ileal L cells after taking the meals. They posses N-terminal having tyrosine moiety and C-terminal having the amide residue of tyrosine.[74] PYY is mostly confined to the endocrine cells of the gut. NPY and Y2 are involved in different activities like appetite and feeding, angiogenesis, carcinogenesis, and DM. NPYergic neurons are inhibitory autoreceptor, can regulate the expression and secretion of NPY and other related neurotransmitters. They are also involved in leptin receptor expression that enables the maintenance of energy homeostasis. Moreover, Y2 receptor deletion in ob/ob mice attenuates the type 2 DM in mice.[75]

Toll-like Receptors (TLR)

Inflammation and its mediators are involved in different types of diseases like atherosclerosis, cancer, and DM.[76] DM is mainly associated with the inflammatory mediators like sialic acid, C-reactive protein, alpha-1 acid glycoprotein etc., suggesting the lack of innate-immunity response.[77] TLRs are expressed specifically at the site of tissue injury and interact with endogenous ligands like HSPs (heat-shock proteins) 60/70, oxLDL (oxidised LDL), fibronectin and fibrinogen which are abundantly seen in DM.[78-83] TLR family consists of 13 different types mammalian receptors. Among them TLR2 and TLR4 are mainly involved in the pathogenesis of insulin resistance (IR), and DM in experimental and clinical conditions.[76] Kim HS et al. found that TLR-2 senses the β-cell death as a mediator of inflammation,[83] and activation of TLR-2 and TLR-4 leads to the downstream cytokine, p38 MAPK and NF-kB production.[76,84,85] In addition to this Song et al.[86] showed increase in TLR4mRNA expression in differentiating adipose tissue of *db/db* mice. TLR-2 is involved in streptozotocin induced inflammation through the MyD88-dependent pathway, and TLR-4 also involved in MyD88-independent pathway along with NF-kB pathway.[87] Lastly by inhibiting the TLR pathway, we can control the inflammation. But an in-depth further experimental and clinical research is required to develop the novel therapeutic drugs in this area.

Protein Tyrosine Phosphatase (PTP)-1B Inhibitors

Tyrosine phosphorylation is one of the basic mechanism involved in cell growth and differentiation. Insulin upon binding to its receptor activates the insulin receptor tyrosine kinase (IRTK) through auto phosphorylation mechanism. This leads to the activation of recruitment of insulin receptor substrate (IRS)-1, followed by the activation of phosphatidyl inositol 3 kinase (PI3K) and subsequent translocation of glucose transporter-4 (GLUT-4).[88] In contrast, tyrosine phosphatase enzymes dephosphorylate them, and inactivates the fundamental cellular process like cell differentiation, metabolism, and cell apoptosis.[89] Along with this, other PTPs which are involved in negative regulation of the insulin secretion are leukocyte antigen-related tyrosine phosphatase(LAR), SH2-domain-containing phosphotyrosine phosphatase (SHP2), receptor protein tyrosine phosphatase (rPTP), and protein tyrosine phosphatase 1B (PTP1B). Certainly, PTP1B seemed to be a key regulator in insulin receptor signalling[90] and inhibition of PTP1B is a novel receptor target in the treatment of DM.

Conclusion

Receptors always play a prominent role in physiology and pathology of various disease conditions in humans as well as in animals. Due to interdependency and complexity of receptors in their mechanism, one can't corroborate their involvement in the pathophysiological event of the disease. However, we can conclude that receptor-ligand interaction mechanism can be used in development of new therapeutic agents by gaining sufficient knowledge on it, and thereby, designing the new drugs based on ligand-receptor interaction for better optimal drug discovery. The researchers have to develop the alternative chemical moieties that retain its affinity to receptor and efficacy. So, one can utilise these preliminary findings to develop novel therapeutic agents that target the selective receptor providing better therapy for DM. Finally, DM is a metabolic disorder due to the glucose surfeit, it alarms the need to maintain it levels by optimising medications along with regular excercise and changes in diet.

Acknowledgements

Authors would like to say deep gratitude of thanks to Ms. V. Rajani Sekhar for her support in editing the manuscript.

Conflict of Interest

We don't have any potential conflicts of Interest.

References

1. Samadder A, Chakraborty D, De A, Bhattacharyya SS, Bhadra K, Khuda-Bukhsh AR. Possible signaling cascades involved in attenuation of alloxan-induced oxidative stress and hyperglycemia in mice by ethanolic extract of Syzygium jambolanum: drug-DNA interaction with calf thymus DNA as target. *Eur J Pharm Sci* 2011;44(3):207-17.

2. Barathmanikanth S, Kalishwaralal K, Sriram M, Pandiyan SR, Youn HS, Eom S, et al. Anti-oxidant effect of gold nanoparticles restrains hyperglycaemic conditions in diabetic mice. *J Nanobiotechnology* 2010;8:16.

3. Shaw JE, Sicree RA, Zimmet PZ. Global estimates of the prevalence of diabetes for 2010 and 2030. *Diabetes Res Clin Pract* 2010;87(1):4-14.

4. Gonzalez EL, Johansson S, Wallander MA, Rodriguez LA. Trends in the prevalence and incidence of diabetes in the UK: 1996-2005. *J Epidemiol Community Health* 2009;63(4):332-6.

5. Ginsberg HN. Insulin resistance and cardiovascular disease. *J Clin Invest* 2000;106(4):453-8.

6. Saini V. Molecular mechanisms of insulin resistance in type 2 diabetes mellitus. *World J Diabetes* 2010;1(3):68-75.

7. Shah K, DeSilva S, Abbruscato T. The Role of Glucose Transporters in Brain Disease: Diabetes and Alzheimer's Disease. *Int J Mol Sci* 2012;13(10):12629-55.

8. Genetics Home Reference. U.S. National Library of Medicine; 2013 [cited December 23, 2013]; Available from: http://ghr.nlm.nih.gov.

9. Wood IS, Trayhurn P. Glucose transporters (GLUT and SGLT): expanded families of sugar transport proteins. *Br J Nutr* 2003;89(1):3-9.

10. Vestri S, Okamoto MM, De Freitas HS, Aparecida Dos Santos R, Nunes MT, Morimatsu M, et al. Changes in sodium or glucose filtration rate modulate expression of glucose transporters in renal proximal tubular cells of rat. *J Membr Biol* 2001;182(2):105-12.

11. Marks J, Carvou NJ, Debnam ES, Srai SK, Unwin RJ. Diabetes increases facilitative glucose uptake and GLUT2 expression at the rat proximal tubule brush border membrane. *J Physiol* 2003;553(Pt 1):137-45.

12. Adachi T, Yasuda K, Okamoto Y, Shihara N, Oku A, Ueta K, et al. T-1095, a renal Na+-glucose transporter inhibitor, improves hyperglycemia in streptozotocin-induced diabetic rats. *Metabolism* 2000;49(8):990-5.

13. Vallon V, Sharma K. Sodium-glucose transport: role in diabetes mellitus and potential clinical implications. *Curr Opin Nephrol Hypertens* 2010;19(5):425-31.

14. Magno AL, Ward BK, Ratajczak T. The calcium-sensing receptor: a molecular perspective. *Endocr Rev* 2011;32(1):3-30.

15. Gray E, Muller D, Squires PE, Asare-Anane H, Huang GC, Amiel S, et al. Activation of the extracellular calcium-sensing receptor initiates insulin secretion from human islets of Langerhans:

involvement of protein kinases. *J Endocrinol* 2006;190(3):703-10.

16. Pittas AG, Dawson-Hughes B, Li T, Van Dam RM, Willett WC, Manson JE, et al. Vitamin D and calcium intake in relation to type 2 diabetes in women. *Diabetes Care* 2006;29(3):650-6.

17. Belmadani S, Palen DI, Gonzalez-Villalobos RA, Boulares HA, Matrougui K. Elevated epidermal growth factor receptor phosphorylation induces resistance artery dysfunction in diabetic db/db mice. *Diabetes* 2008;57(6):1629-37.

18. Matrougui K. Diabetes and microvascular pathophysiology: role of epidermal growth factor receptor tyrosine kinase. *Diabetes Metab Res Rev* 2010;26(1):13-6.

19. Miettinen P, Ormio P, Hakonen E, Banerjee M, Otonkoski T. EGF receptor in pancreatic beta-cell mass regulation. *Biochem Soc Trans* 2008;36(Pt 3):280-5.

20. White RE. Estrogen and vascular function. *Vascul Pharmacol* 2002;38(2):73-80.

21. Wild S, Roglic G, Green A, Sicree R, King H. Global prevalence of diabetes: estimates for the year 2000 and projections for 2030. *Diabetes Care* 2004;27(5):1047-53.

22. Kumar R, Balhuizen A, Amisten S, Lundquist I, Salehi A. Insulinotropic and antidiabetic effects of 17beta-estradiol and the GPR30 agonist G-1 on human pancreatic islets. *Endocrinology* 2011;152(7):2568-79.

23. Cignarella A, Bolego C, Pelosi V, Meda C, Krust A, Pinna C, et al. Distinct roles of estrogen receptor-alpha and beta in the modulation of vascular inducible nitric-oxide synthase in diabetes. *J Pharmacol Exp Ther* 2009;328(1):174-82.

24. Claudel T, Staels B, Kuipers F. The Farnesoid X receptor: a molecular link between bile acid and lipid and glucose metabolism. *Arterioscler Thromb Vasc Biol* 2005;25(10):2020-30.

25. Garg A, Grundy SM. Cholestyramine therapy for dyslipidemia in non-insulin-dependent diabetes mellitus. A short-term, double-blind, crossover trial. *Ann Intern Med* 1994;121(6):416-22.

26. Renga B, Mencarelli A, Vavassori P, Brancaleone V, Fiorucci S. The bile acid sensor FXR regulates insulin transcription and secretion. *Biochim Biophys Acta* 2010;1802(3):363-72.

27. Yamagata K, Daitoku H, Shimamoto Y, Matsuzaki H, Hirota K, Ishida J, et al. Bile acids regulate gluconeogenic gene expression via small heterodimer partner-mediated repression of hepatocyte nuclear factor 4 and Foxo1. *J Biol Chem* 2004;279(22):23158-65.

28. Ma K, Saha PK , Chan L, Moore DD. Farnesoid X receptor is essential for normal glucose homeostasis. *J Clin Invest* 2006;116(4):1102-9.

29. Cariou B, Van Harmelen K, Duran-Sandoval D, Van Dijk TH, Grefhorst A, Abdelkarim M, et al. The farnesoid X receptor modulates adiposity and peripheral insulin sensitivity in mice. *J Biol Chem* 2006;281(16):11039-49.

30. Persson K, Pacini G, Sundler F, Ahren B. Islet function phenotype in gastrin-releasing peptide receptor gene-deficient mice. *Endocrinology* 2002;143(10):3717-26.

31. Nemoz-Gaillard E, Cordier-Bussat M, Filloux C, Cuber JC, Van Obberghen E, Chayvialle JA, et al. Bombesin stimulates cholecystokinin secretion through mitogen-activated protein-kinase-dependent and -independent mechanisms in the enteroendocrine STC-1 cell line. *Biochem J* 1998;331 (Pt 1):129-35.

32. Gregersen S, Ahren B. Studies on the mechanisms by which gastrin releasing peptide potentiates glucose-induced insulin secretion from mouse islets. *Pancreas* 1996;12(1):48-57.

33. Zhang H, Bialkowska A, Rusovici R, Chanchevalap S, Shim H, Katz JP, et al. Lysophosphatidic acid facilitates proliferation of colon cancer cells via induction of Kruppel-like factor 5. *J Biol Chem* 2007;282(21):15541-9.

34. Umezu-Goto M, Kishi Y, Taira A, Hama K, Dohmae N, Takio K, et al. Autotaxin has lysophospholipase D activity leading to tumor cell growth and motility by lysophosphatidic acid production. *J Cell Biol* 2002;158(2):227-33.

35. Yea K, Kim J, Lim S, Park HS, Park KS, Suh PG, et al. Lysophosphatidic acid regulates blood glucose by stimulating myotube and adipocyte glucose uptake. *J Mol Med (Berl)* 2008;86(2):211-20.

36. Gilman AG. G proteins and dual control of adenylate cyclase. *Cell* 1984;36(3):577-9.

37. Weston-Green K, Huang XF, Lian J, Deng C. Effects of olanzapine on muscarinic M3 receptor binding density in the brain relates to weight gain, plasma insulin and metabolic hormone levels. *Eur Neuropsychopharmacol* 2012;22(5):364-73.

38. Gilon P, Henquin JC. Mechanisms and physiological significance of the cholinergic control of pancreatic beta-cell function. *Endocr Rev* 2001;22(2):565-604.

39. Kong KC, Butcher AJ, Mcwilliams P, Jones D, Wess J, Hamdan FF, et al. M3-muscarinic receptor promotes insulin release via receptor phosphorylation/arrestin-dependent activation of protein kinase D1. *Proc Natl Acad Sci U S A* 2010;107(49):21181-6.

40. Swayne LA, Mezghrani A, Varrault A, Chemin J, Bertrand G, Dalle S, et al. The NALCN ion channel is activated by M3 muscarinic receptors in a pancreatic beta-cell line. *EMBO Rep* 2009;10(8):873-80.

41. Bayer VE, Towle AC, Pickel VM. Vesicular and cytoplasmic localization of neurotensin-like immunoreactivity (NTLI) in neurons postsynaptic to terminals containing NTLI and/or tyrosine hydroxylase in the rat central nucleus of the amygdala. *J Neurosci Res* 1991;30(2):398-413.

42. Wang X, Jackson LN, Johnson SM, Wang Q, Evers BM. Suppression of neurotensin receptor type 1 expression and function by histone deacetylase inhibitors in human colorectal cancers. *Mol Cancer Ther* 2010;9(8):2389-98.

43. Mazella J, Beraud-Dufour S, Devader C, Massa F, Coppola T. Neurotensin and its receptors in the control of glucose homeostasis. *Front Endocrinol (Lausanne)* 2012;3:143.

44. Martinasso G, Oraldi M, Trombetta A, Maggiora M, Bertetto O, Canuto RA, et al. Involvement of PPARs in Cell Proliferation and Apoptosis in Human Colon Cancer Specimens and in Normal and Cancer Cell Lines. *PPAR Res* 2007;2007:93416.

45. Kim HI, Ahn YH. Role of peroxisome proliferator-activated receptor-gamma in the glucose-sensing apparatus of liver and beta-cells. *Diabetes* 2004;53 Suppl 1:S60-5.

46. Iwata M, Haruta T, Usui I, Takata Y, Takano A, Uno T, et al. Pioglitazone ameliorates tumor necrosis factor-alpha-induced insulin resistance by a mechanism independent of adipogenic activity of peroxisome proliferator--activated receptor-gamma. *Diabetes* 2001;50(5):1083-92.

47. Smith U, Gogg S, Johansson A, Olausson T, Rotter V, Svalstedt B. Thiazolidinediones (PPARgamma agonists) but not PPARalpha agonists increase IRS-2 gene expression in 3T3-L1 and human adipocytes. *FASEB J* 2001;15(1):215-20.

48. Ribon V, Johnson JH, Camp HS, Saltiel AR. Thiazolidinediones and insulin resistance: peroxisome proliferatoractivated receptor gamma activation stimulates expression of the CAP gene. *Proc Natl Acad Sci U S A* 1998;95(25):14751-6.

49. Rieusset J, Auwerx J, Vidal H. Regulation of gene expression by activation of the peroxisome proliferator-activated receptor gamma with rosiglitazone (BRL 49653) in human adipocytes. *Biochem Biophys Res Commun* 1999;265(1):265-71.

50. Hubbard SR, Wei L, Ellis L, Hendrickson WA. Crystal structure of the tyrosine kinase domain of the human insulin receptor. *Nature* 1994;372(6508):746-54.

51. Hubbard SR. Crystal structure of the activated insulin receptor tyrosine kinase in complex with peptide substrate and ATP analog. *EMBO J* 1997;16(18):5572-81.

52. Kido Y, Nakae J, Accili D. Clinical review 125: The insulin receptor and its cellular targets. *J Clin Endocrinol Metab* 2001;86(3):972-9.

53. White MF. The IRS-signalling system: a network of docking proteins that mediate insulin action. *Mol Cell Biochem* 1998;182(1-2):3-11.

54. Fujisawa T, Endo H, Tomimoto A, Sugiyama M, Takahashi H, Saito S, et al. Adiponectin suppresses colorectal carcinogenesis under the high-fat diet condition. *Gut* 2008;57(11):1531-8.

55. Scherer PE, Williams S, Fogliano M, Baldini G, Lodish HF. A novel serum protein similar to C1q, produced exclusively in adipocytes. *J Biol Chem* 1995;270(45):26746-9.

56. Osei K, Gaillard T, Schuster D. Plasma adiponectin levels in high risk African-Americans with normal glucose tolerance, impaired glucose tolerance, and type 2 diabetes. *Obes Res* 2005;13(1):179-85.

57. Pereira RI, Snell-Bergeon JK, Erickson C, Schauer IE, Bergman BC, Rewers M, et al. Adiponectin dysregulation and insulin resistance in type 1 diabetes. *J Clin Endocrinol Metab* 2012;97(4):E642-7.

58. Maeda N, Takahashi M, Funahashi T, Kihara S, Nishizawa H, Kishida K, et al. PPARgamma ligands increase expression and plasma concentrations of adiponectin, an adipose derived protein. *Diabetes* 2001;50(9):2094-9.

59. Spranger J, Kroke A, Mohlig M, Bergmann MM, Ristow M, Boeing H, et al. Adiponectin and protection against type 2 diabetes mellitus. *Lancet* 2002;361(9353):226-8.

60. Fredholm BB. Adenosine, an endogenous distress signal, modulates tissue damage and repair. *Cell Death Differ* 2007;14(7):1315-23.

61. Johnston-Cox H, Koupenova M, Yang D, Corkey B, Gokce N, Farb MG, et al. The A2b adenosine receptor modulates glucose homeostasis and obesity. *PloS one* 2012;7(7):e40584.

62. Niederau C, Liddle RA, Williams JA, Grendell JH. Pancreatic growth: interaction of exogenous cholecystokinin, a protease inhibitor, and a cholecystokinin receptor antagonist in mice. *Gut* 1987;28 Suppl:63-9.

63. Solomon TE, Vanier M, Morisset J. Cell site and time course of DNA synthesis in pancreas after caerulein and secretin. *Am J Physiol* 1983;245(1):G99-105.

64. Wisner JR, Jr., Mclaughlin RE, Rich KA, Ozawa S, Renner IG. Effects of L-364,718, a new cholecystokinin receptor antagonist, on camostate-induced growth of the rat pancreas. *Gastroenterology* 1988;94(1):109-13.

65. Sato N, Suzuki S, Kanai S, Ohta M, Jimi A, Noda T, et al. Different effects of oral administration of synthetic trypsin inhibitor on the pancreas between cholecystokinin-A receptor gene knockout mice and wild type mice. *Jpn J Pharmacol* 2002;89(3):290-5.

66. Gurda GT, Guo L, Lee SH, Molkentin JD, Williams JA. Cholecystokinin activates pancreatic calcineurin-NFAT signaling in vitro and in vivo. *Mol Bio Cell* 2008;19(1):198-206.

67. Horvath B, Mukhopadhyay P, Hasko G, Pacher P. The endocannabinoid system and plant-derived cannabinoids in diabetes and diabetic complications. *Am J Pathol* 2012;180(2):432-42.

68. Weiss L, Zeira M, Reich S, Har-Noy M, Mechoulam R, Slavin S, et al. Cannabidiol lowers

incidence of diabetes in non-obese diabetic mice. *Autoimmunity* 2006;39(2):143-51.

69. O'sullivan SE. Cannabinoids go nuclear: evidence for activation of peroxisome proliferator-activated receptors. *Br J Pharmacol* 2007;152(5):576-82.

70. Scheen AJ. The endocannabinoid system: a promising target for the management of type 2 diabetes. *Curr Protein Pept Sci* 2009;10(1):56-74.

71. Khandwala HM, McCutcheon IE, Flyvbjerg A, Friend KE. The effects of insulin-like growth factors on tumorigenesis and neoplastic growth. *Endocr Rev* 2000;21(3):215-44.

72. Kido Y, Nakae J, Hribal ML, Xuan S, Efstratiadis A, Accili D. Effects of mutations in the insulin-like growth factor signaling system on embryonic pancreas development and beta-cell compensation to insulin resistance. *J Biol Chem* 2002;277(39):36740-7.

73. Jacob R, Barrett E, Plewe G, Fagin KD, Sherwin RS. Acute effects of insulin-like growth factor I on glucose and amino acid metabolism in the awake fasted rat. Comparison with insulin. *J Clin Invest* 1989;83(5):1717-23.

74. Renshaw D, Hinson JP. Neuropeptide Y and the adrenal gland: a review. *Peptides* 2001;22(3):429-38.

75. Sainsbury A, Schwarzer C, Couzens M, Herzog H. Y2 receptor deletion attenuates the type 2 diabetic syndrome of ob/ob mice. *Diabetes* 2002;51(12):3420-7.

76. Dasu MR, Ramirez S, Isseroff RR. Toll-like receptors and diabetes: a therapeutic perspective. *Clin Sci (Lond)* 2012;122(5):203-14.

77. Browning LM, Jebb SA, Mishra GD, Cooke JH, O'connell MA, Crook MA, et al. Elevated sialic acid, but not CRP, predicts features of the metabolic syndrome independently of BMI in women. *Int J Obes Relat Metab Disord* 2004;28(8):1004-10.

78. Wagner H. Endogenous TLR ligands and autoimmunity. *Adv Immunol* 2006;91:159-73.

79. Tsan MF, Gao B. Endogenous ligands of Toll-like receptors. *J Leukoc Biol* 2004;76(3):514-9.

80. Taylor KR, Trowbridge JM, Rudisill JA, Termeer CC, Simon JC, Gallo RL. Hyaluronan fragments stimulate endothelial recognition of injury through TLR4. *J Biol Chem* 2004;279(17):17079-84.

81. Osterloh A, Breloer M. Heat shock proteins: linking danger and pathogen recognition. *Med Microbiol Immunol* 2008;197(1):1-8.

82. Chiu YC, Lin CY, Chen CP, Huang KC, Tong KM, Tzeng CY, et al. Peptidoglycan enhances IL-6 production in human synovial fibroblasts via TLR2 receptor, focal adhesion kinase, Akt, and AP-1-dependent pathway. *J Immunol* 2009;183(4):2785-92.

83. Hreggvidsdottir HS, Ostberg T, Wahamaa H, Schierbeck H, Aveberger AC, Klevenvall L, et al. The alarmin HMGB1 acts in synergy with endogenous and exogenous danger signals to promote inflammation. *J Leukoc Biol* 2009;86(3):655-62.

84. Kim HS, Han MS, Chung KW, Kim S, Kim E, Kim MJ, et al. Toll-like receptor 2 senses beta-cell death and contributes to the initiation of autoimmune diabetes. *Immunity* 2007;27(2):321-33.

85. Yan SF, Ramasamy R, Schmidt AM. Mechanisms of disease: advanced glycation end-products and their receptor in inflammation and diabetes complications. *Nat Clin Pract Endocrinol Metab* 2008;4(5):285-93.

86. Song MJ, Kim KH, Yoon JM, Kim JB. Activation of Toll-like receptor 4 is associated with insulin resistance in adipocytes. *Biochem Biophys Res Commun* 2006;346(3):739-45.

87. Dasu MR, Thangappan RK, Bourgette A, Dipietro LA, Isseroff R, Jialal I. TLR2 expression and signaling-dependent inflammation impair wound healing in diabetic mice. *Lab Invest* 2010;90(11):1628-36.

88. Vats RK, Kumar V, Kothari A, Mital A, Ramachandran U. Emerging targets for diabetes. *Curr Sci* 2005;88:241-9.

89. Reddy SV, Chakshusmathi G, Narasu LM. Small Molecule Inhibitors of PTP1B and TCPTP. *Int J Pharm Phytopharmacol Res* 2012;1(5):287-91.

90. Johnson TO, Ermolieff J, Jirousek MR. Protein tyrosine phosphatase 1B inhibitors for Diabetes. *Nat Rev Drug Discov* 2002;1(9):696-709.

24

Induction of Apoptosis and Cytotoxic Activities of Iranian Orthodox Black Tea Extract (BTE) using in vitro Models

Amirala Aghbali[1,2], Faranak Moradi Abbasabadi[3], Abbas Delazar[1], Behzad Baradaran[1,4]*

[1] Drug Applied Research Center, Tabriz University of Medical Sciences, Tabriz, Iran.

[2] Department of Oral and Maxillofacial Pathology, Faculty of Dentistry, Tabriz University of Medical Sciences, Tabriz, Iran.

[3] Department of Oral and Maxillofacial Pathology, Faculty of Dentistry, Qom University of Medical Sciences, Qom, Iran.

[4] Immunology Research Center, Tabriz University of Medical Sciences, Tabriz, Iran.

ARTICLE INFO

Keywords:
Cytotoxic
Apoptosis
Anticancer
Oral squamous cell carcinoma
Iranian orthodox black tea extract

ABSTRACT

Purpose: Plant-derivate therapeutic agents can perform cancer chemotherapeutic activity through triggering apoptotic cell death. Our aim was to investigate the cytotoxic effects, induction of apoptosis, and the mechanism of cell death of Iranian orthodox black tea extracts (BTEs) and hydro methanolic purified fractions (40, 60, 80 and 100%) in KB cells (oral squamous cell carcinoma).

Methods: In order to analyze the cytotoxic activity of the BTEs, MTT (3-(4, 5-dimetylthiazol-2-yl)-2, 5 diphenyltetrazolium bromide) and Trypan-blue assays were performed in oral squamous cell carcinoma (KB). Furthermore, the apoptosis inducing action of the extracts was determined by TUNEL, DNA fragmentation and cell death detection analysis.

Results: Dichloromethane BTE and hydro methanol fractions (40 and 60%) extract showed no cytotoxic effects; however, hydro methanol crude and hydro methanol fractions of BTE (80 and 100%) significantly inhibited cell growth and viability in a dose and time dependent manner. In addition, Cell death assay, TUNEL, and DNA fragmentation indicated induction of apoptosis by hydro methanol 80 and 100% fractions of BTE in KB cells. Statistical significance was determined by analysis of variance (ANOVA), followed by Duncan test and p value ≤0.05 was considered significant.

Conclusion: The results from the present study suggests that the hydro methanol crude and hydro methanol fractions of BTE (80 and 100%) are significant source of compounds with the anti proliferative and cytotoxic activities, and this may be useful for developing potential chemo preventive substances.

Introduction

Oral squamous cell carcinoma (OSCC), which is a knotty health setback, leads to a wide range of mortality and morbidity in developing countries.[1] Conventional therapeutic modalities (e.g., surgery, radiotherapy, chemotherapy and drugs) have been utilized for tackling OSCC. In spite of advances in surgery and radiotherapy, these approaches cause unwanted side effects by the non-specific targeting on both normal and cancer cells.[2] Currently, chemotherapy has been applied for oral cancer patients. For example, cisplatin-based chemo radiation has been used for loco regionally advanced head and neck SCC.[3]

One of the approaches used in drug discovery, is herbal medicine as an alternative cancer therapy due to their low toxicity or damage to normal cells. Most therapeutic agents exert their cancer chemotherapeutic activity by triggering apoptotic cell death.[4] Therefore, induction of apoptosis in tumor cells has become an indicator of the tumor treatment response in employing a plant derived-bioactive substance to reduce and control human mortality resulting from cancer. Individual cells in apoptosis, as a programmed cell suicide, are destroyed, while the integrity and architecture of surrounding tissue is preserved.[5]

Black Tea from the young tender leaves of *Camellia sinensis* (L) is one of the most popular non-alcoholic beverages in the world. In the recent decades, therapeutic effects of various type of tea has been revealed in many studies.[6] The chemical composition of Black tea includes poly phenols, alkaloids (caffeine, theophyllineand theobromine), amino acids, carbohydrates, proteins, chlorophyll, volatile

*Corresponding author: Behzad Baradaran, Assistant Professor of Immunology, Immunology Research Center, Tabriz University of Medical Sciences, Tabriz, Iran. Email: baradaranb@tbzmed.ac.ir

compounds, minerals, and trace elements.[7] The toxicity of Iranian orthodox black tea extract (BTE) has not been intensively studied yet. Accordingly, the toxicity of BTE was investigated in the present research. The objective of this study was to examine the *in vitro* cytotoxic activities of a wild Iranian orthodox black tea extracts (BTEs) and hydro methanolic purified fractions (40, 60, 80 and 100%) using a MTT cytotoxicity assay. The study also tested whether the mechanism of action involves induction of apoptosis. Cell death ELISA, TUNEL and DNA fragmentation gel agarose were employed to quantify the nucleosome production resulting from nuclear DNA fragmentation during apoptosis.

Materials and Methods
Preparation of extracts
For preparation of the hydro methanol extract of Iranian black tea, *Camellia sinensis*, Var sinensis leaves were collected from North of Iran, in April 2012. A voucher specimen was deposited at the Herbarium of the Faculty of Pharmacy, Tabriz University of Medical Sciences and processed in orthodox method. The leaves were washed, dried and ground to get powder using a blender. Extractions were performed in a Soxhlet apparatus with hydro methanol. The black tea extract (BTE) was concentrated by rotary evaporator (Heildolph, Germany) at about 45 °C and then dried in very low pressure. The dried extracts were stored at –20 °C. In order to localize the active fraction, hydro methanolic extract of Iranian orthodox BTE was purified using C18 cartridges (Sep-pack, Supelco), by gradient elution with Hydro methanol mixture (40%, 60%, 80 and 80% Hydro methanol) to give 4 fractions. Hydro methanol solvent was removed from fractions by using rotating evaporator at 35°C and distilled water was then added to the residues and the aqueous phases were lyophilized. The powdered fractions were stored at −20°C until use. Twenty mg of each extract and purified fractions (40, 60, 80 and 100%) were dissolved in 100 µL dimethyl sulfoxide (DMSO) and were diluted with RPMI-1640 medium. Then, test solutions were sterilized using 0.22 µm Syringe filters (Nunc, Denmark) and used as stock solution for further experiments.

Cell culture
KB cell (oral squamous cell carcinoma cell line and HUVEC (Human umbilical vein endothelial cells)) were purchased from National Cell Bank of Iran (Pasteur Institute, Tehran, Iran). Cells were grown in RPMI- 1640 medium (Sigma, Germany) supplemented with 10% fetal bovine serum (FBS) (Sigma, Germany), 100 U/ml penicillin and 100 µg/ml streptomycin (Sigma, Germany). The cells were then incubated in a humidified incubator containing 5% CO2 at 37 °C. At 80% confluence, cells were rinsed with PBS/0.5% EDTA and harvested from 25 cm² flasks using 0.25 % trypsin/ EDTA solution (Gibco, U.K). Then, the cells were sub cultured into 75cm2 flasks, 96-well plates or

6-well plates (Nunc, Denmark) according to our researches. The experiments were performed in triplicate.

MTT assay
Cytotoxicity of hydro methanolic extract from Iranian orthodox black tea extracts (BTEs) and hydro methanolic purified fractions (40, 60, 80, and 100%) were assessed in KB cells as well as HUVEC by measuring the amount of insoluble formazan formed in live cells based on the reduction of 3-(4, 5 dimethylthiazol-2-yl)-2, 5-diphenyltetrazolium bromide (MTT) salt (Roche Diagnostics GmbH, Germany) according to the manufacturer's protocol. The cells were seeded in 96-well plates with a density of 10^4 cells/well incubated for 24 h at 37°C and 5% CO2. The cells were treated with different concentrations of BTE extracts (50, 100, 150, 200, 300, 400, 500, 600 µg/ml) and 0.2 % (v/v) DMSO (Merck, Germany) as a negative control. After 24 h treatment, 50 µl of MTT labeling reagent (2µg/ml) was added to each well. The plates were incubated at 37°C in a humidified atmosphere with 5% CO2 for 4 hours. Thereafter, 100 µl of the solubilization solution was added to each well and followed by incubation overnight at 37°C to dissolve formazan crystals. Absorbance was ultimately read using an ELISA plate reader (Bio Teck, Germany) at a wavelength of 570 nm.[8] The percentage of cytotoxicity was calculated using the following equation:

$$\% \, Cytotoxicity = 1 - \frac{AB_T}{AB_N}$$

Where, AB_T and AB_N are mean absorbance of treated cells and negative control, respectively.

The dose-response curve was plotted and concentration which gave 50% inhibition of cell growth (IC50) was calculated. Concentration that inhibits 50% of cell viability was used as a parameter for cytotoxicity.

Trypan blue assay
Cell membrane integrity and direct counting of living and dead cells were evaluated by trypan blue dye exclusion. This dye does not enter living cells, but it passes through the membranes of dead cells. KB cells (10^4) in 96 well-plates were exposed to same different concentrations of Iranian orthodox black tea extracts (BTEs) and hydro methanolic purified fractions (40, 60, 80 and 100%) and 0.2 % (v/v) DMSO for 24 h. The medium was then removed from the wells, and the cells were washed with 200 µL of PBS. The cells were detached by adding100 µL of 0.5 % trypsin/EDTA. RPMI-1640 medium supplement with 10% FBS (50 µL) and 0.5 % trypan blue (50 µL) (Merck, Germany) were added to each well, and the plates were incubated for 5 min. Subsequently, a 20 µL aliquot was removed and placed on a Neubauer hemacytometer. The numbers of viable and nonviable cells were finally counted under a microscope. The number of viable cells was calculated according to the following formula:

$$\frac{\text{viable cell count} \times \text{dilution} \times 104}{n}$$

Where n is the number of hemacytometer squares that were counted. The percent viability was calculated as:

$$\frac{\text{viable cell count}}{\text{total cell count}} \times 100$$

Morphological changes of cells

After treating of cells with BTE, cells morphological appearance was observed under inverted microscopy. Morphologic alteration was considered including detachment, cell shrinkage, nuclear condensation, fragmentation, margination, cell blebbing and presence of apoptotic bodies.

Assessment of necrosis and apoptosis

Apoptosis and necrosis of cells were measured using the Cell Death Detection ELISA and a kit (Roche Diagnostics GmbH, Germany) that quantified histone associated DNA fragments (mono and oligonucleosomes). KB cells (10^4) were treated with the same different concentrations of hydro methanol and 80 and 100% fractions of BTE and 0.2 % (v/v) DMSO at 37°C for 24 hrs. The procedure was performed according to the manufacturer's protocol. Briefly, the culture supernatants and lysate of cells were prepared and incubated in the microtiter plate coated with anti-histone antibody. Subsequent to color development, the results were analyzed spectrophotometrically using an ELISA plate reader at 405 nm.[9]

TUNEL assay

DNA fragmentation was detected by terminal deoxy transferase (TdT)-mediated dUTP nick- end labeling (TUNEL) with the In Situ Cell Death Detection Kit, POD (Roche Diagnostics GmbH, Germany) as described by the manufacturer's protocol. Briefly, (1.5×10^5) KB cells were sub-cultured into 6 well-plates and incubated for 24 h at 37°C and 5% CO2. The cells were treated with hydro methanol 80 and 100% fractions of BTE at concentrations required for 50% inhibition of growth of KB cells (IC50) for 24h. Negative control cells were treated with the same final concentration of DMSO present in treated wells [0.2% (v/v)]. Having treated, the cells were fixed with 4% (w/v) paraformaldehyde in PBS (pH 7.4) for 1 h at room temperature and rinsed twice with PBS. Then, the fixed cells were incubated with blocking solution (3% H2O2 in methanol) for 10 min and rinsed with PBS. The cells were then incubated in permeabilisation solution (0.1% Triton X-100 in 0.1% sodium citrate) for 2 min on ice. Subsequently, 50 μl of reaction mixture containing TdT enzyme and nucleotide was added to the cells and they were all incubated for 1 h at 37°C. After washing three times with PBS, the slides were incubated with 50 μl converter-POD sterptavidin HRP solution for 30 min, and rinsed three times with PBS. Finally, the cells incubated with DAB and stained cells were analyzed with the light microscopy.[10]

DNA Fragmentation assay

Apoptosis has been characterized biochemically by the activation of a nuclear endonuclease that cleaves the DNA into multimers of 180-200 base pairs and can be visualized as an oligosomal ladder by standard agarose gel electrophoresis. KB cells were seeded in 6 wells plates and kept in CO2 incubator. KB cells were treated by hydro methanol and 80 and 100% fractions of BTE in IC50 concentrations (μg/ml) for 24 h. At the end of incubation period, the cells were centrifuged for 1000 rpm for 3 mins at 14°C. The pellet was re suspended in a lysis buffer (10 mM Tris-HCI, pH 8.0, 10 mM NaCl, I0 mM EDTA, 20mg/ml Proteinase K, 10% SDS), and incubated at 37°C. The pellet was dissolved in TE buffer (0.1 M Tris-HCl, pH 8.0, 10 mM EDTA). DNA samples were electrophoretically separated on 1.8 % agarose gel containing ethidium bromide (0.4μg/mL). DNA was visualized by a UV (302 nm) transilluminator. Untreated cells were used as control.[11]

Statistical analysis

All the data represented in this study were based on means ± SEM of three identical experiments made in three replicates. Statistical significance was determined by analysis of variance (ANOVA), followed by Duncan test. P value ≤ 0.05 was considered statistically significant. LC50 values were derived from prohibit analysis. All analyses were conducted using the SPSS 20.

Results

The cytotoxic effects of Iranian orthodox black tea extracts (BTEs) on the growth of oral squamous cell carcinoma (KB cell line) were determined by MTT and trypan blue assays shown in Figure 1 and 2. As illustrated in Figure 1, the treated cells with hydromethanol and 80 and 100% fractions of BTE exhibited significant decline in viability, in comparison with the untreated control cells. Moreover, the dichloromethane BTE and hydromethanol fractions (40 and 60%) extract had no cytotoxic effects on KB cell.

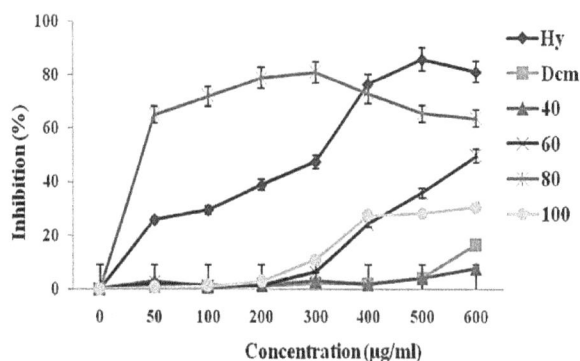

Figure 1. Effects of Iranian orthodox black tea extracts (BTEs) and hydromethanolic purified fractions (40, 60, 80 and 100%) with increasing concentrations (50–600 μg/mL) on proliferation of KB cells (b) for 24 h, the proliferative response was assessed by MTT assay.

Moreover, treatment of KB cells with hydro methanol crude and hydro methanol fractions of BTE (80 and 100%) showed cell growth inhibition in a time and dose dependent response. In the higher concentrations and longer time of the hydro methanol crude and hydro methanol 80% fractions of BTE treatment on KB cells, higher significant cytotoxicity was observed. Data analysis of cytotoxicity assay showed that IC50 (dose required for 50% inhibition) of hydro methanol crude and hydro methanol 80% fractions of BTE on KB cells were 446.08± 12.4 and 280.4 ± 33.1 μg/ml for 24 h, respectively.

Direct counting for viable cells using the trypan blue exclusion test showed that 86% hydro methanol BTE-treated cells with the highest concentration (600 μg/ml) absorbed the dye at 24 h (Figure 2).

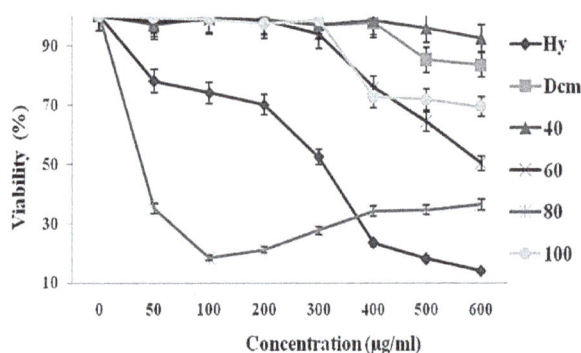

Figure 2. Results are expressed as the mean percentage of viable cells with 3 wells each. Percentage of viable cells was calculated from the ratio of viable cells to total number of cells using trypan blue exclusion test.

After incubation with IC50 of hydro methanol crude and hydro methanol 80 and 100% fractions of BTE, morphological alteration in KB cells were illustrated compared to the control cells (Figure 3). Sensitive cells were detached roundly from the surface. In order to determine the mechanism of the cytotoxic effects of hydro methanol and purified fractions (80 and 100%), apoptosis of cells were measured by cell death detection ELISA kit.

The ratio of apoptotic effect in hydro methanol and 80 and 100% purified fraction was 48%, 73% and 89%, respectively. In comparison with the hydro methanol and their fractions of BTE and the purified fractions extract induced the greatest apoptotic activity in KB cells.

One of the hallmarks of apoptotic cell death confirmed the presence of nucleosomal DNA fragments in cells treated with Iranian orthodox black tea extracts (BTEs) and hydro methanolic purified fractions (80 and 100%) by TUNEL assay. As shown in Figure 4, after the treatment of KB cells with 24 h IC50 concentration of hydro methanol BTE and their fractions, the apoptotic cells produced dark brown stained nuclei, whereas the non-apoptotic cells were not stained with similar observation was found in the negative control cells treated with 0.2% (v/v) DMSO.

As shown in agarose gel electrophoresis in Figure 5, increased DNA fragmentation was apparent in KB cells after treatment with 300 μg/ml (near to IC50) of BTE. Fragmented DNA was clearly observed in KB cells, whereas untreated cell did not provide ladders. Thereby, hydro methanol BTE and hydro methanolic purified fractions (80 and 100%) possibly cause apoptosis in KB cells.

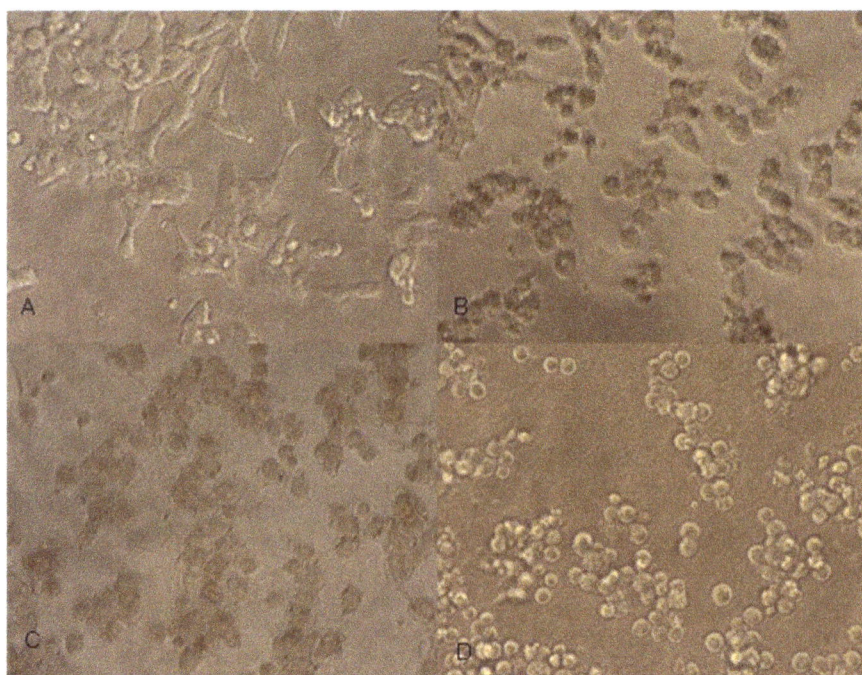

Figure 3. Morphological changes induced after incubation with IC50 of hydro methanol crude and hydro methanol 80 and 100% fractions of BTEon KB cells during 24 h treatment. (A) Untreated controls, (B) hydro methanol crude, (C) hydro methanol 80 and (D) 100% fractions of BTE.

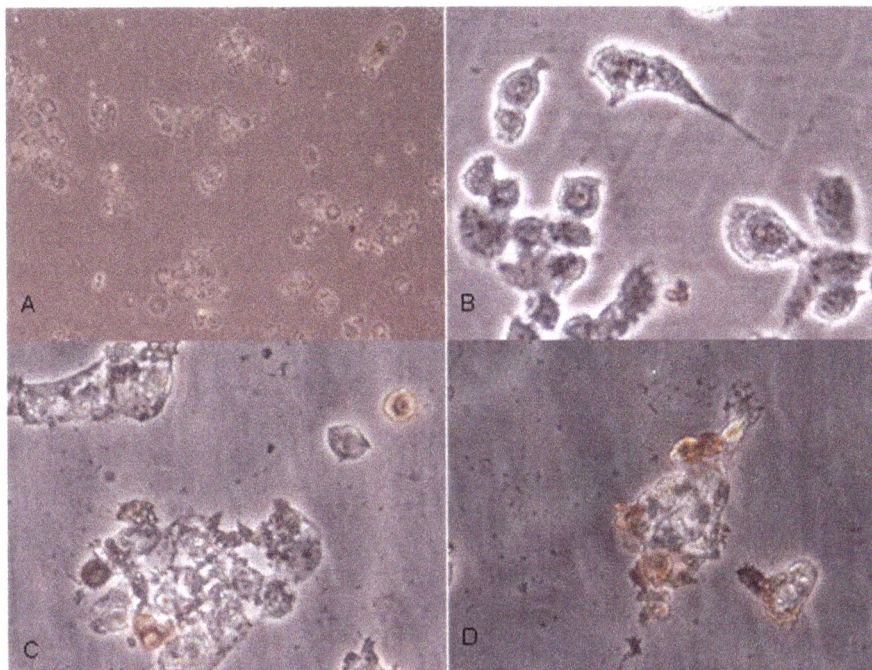

Figure 4. Nuclei morphological changes during hydro methanol BTE and hydro methanolic purified fractions (80 and 100%) induced apoptosis in KB cells detected by TUNEL assay. For KB cells, (a) shows negative control (without treatment) and (b) and (c, d) treated with extract (IC50) for 24 h (*n*: 3). (b), (c) and (d) indicate representative apoptotic cells with nuclei morphological changes.

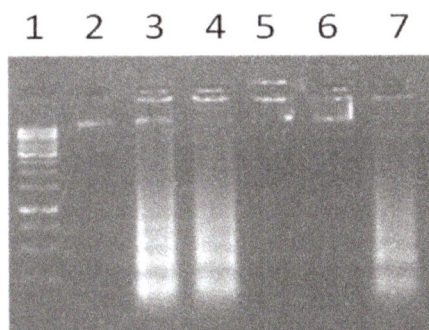

Figure 5. Analysis of DNA fragmentation using agarose gel electrophoresis. **KB** cells were incubated in the presence of IC50 of hydro methanol crude and hydro methanol 80 and 100% fractions of BTE on KB cells during 24 h treatment. Genomic DNA was prepared and analyzed by 2% agarose gel electrophoresis followed by ethidium bromide staining. Lanes show results from 1000 bp marker , Left side(lane 1), untreated sample (lane 2), hydromethanol100% fraction (lane 3), 80% fraction (lane 4), 60% fraction (lane 5), 40% fraction (lane 6), and hydro methanol crude (lane 7) of BTE. The figure is a representative of the results from three independent experiments.

Discussion

Recent in vitro studies have shown that many constituents from Iranian orthodox black tea extracts have a wide range of biological action including antibacterial and antifungal activities. The inhibitory action of the tea against experimental carcinogenesis has been demonstrated in many animal models, including those involving cancers of the lung, skin, esophagus, liver and stomach.[12] For example, the biological activities of purified tea polyphenols, strong growth inhibitory effects were investigated using human lung adenocarcinoma cell lines (NCI-H661,

NCI-H441 and NCIH1299) and a human colon cancer cell line (HT-29).[13] Growth inhibition was measured by [3H] thymidine incorporation after 48 h of treatment. In addition, the induction of apoptosis was investigated using the Apo Alert TM Annexin V and TUNEL methods.[13]

In the present study, the cytotoxic effects, induction of apoptosis, and the mechanism of cell death of Iranian orthodox black tea extracts (BTEs) and hydro methanolic purified fractions (40, 60, 80 and 100%) were investigated in KB cells (oral squamous cell carcinoma) in vitro. Hydro methanol crude and hydro methanol 80 and 100% fractions of BTE significantly inhibited oral squamous cell carcinoma cells after an incubation period of 24 h by MTT reduction assays. The dye exclusion assay showed a concentration-dependent decrease in percentage of cell viability and a 300 μg/ml concentration of BTE was sufficient to effectively inhibit the cell proliferation. To investigate whether apoptosis is involved in the cell death caused by hydro methanol crude and 80 and 100% fractions of BTE on KB cells, cell death detection ELISA, morphological changes, TUNEL, DNA ladder patterns on agarose gel electrophoresis were done. Morphological changes were observed by convert microscopy which exhibited cytoplasmic membrane, loss of contact with neighboring cells and membrane belbbing. TUNEL assay based on labeling of DNA strand breaks generated during apoptosis revealed that hydro methanol crude and 80 and 100% fractions of BTE induces apoptosis in KB cells. Due to degradation of DNA that resulted from the activation of Ca/ Mg-dependent endonucleases in apoptotic cells, DNA cleavage occurred and led to breaking of strand within the DNA. In addition, oligonucleosomal DNA fragment (ladders) from cells were exhibited by 1.8% agarose gel electrophoresis after incubation with IC50 of hydro methanol crude and 80 and 100% fractions of BTE. These hallmark features of morphological changes suggest that hydro methanol crude and 80 and 100% fractions of BTE caused apoptosis of KB oral squamous cell carcinoma cells.[14,15]

These probable properties of hydro methanol crude and 80 and 100% fractions of BTE need further detailed evaluation. In order to elucidate the cytotoxic activities of hydro methanol crude and 80 and 100% fractions of BTE extract on the growth of different cell lines may become the target cells used in our future studies. In addition, mechanistic studies on cell cycle arrest and early apoptotic events may be conducted to delineate other possible anti-tumor mechanisms of the hydro methanol crude and 80 and 100% fractions of BTE extract. Besides, future in vivo anti-tumor studies are suggested in order to confirm these in vitro results.

Conclusion

In conclusion, the present study, perhaps for the first time, showed cytotoxicity of Iranian orthodox black tea extracts in oral squamous cell carcinoma in which apoptosis or programmed cell death plays an important role. In addition, mechanisms underlying this cytotoxicity were further clarified. Iranian orthodox black tea extracts could be also considered as a promising chemotherapeutic agent in cancer treatment.

Conflict of Interest

The authors report no conflicts of interest.

References

1. Bagan JV, Scully C. Recent advances in Oral Oncology 2007: epidemiology, aetiopathogenesis, diagnosis and prognostication. *Oral Oncol* 2008;44(2):103-8.
2. Warnakulasuriya S. Global epidemiology of oral and oropharyngeal cancer. *Oral Oncol* 2009;45(4-5):309-16.
3. Mehrotra R, Yadav S. Oral squamous cell carcinoma: etiology, pathogenesis and prognostic value of genomic alterations. *Indian J Cancer* 2006;43(2):60-6.
4. Mehta RG, Murillo G, Naithani R, Peng X. Cancer chemoprevention by natural products: How far have we come? *Pharm Res* 2010;27(6):950-61.
5. Cragg GM, Newman DJ. Plants as a source of anticancer agents. *J Ethnopharmacol* 2005;100(1-2):72-9.
6. Yang CS, Wang ZY. Tea and cancer. *J Natl Cancer Inst* 1993;58(13):1038-49.
7. Katiyar SK, Mukhtar H. Tea in chemoprevention of cancer: epidemiological and experimental studies. *Int J Oncol* 1996;8:221-38.
8. Mosmann T. Rapid colorimetric assay for cellular growth and survival: application to proliferation and cytotoxicity assays. *J Immunol Methods* 1983;65(1-2):55-63.
9. Frankfurt OS, Krishan A. Enzyme-linked immunosorbent assay (ELISA) for the specific detection of apoptotic cells and its application to rapid drug screening. *J Immunol Methods* 2001;253(1-2):133-44.
10. Rogakou EP, Nieves-Neira W, Boon C, Pommier Y, Bonner WM. Initiation of DNA fragmentation during apoptosis induces phosphorylation of H2AX histone at serine 139. *J Biol Chem* 2000;275(13):9390-5.
11. Basnakian AG, James SJ. A rapid and sensitive assay for the detection of DNA fragmentation during early phases of apoptosis. *Nucleic Acids Res* 1994;22(13):2714-5.
12. Bhattacharyya A, Choudhuri T, Pal S, Chattopadhyay S, K Datta G, Sa G, et al. Apoptogenic effects of black tea on Ehrlich's ascites carcinoma cell. *Carcinogenesis* 2003;24(1):75-80.
13. Yang GY, Liao J, Kim K, Yurkow EJ, Yang CS. Inhibition of growth and induction of apoptosis in human cancer cell lines by tea polyphenols. *Carcinogenesis* 1998;19(4):611-6.
14. Hanahan D, Weinberg RA. The hallmarks of cancer. *Cell* 2000;100(1):57-70.
15. Brown JM, Attardi LD. The role of apoptosis in cancer development and treatment response. *Nat Rev Cancer* 2005;5(3):231-7.

25

Perindopril may Improve the Hippocampal Reduced Glutathione Content in Rats

Tahereh Mashhoody[1], Karim Rastegar[1], Fatemeh Zal[2,3]*

[1] Physiology Department, School of Medicine, Shiraz University of Medical Sciences, Shiraz, Iran.

[2] Reproductive Biology Department, School of Advanced Medical Sciences and Technologies, Shiraz University of Medical Sciences, Shiraz, Iran.

[3] Infertility Research Center, Shiraz University of Medical Sciences, Shiraz, Iran.

ARTICLE INFO

Keywords:
ACE inhibitor
Rat
Perindopril
Glutathione
Hippocampus

ABSTRACT

Purpose: Oxidative stress and renin- angiotensin system are both involved in the pathophysiology of most of the systemic and central disorders as well as in aging. Angiotensin converting enzyme (ACE) inhibitors, well known for their cardiovascular beneficial effects, have also shown antioxidant properties in pathologic conditions. This study aimed to evaluate the central effect of ACE inhibitors on oxidative status under no pathologic condition.

Methods: Adult male rats were divided into four groups of 9 rats each. Groups were treated orally by perindopril at the doses of 1, 2, 4 mg/kg/day or normal saline as the control for four consecutive weeks. At the end of the treatment period the reduced and oxidized glutathione (GSH and GSSG respectively) and malondialdehyde (MDA), the product of lipid peroxidation, were measured in the rats' hippocampus.

Results: The GSH increased dose dependently and was significantly higher in the 2 mg/kg perindopril treated group than the control group ($p < 0.05$) while the GSSG level remained unchanged. As a consequent, the ratio of GSH to GSSG increased significantly in a dose dependent manner. There was not any significant change in MDA.

Conclusion: This study demonstrated that ACE inhibition may cause an increase in GSH as an anti- oxidant defense in the hippocampus.

Introduction

Free radicals generated mainly from mitochondria induce oxidative stress, being involved in pathogenesis of several organ diseases. In the central nervous system, oxidative stress was found to be associated with a lot of brain disorders such as, depression,[1] mental disorders due to severe life stress,[2] Parkinson's and Alzheimer's diseases.[3,4] In addition, oxidative stress is a well-documented cause of tissue damages leading to aging.[5] Oxidative stress also hypothesized to lie in the upstream of neurodegenerative processes ending in Parkinson's and Alzheimer's diseases during normal life time.[6]

Angiotensin converting enzyme (ACE) inhibitors are common drugs used in treatment of hypertension and heart failure. They reduced high blood pressure and vascular resistance by decreasing angiotensin II (Ang II) production.[7] Due to the existence of a unique renin-angiotensin system in the brain, ACE inhibitors have recently revealed neuroprotective effects in the central nervous system disorders including neurodegenerative diseases.[8-10] In some tissues including the brain, it has been found that ACE inhibitors interfere with oxidative damages induced experimentally.[11,12] However, to date it is not clear if the oxidative status under normal circumstances can also be affected by ACE inhibitors. Chronically administration of ACE inhibitors demonstrated through unknown mechanism an improvement in learning and memory of rats.[13] Considering the unknown mechanisms of ACE on improvement of physiologic behavioral functions like learning and memory,[13] together with the existence of oxidative stress in the upstream of neurodegenerative processes leading to aging,[5] Alzheimer's and Parkinson's diseases,[6] this study aimed to evaluate the basal oxidative status and anti-oxidant defense of neuronal tissue under ACE inhibition. For this purpose, we chronically administered different doses of perindopril to adult male rats and analyzed the oxidative parameters in their hippocampus.

Materials and Methods
Chemicals
Tricloroacetic acid (TCA), 2,3 thiobarbitoric acid (TBA), 1, 1, 3, 3-tetraethoxy propane (TEP), Coomassie brilliant

*Corresponding author: Fatemeh Zal, School of Advanced Medical Sciences and Technologies, Shiraz University of Medical Sciences, Shiraz, Iran. Postal code: 7134845794, Email: zalf@sums.ac.ir

blue G-250, bovine serum albumin (BSA), and phosphate buffer saline (PBS) tablets were purchased from Sigma-Aldrich St. Louis, MO, USA. Ellman's reagent (5-5'-dithiobis-(2-nitrobenzoic acid; DTNB), NADPH, reductase, scavenger, glutathione standard, meta phosphoric acid, and assay buffer provided by a Reduced/Oxidized Glutathione Cuvette Assay kit # GSH39-K01 purchased from Eagle Biosciences Inc., Boston, USA. Other chemicals were commercially available.

Animals

Male Sprague–Dawley rats aging three to four months were obtained from Animal Care Center of Shiraz University of Medical Sciences. The rats were housed two per cage under controlled (12 h/12 h) light/dark cycle and constant temperature of 24±2 °C; they had free access to food and water. All experiments were carried out during the light phase and in accordance to the guideline of the animal ethics committee of Shiraz University of Medical Sciences.

Drug treatments

The rats were randomly divided into four groups containing nine animals each. Test groups received perindopril (Coversyl®, Servier, Cedex, France) at a dose of 1, 2 or 4 mg/kg/ml. Control group received normal saline at the same volume. Drugs were administered orally via an intragastric gavage tube once daily for four consecutive weeks.

Tissue preparation

The rats were decapitated under light ether anesthesia. The skull was cut open and the whole brain was quickly removed. The hippocampi were dissected and cleaned with chilled normal saline on the ice, frozen quickly in liquid nitrogen and stored separately under -70 °C for future use.

Biochemical assay

Estimation of malondialdehyde (MDA) and protein

One of the right or left hippocampus of each rat was selected randomly (n=9) and homogenized in 10% (w/v) of PBS (pH 7.4) with an ultrasonic homogenizer (BANDELIN, Sonoplus, Berlin) for 20 seconds with 3/2 seconds on/off periods. The homogenate was centrifuged at 10000 g for 20 min at 4°C and the supernatant was used for the measurement of MDA and protein. The concentration of protein in the supernatant was measured by spectrophotometer at 595 nm by the Coomassie brilliant blue G-250 dye-binding technique of Bradford[14] using serial dilution of BSA (1mg/1ml) as standard.

MDA as a marker of lipid peroxidation was estimated according to its reaction with TBA as a TBA reactive substance[15] with modification. Briefly, 0.5 ml of the supernatant was added to 2 ml TBA reagent containing 0.375% TBA, 15% TCA and 0.25 mol/L HCl. The mixture was boiled in a water bath at 95°C for 30 minutes and after fast cooling it was centrifuged at 8000 g for 15 min at 4°C. The absorbance of the pink color supernatant

was measured at 532 nm. MDA concentration was calculated using TEP as standard and expressed as nmol/mg protein.

Glutathione analyses

The second hippocampus of the corresponding rat (n=7) was weighed precisely and homogenized the same way as that for MDA. The reduced and the oxidized glutathione content, GSH and GSSG respectively, and the ratio of GSH to GSSG were measured according to an eagle bioscience GSH/GSSG cuvette assay kit. Briefly, two samples were prepared from the homogenate, one for GSH and the second mixed with scavenger for GSSG assessment. After protein denaturation by metaphosphoric acid, the samples were centrifuged at 10000 g for 10 minutes at 4°C and the supernatant was diluted with assay buffer. The samples were then mixed with DTNB, reductase and NADPH at equal volumes (200μL) to yield a yellowish color as a result of thiol-DTNB enzymatic reaction. The absorbance was measured kinetically at 412 nm for 5 minutes. The glutathione concentrations were calculated using GSH and GSSG standard curves and the ratio of GSH/GSSG was calculated by (GSH-2*GSSG)/GSSG equation. All reagents and formulas were provided by the kit. The results were expressed as μmol/ gram wet tissue.

Data analysis

All statistical analyses were performed by SPSS version 15. Data were presented as mean ±SEM. Because of the normal distribution of data confirmed by Kolmogrov Esmirnov test; comparisons between the studied groups were made using one way ANOVA followed by Tukey's post hoc test. The P values less than 0.05 were considered as significant.

Results

Table 1 shows the results of GSH and GSSG analyses in the hippocampus of perindopril and normal saline treated rats. The data indicate that treatment of rats with perindopril induced enhancement of GSH in a dose dependent manner [$F (3, 24) = 4.34$ P=0.014] that was significantly about 66.6 % higher (p<0.01) in 2 mg/kg perindopril treated group in comparison to the control rats.

Table 1. Effect of normal saline (N/S) or perindopril (P) on GSH and GSSG

Treatments	GSH(μMol/mg tissue)	GSSG(μMol/mg tissue)
N/S as control	1.8±0.2	0.04±0.004
P 1 mg/kg	2.5±0.2	0.04±0.005
P 2 mg/kg	3±0.25*	0.035±0.003
P 4 mg/kg	2.6±0.25	0.04±0.005

Effect of perindopril (P 1, 2, 4 mg/kg/day orally) compared to normal saline (N/S) as controlon GSH and GSSG (n= 7). Results are expressed as mean± SEM and data were analyzed by one way ANOVA followed by Tukey multiple comparison test. * Significantly different from the control, *p<0.05*

On the other hand the data in Table 1 demonstrate that the GSSG level remained unchanged in all groups as compared to the control groups [F (3,24)= 0.74 P=0.538]. Therefore the GSH/GSSG ratio showed a significant increase [F (3,24) = 3.16 P=0.043] as an antioxidant marker and this ratio was higher in 2 mg/kg perindopril treated group, showing 82.8 % enhancement as compared to the control group (P<0.05) as shown in Figure 1.

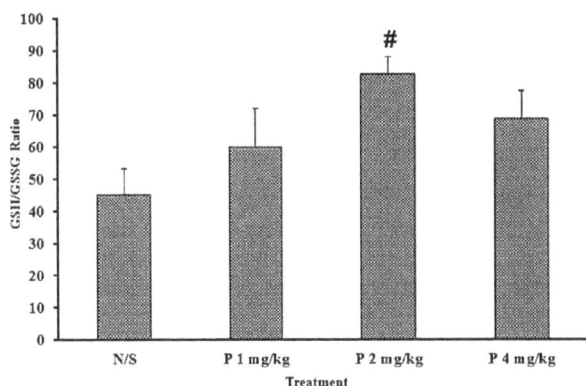

Figure 1. Effect of perindopril (P 1, 2, 4 mg/kg/day orally) compared to normal saline (N/S) as control on GSH/GSSG ratio (n= 7). Results are expressed as mean± SEM and data were analyzed by one way ANOVA followed by Tukey multiple comparison test. # Significantly different from the control, *p<0.05*

The data in Figure 2 demonstrate that treatment of normal rats with perindopril recorded an insignificant reduction in brain MDA level [F (3, 30) = 1.693, P=0.19] from 2.6±0.5 in control group to 1.7±0.2 in 1 mg/kg perindopril treated group. However the MDA level rises again, although not significant, to 2.9±0.4 in 4 mg/kg perindopril treated group.

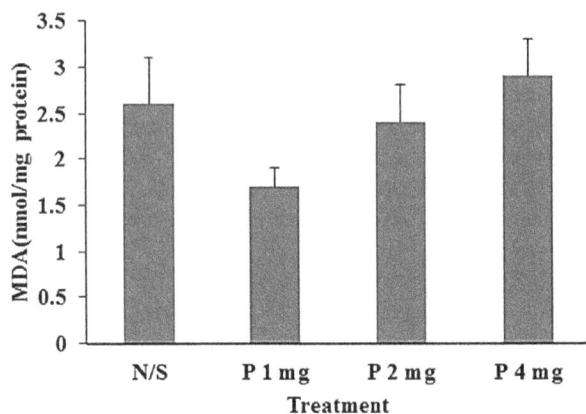

Figure 2. Effect of perindopril (P 1, 2, 4 mg/kg/day orally) compared to normal saline (N/S) as control on MDA (n=8-9). Results are expressed as mean± SEM and data were analyzed by one way ANOVA followed by Tukey multiple comparison test.

Discussion
In the present study GSH and GSH/GSSG ratio increased dose dependently in the hippocampus of

perindopril treated groups. Brain is a susceptible organ to oxidative stress due to high metabolic rate, high poly-unsaturated fatty acids and low antioxidant demand.[16] To combat with oxidative conditions the cells are provided with several antioxidants such as GSH which is a major and strong intracellular antioxidant. GSH acts as a donor of electron to free radicals, giving rise to GSSG which then reduced and recycled again to GSH through enzymatic reactions.[17] GSH also acts as a scavenger of reactive oxygen species (ROS) and an inhibitor of H_2O_2-induced hydroxyl radical formation. Thereby, GSH and the GSH/GSSG ratio levels determine the defensive potency of the cells against oxidative stress in tissues like the brain.[18]

The glutathione analysis technique in this study support directly analysis of both reduced and oxidized glutathione. Previous studies showed that the inappropriate changes of total or oxidized glutathione recovered by ACE inhibitors such as ramipril or captopril in the experimentally models of oxidative damages.[12,19] In our study although perindopril did not exert any beneficial effect on physiologic amount of GSSG, but it suggested that even physiologic amounts of GSH, the reduced form, may increase in response to ACE inhibitors. In the current study, all of the perindopril –treated groups showed higher amounts of GSH and GSH/GSSG ratio. However, a significant rise was only seen in 2 mg/kg perindopril-treated group indicating that there might be an optimum dose for perindopril to effectively cause an increase in the reduced glutathione level.

An insignificant decrease was observed in MDA analysis which was recovered as the dose of perindopril increased. MDA, a by-product of lipid peroxidation, is a major biomarker of the membrane lipid peroxidation by excessive ROS in the brain tissue that composes high poly unsaturated fatty acids.[16] In the oxidative condition induced by chronic cerebral hypoperfusion in rats, the elevated MDA decreased after captopril treatment.[11] In the present study there was also a tendency for MDA to be lessened in 1 mg/kg perindopril treated group. MDA then increased progressively to a higher level than control in 4 mg/kg perindopril treated group, indicating a probable dual action of perindopril: the antioxidant effects at low doses and oxidative effects at high doses. The insignificant decrease in GSH level in 4 mg/kg perindopril treated group, in accordance with enhancement of MDA level at 4 mg//kg perindopril treated group, also may result from conversion of benefit to toxic effects of perindopril through increasing the dose that should be confirmed by further studies.

In another point of view, the insignificant alteration in MDA and GSSG in this study may also indicate first: under physiologic condition, the basal lipid peroxidation may be continued normally and might not be changed prominently by perindopril. Second: the increase of reduced glutathione may not be the outcome of a compensatory response to increased free radicals as indicated previously,[20] but it is potentially an improvement in anti-oxidant defense in response to perindopril. This may strengthen the antioxidant pool of the tissues like the brain as a sensitive organ to oxidative stress.

The main mechanism by which perindopril caused the increase of reduced glutathione in this study might be the inhibition of ACE. Hippocampus is a large structure in the brain and involved in advanced brain functions like learning and memory.[21] It has been found to possess all of the renin-angiotensin components including ACE, which is abundant both in the vessels and neuronal cells, its active product, angiotensin II, and all of the angiotensin receptors.[22] Perindopril is a lipophilic brain penetrating ACE inhibitor with an effective potency of ACE inhibition in structures like hippocampus. In this study we used the similar doses of perindopril which have been demonstrated previously to inhibit more than 50% of hippocampal ACE.[10,23]

ACE inhibition by perindopril in turn leads to attenuation of Ang II formation and AT1 receptor expression.[11] Ang II through stimulation of AT1 receptor exerts its potent vasoconstrictory activity.[7] Circulatory disturbance, as seen in hypo-perfusion or ischemia reperfusion, resulted in severe oxidative stress in several tissues as well as the brain.[12,24,25] Therefore, ACE inhibition may lead to better circulation and prevent minor oxidative stresses caused by transient vasoconstrictions that may happen during normal life or probably during one month treating with perindopril in this study. Attenuation of Ang II by ACE inhibition, additionally, may diminish the activation of NADPH oxidase[26] which is a pivotal enzyme in the production of free radicals.[27] ACE inhibitors were also evidenced to directly act as a scavenger of free radicals.[28,29] All these mechanisms may lower the amount of free radicals and the consequent GSH consumption. On the other hand, ACE inhibitors was found to augment the activity of glutathione reductase, the enzyme that catalyze recycling of GSSG to GSH[19] and may result in more GSH production. Further studies should address this issue and also the probable effect of ACE inhibitors on the activity of the enzymes that catalyze GSH synthesis reactions and/ or intestinal absorption of GSH which are other GSH supplementary pathways.[30]

Conclusion
This study reports that ACE inhibition can improve the cellular anti-oxidant defense and may suggest ACE inhibitors, especially those that penetrate blood-brain barrier, as worthy drugs for prevention of neural damages induced by oxidative stress.

Acknowledgments
The results described in this paper were part of student thesis written by Tahereh Mashhoody and was financially supported by the office of Vice Chancellor of Research Affair, Shiraz University of Medical Sciences (Grant No. 89-5231).

Conflict of Interest
The authors declare that they have no conflict of interest.

Abbreviations
Angiotensin II (Ang II), Angiotensin converting enzyme (ACE), malondialdehyde (MDA), reduced (GSH), oxidized glutathione (GSSG), angiotensin (Ang II), Tricloroacetic acid (TCA), thiobarbitoric acid (TBA), 1, 1, 3, 3-tetraethoxy propane (TEP), Ang II type1 (AT1)

References
1. Wang C, Wu HM, Jing XR, Meng Q, Liu B, Zhang H, et al. Oxidative parameters in the rat brain of chronic mild stress model for depression: relation to anhedonia-like responses. *J Membr Biol* 2012;245(11):675-81.
2. Schiavone S, Jaquet V, Trabace L, Krause KH. Severe life stress and oxidative stress in the brain: from animal models to human pathology. *Antioxid Redox Signal* 2013;18(12):1475-90.
3. Kumar H, Lim HW, More SV, Kim BW, Koppula S, Kim IS, et al. The role of free radicals in the aging brain and Parkinson's disease: convergence and parallelism. *Int J Mol Sci* 2012;13(8):10478-504.
4. Gandhi S, Abramov AY. Mechanism of oxidative stress in neurodegeneration. *Oxid Med Cell Longev* 2012;2012:428010.
5. Labunskyy VM, Gladyshev VN. Role of Reactive Oxygen Species-Mediated Signaling in Aging. *Antioxid Redox Signal* 2012.
6. Federico A, Cardaioli E, Da Pozzo P, Formichi P, Gallus GN, Radi E. Mitochondria, oxidative stress and neurodegeneration. *J Neurol Sci* 2012;322(1-2):254-62.
7. Ruilope LM, Rosei EA, Bakris GL, Mancia G, Poulter NR, Taddei S, et al. Angiotensin receptor blockers: therapeutic targets and cardiovascular protection. *Blood Press* 2005;14(4):196-209.
8. Mertens B, Vanderheyden P, Michotte Y, Sarre S. The role of the central renin-angiotensin system in Parkinson's disease. *J Renin Angiotensin Aldosterone Syst* 2010;11(1):49-56.
9. Duron E, Hanon O. Antihypertensive treatments, cognitive decline, and dementia. *J Alzheimers Dis* 2010;20(3):903-14.
10. Yamada K, Uchida S, Takahashi S, Takayama M, Nagata Y, Suzuki N, et al. Effect of a centrally active angiotensin-converting enzyme inhibitor, perindopril, on cognitive performance in a mouse model of Alzheimer's disease. *Brain Res* 2010;1352:176-86.
11. Kumaran D, Udayabanu M, Kumar M, Aneja R, Katyal A. Involvement of angiotensin converting enzyme in cerebral hypoperfusion induced

anterograde memory impairment and cholinergic dysfunction in rats. *Neuroscience* 2008;155(3):626-39.

12. Kim JS, Yun I, Choi YB, Lee KS, Kim YI. Ramipril protects from free radical induced white matter damage in chronic hypoperfusion in the rat. *J Clin Neurosci* 2008;15(2):174-8.

13. Jenkins TA, Chai SY. Effect of chronic angiotensin converting enzyme inhibition on spatial memory and anxiety-like behaviours in rats. *Neurobiol Learn Mem* 2007;87(2):218-24.

14. Bradford MM. A rapid and sensitive method for the quantitation of microgram quantities of protein utilizing the principle of protein-dye binding. *Anal Biochem* 1976;72:248-54.

15. Colado MI, O'shea E, Granados R, Misra A, Murray TK, Green AR. A study of the neurotoxic effect of MDMA ('ecstasy') on 5-HT neurones in the brains of mothers and neonates following administration of the drug during pregnancy. *Br J Pharmacol* 1997;121(4):827-33.

16. Evans PH. Free radicals in brain metabolism and pathology. *Br Med Bull* 1993;49(3):577-87.

17. Dringen R, Gutterer JM, Hirrlinger J. Glutathione metabolism in brain metabolic interaction between astrocytes and neurons in the defense against reactive oxygen species. *Eur J Biochem* 2000;267(16):4912-6.

18. Woltjer RL, Nghiem W, Maezawa I, Milatovic D, Vaisar T, Montine KS, et al. Role of glutathione in intracellular amyloid-alpha precursor protein/carboxy-terminal fragment aggregation and associated cytotoxicity. *J Neurochem* 2005;93(4):1047-56.

19. De Cavanagh EM, Inserra F, Ferder L, Fraga CG. Enalapril and captopril enhance glutathione-dependent antioxidant defenses in mouse tissues. *Am J Physiol Regul Integr Comp Physiol* 2000;278(3):R572-7.

20. Sinha K, Degaonkar MN, Jagannathan NR, Gupta YK. Effect of melatonin on ischemia reperfusion injury induced by middle cerebral artery occlusion in rats. *Eur J Pharmacol* 2001;428(2):185-92.

21. Turgut YB, Turgut M. A mysterious term hippocampus involved in learning and memory. *Childs Nerv Syst* 2011;27(12):2023-5.

22. Von Bohlen Und Halbach O, Albrecht D. The CNS renin-angiotensin system. *Cell Tissue Res* 2006;326(2):599-616.

23. Jenkins TA, Mendelsohn FA, Chai SY. Angiotensin-converting enzyme modulates dopamine turnover in the striatum. *J Neurochem* 1997;68(3):1304-11.

24. Allen CL, Bayraktutan U. Oxidative stress and its role in the pathogenesis of ischaemic stroke. *Int J Stroke* 2009;4(6):461-70.

25. Wong CH, Crack PJ. Modulation of neuro-inflammation and vascular response by oxidative stress following cerebral ischemia-reperfusion injury. *Curr Med Chem* 2008;15(1):1-14.

26. Griendling KK, Minieri CA, Ollerenshaw JD, Alexander RW. Angiotensin II stimulates NADH and NADPH oxidase activity in cultured vascular smooth muscle cells. *Circ Res* 1994;74(6):1141-8.

27. Griendling KK, Sorescu D, Ushio-Fukai M. NAD(P)H oxidase: role in cardiovascular biology and disease. *Circ Res* 2000;86(5):494-501.

28. Suzuki S, Sato H, Shimada H, Takashima N, Arakawa M. Comparative free radical scavenging action of angiotensin-converting enzyme inhibitors with and without the sulfhydryl radical. *Pharmacology* 1993;47(1):61-5.

29. Mira ML, Silva MM, Queiroz MJ, Manso CF. Angiotensin converting enzyme inhibitors as oxygen free radical scavengers. *Free Radic Res Commun* 1993;19(3):173-81.

30. Sies H. Glutathione and its role in cellular functions. *Free Radic Biol Med* 1999;27(9-10):916-21.

26

Protective Effects of *Nigella sativa* on Metabolic Syndrome in Menopausal Women

Ramlah Mohamad Ibrahim[1], Nurul Syima Hamdan[1], Maznah Ismail[1,2], Suraini Mohd Saini[3], Saiful Nizam Abd Rashid[3], Latiffah Abd Latiff[4], Rozi Mahmud[3]*

[1] *Department of Nutrition and Dietetics, Faculty of Medicine and Health Sciences, Universiti Putra Malaysia, 43400 Serdang, Selangor Darul Ehsan, Malaysia.*

[2] *Nutrigenomic Programme, Laboratory of Molecular Biomedicine, Institute of Bioscience, Universiti Putra Malaysia, 43400 Serdang, Selangor Darul Ehsan, Malaysia.*

[3] *Department of Imaging, Faculty of Medicine and Health Sciences, Universiti Putra Malaysia, 43400 Serdang, Selangor Darul Ehsan, Malaysia.*

[4] *Department of Community Health, Faculty of Medicine and Health Sciences, Universiti Putra Malaysia, 43400 Serdang, Selangor Darul Ehsan, Malaysia.*

ARTICLE INFO

Keywords:
Nigella sativa
Menopause
Metabolic syndrome
Hyperlipidemic
Hyperglycemia

ABSTRACT

Purpose: This study was conducted in menopausal women to determine the metabolic impact of *Nigella sativa.*

Methods: Thirty subjects who were menopausal women within the age limit of 45-60 were participated in this study and randomly allotted into two experimental groups. The treatment group was orally administered with *N. sativa* seeds powder in the form of capsules at a dose of 1g per day after breakfast for period of two months and compared to control group given placebo. Anthropometric and biochemical parameters were measured at baseline, 1st month, 2nd month and a month after treatment completed to determine their body weight, serum lipid profile and fasting blood glucose (FBG).

Results: The treatment group showed slight reduction with no significant difference in body weight changes of the respondents. However, significant ($p<0.05$) improvement was observed in total cholesterol (TC), triglycerides (TG), low density lipoprotein cholesterol (LDL-C), high density lipoprotein cholesterol (HDL-C), and blood glucose ($p<0.05$).

Conclusion: These results suggested that treatment with *N. sativa* exert a protective effect by improving lipid profile and blood glucose which are in higher risk to be elevated during menopausal period.

Introduction

Menopause is an important physiological event, with the cessation of menstruation indicating the end of a woman's reproductive lifespan.[1] Menopause is associated with a fall in estrogen levels which accompanied with many health changes. Changes in the hormone levels at menopause, in particular estrogen deficiency are associated with an increase in body fat.[2] Additionally, it sounds an alarm for women's health since it leads to elevated blood pressure, insulin resistance and dyslipidemia.[3] These changes may contribute to increased risks of metabolic syndrome (MetS) in menopause women. The features of the metabolic syndrome include the accumulation of visceral (abdominal) adiposity, insulin resistance, hypertension, and dyslipidemia (hypertriglyceridemia, reduced high density lipoprotein (HDL), and small dense LDL particles based on a set of diagnostic criteria suggested by National Cholesterol Education Program Adult Treatment Panel III (NCEP-ATP III).[4] To date, several previous studies found significant difference in prevalence of MetS among pre- and postmenopausal women.[5-8] The prevalence of MetS in menopausal women was found to be 36.7% in one of the states, Kelantan in Malaysia.[9]

Nowadays there is an increased demand for using plants in therapy instead of using synthetic drugs which may have adverse effects. Traditional medicinal plants are often cheaper, locally available, and easily consumable (raw or as simple medicinal preparations). The seeds of Nigella sativa (*N. sativa*) plant have been used to promote health and fight disease for centuries especially in the Middle East and Southeast Asia.[10]

*Corresponding author: Rozi Mahmud, Department of Imaging, Faculty of Medicine and Health Sciences, Universiti Putra Malaysia, Malaysia.
Email: rozi@medic.upm.edu.my

Locally, it is called Habattus Sauda and referred as Black cumin in English. This plant has been a great focus of research and has several traditional uses and consequently has been extensively studied for its chemical constituents and biological activities. A lot of studies have been done to determine the various activities of *N. sativa* on different components of the metabolic syndrome for example blood sugar, lipid profile, hypertension and etc.[11,12] In spite of large number of pharmacological studies carried out worldwide on *N. sativa* seeds, only few experimental studies have been done in menopausal women especially in Malaysia. Moreover, many Malaysian women were consuming *N. sativa* in the form of coffee mix, oil products as a source of supplement which they believe can help to boost energy level. However, not many aware neither the actual benefits nor toxicity effect of those *N. sativa* products. Previous studies on the various effect of *N. sativa* in individuals have been performed on a heterogeneous population and only limited data are available for the effect of *N. sativa* on metabolic syndrome in menopausal women. Thus, this study was undertaken with the aim to know the adjuvant effect of *N. sativa* on clinical and biochemical parameters of the metabolic syndrome in menopausal women in Klang Valley, Malaysia.

Materials and Methods
Plant materials
N. sativa seeds samples imported from three different countries like Iran, India and Yemen were purchased through a local company named Sari Tani Desa SDN. BHD located in Shah Alam, Malaysia which has health accreditation from Ministry of Health, Malaysia. The seeds were identified and authenticated by Professor Dr. Maznah Ismail, Head of the Laboratory of Molecular Biomedicine, Institute of Bioscience, Universiti Putra Malaysia and the voucher specimens of the seeds were kept there. The identified seeds were analyzed for its thymoquinone (active compound) content and among the seeds that contained high thymoquinone were sent back to the company for cleaning and capsulation process according to Good Manufacturing Practices (GMP). The *N. sativa* seeds were crushed into fine powder and capsulated at a dose of 500mg per capsule and further bottled with an amount of 60 capsules per bottle. The bottles then were sealed and kept under room temperature until further use.

Study Subjects
Ethical clearance for this study was reviewed and approved by the Faculty of Medicine and Health Sciences Medical Research Ethics Committee, Universiti Putra Malaysia. Respondents for the study were selected based on the inclusion and exclusion criteria to ensure the accurately associated factors of metabolic syndrome. The inclusion criteria were women aged 45-60, menopause for a period$\geq$12 months since the last regular menstruation, presenting one or more features of the MetS based on the NCEP-ATP III definition. The exclusion criteria were women having endocrine or other chronic diseases, taking medication for chronic diseases, herbal or supplementation.

Experimental design
The respondents were randomly allotted into two experimental groups. A co-investigator was selected to create subject identification numbers to assign respondents into the groups. A total of 18 respondents were assigned to *N. sativa* group and 17 respondents to placebo group. After a 2-two week's washout period, the respondents received the alternative treatment for 2 months. Capsules of *N. sativa* powder were orally administered at a dose of 1g after breakfast every day for period of two months. A follow- up assessment a month later has been done after the subjects completed the two months treatment. The physical and pathological histories of these subjects were recorded. All subjects requested to maintain their regular lifestyles including their dietary intake and physical activity during the intervention period. Venous blood was drawn from the subjects before and after treatment for further analysis on the effects of *N. sativa*.

Biochemical analysis
Whole blood was collected in plain tube and further centrifuged at 2500rpm for 15min under 25 °C. Serum was collected in order to run the analysis of TC, TG, HDL-C and LDL-C levels, and FBG using commercial diagnostic kits (Randox Laboratories Limited, UK) on *Selectra XL* chemical analyzer (Vital Scientific, Netherlands)

Statistical analysis
All experimental values are presented as means ± standard deviation (SD). Statistical analysis was performed using SPSS windows program version 18 (SPSS Institute, Inc., Chicago, IL, USA). The One-way Analysis of Variance (ANOVA) with Bonferroni correction was used for analysis of data. Difference was considered to be significant if the probability value was less than 0.05 ($p<0.05$).

Results
Body weight
Over the period of treatment, the body weight of *N. sativa* group reduced slightly 0.32% compare to baseline (Figure 1). The body weight of placebo group had no changes. Supplementation with *N. sativa* for eight weeks tended to reduce the body weight of *N. sativa* groups as compared to control group, however no significant reduction was noticed, ($p>0.05$). To be noted, a month after treatment ends body weight of *N. sativa* group showed significant increase ($p<0.05$).

Fasting blood glucose
Supplementation of *N. sativa* for eight weeks was able to reduce fasting blood glucose significantly ($p<0.05$)

by 9.271% at the end of treatment. In contrast, placebo groups showed an elevation in blood glucose, where it increased significantly by 3.796% ($p<0.05$) over the period of treatment (Figure 2).

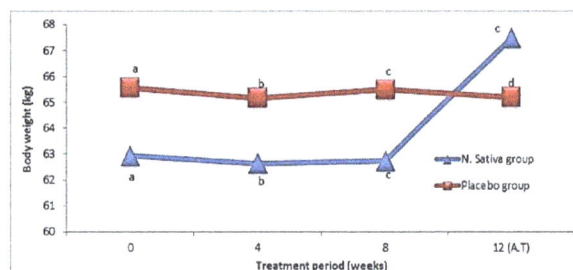

Figure 1. Treatment effect of *N. sativa* and placebo on body weight (kg). Values are expressed as mean ± SD. Same and different lower case letters indicates significant and no significant difference within group, respectively. A.T= one month after treatment ends

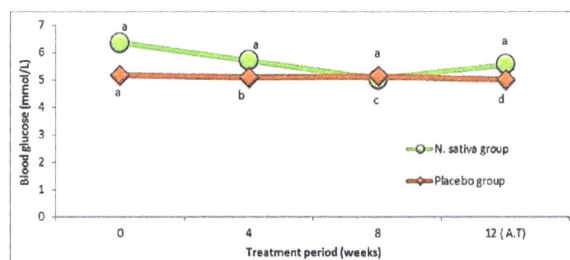

Figure 2. Treatment effect of *N. sativa* and placebo on FBG level (mmol/L). Values are expressed as mean ± SD. Same and different lower case letters indicates significant and no significant difference within group, respectively. A.T= one month after treatment ends

Lipid profile

The sequential changes in serum TC, TG, LDL-C and HDL-C are summarized in Table 1. *N. sativa* supplementations for eight weeks in menopausal women significantly improved TC, TG and LDL-C which was reduced significantly by 9.52%, 35.10% and 26.60%, respectively. HDL-C levels were increased by 8.13% at the end of treatments; however no significant effect was observed ($p > 0.05$). Whereas, in placebo groups, serum TC and LDL-C were found to decreased significantly ($p<0.05$) by 4.36% and 10.02%, respectively. HDL-C was reduced by 2.25% at the end of treatment with no significant difference ($p<0.05$). In contrast, TG was increased by 9.15% at the end of treatment without significant difference ($p<0.05$).

Discussion

The present study was designed to investigate the effect of *N. sativa* on some of the MetS parameters such as body weight, lipid profile and blood glucose level. It is well documented menopause often contribute to increase in body weight due to hormonal changes. Fat substitution in different tissues (fat accumulation in visceral tissues) with menopausal transition due to decrease in estrogen secretion is one of the theories

about the high prevalence of MetS in menopause women.[13] In this study, body weight of the respondents in *N. sativa* group showed slight reduction compared to placebo group throughout the two months of treatment however, not significant reduction was noticed ($p>0.05$). In the same way from another study, body weight was observed to reduce more in *N. sativa* group as compared to the standard group but the difference was not significant.[14] The metabolic pathway of the effect of *N. sativa* on weight reduction is yet to be explored and further studies are needed.

Table 1. Treatment effect of *N. sativa* and placebo on lipid profile changes. Values are expressed as mean ± SD. Same and different lower case letters (abcd) indicates significant and no significant difference within group, respectively. Same and different uppercase letters (AB) indicate significant difference between the groups by weeks, $p<0.05$.

Parameters	Weeks	*Nigella sativa*	Placebo
TC	0	6.027 ± 1.045aA	1.053 ± 6.057aB
	4	5.613 ± 0.971aA	0.796 ± 5.880bA
	8	5.453 ± 1.014aA	0.702 ± 5.793cA
	12	5.973 ± 0.830aA	0.498 ± 5.873dB
TG	0	0.357 ± 1.510aA	0.483 ± 1.497aB
	4	0.320 ± 1.000aA	0.369 ± 1.207bB
	8	0.370 ± 0.980aA	0.398 ± 1.360cA
	12	0.577 ± 1.187bA	0.568 ± 1.393dA
LDL-C	0	0.925 ± 4.647aA	0.597 ± 4.827aB
	4	0.863 ± 3.890bA	0.655 ± 4.553bA
	8	0.784 ± 3.413bA	0.606 ± 4.343bA
	12	0.836 ± 4.037bA	0.284 ± 4.393cB
HDL-C	0	0.258 ± 1.575aA	0.281 ± 1.357aA
	4	0.355 ± 1.620bA	0.207 ± 1.347bA
	8	0.330 ± 1.703bA	0.255 ± 1.327cA
	12	0.253 ± 1.487bA	0.275 ± 1.353dB

The results showed significant decrease in the development of hyperlipidemia among menopausal women in *N. sativa* treatment group compared to placebo group. This result was comparable with a study on oral administration of *N. sativa* seeds powder at a dose of 500 mg/ daily along with statin for 180 days had improved lipid profile in patients who's having stable coronary artery disease in Multan, Pakistan. That study demonstrated the TC, LDL-C and triglycerides decreased by 14.58%, 23.0% and 15.16% respectively whereas HDL-C increased 3.18% significantly when compared with control group taking statin only.[15] Another study showed positive impact ($p<0.05$) of 2 g powdered *N. sativa* seeds intake daily for 4 weeks on lipid profile of hypercholesterolemic patients in Isfahan city, Iran. The study reported a significant decrease in the concentration of TC (4.78%), LDL-C (7.6%) and

TG (16.65%) compared to control group receiving wheat powder.[16]

The possible mechanisms of hypolipidemic action of *N. sativa* as suggested from previous study were most probably due to an up-regulation of LDL-C molecules through receptor mediated endocytosis. The endocytosed membrane vesicles fused with lysosomes and in which the apoproteins were degraded and the cholesterol esters were hydrolyzed to yield free cholesterol. The cholesterol was then incorporated into plasma as necessary and excreted from the body.[17] Indeed, lipid lowering activity of *N. sativa* through decreased dietary cholesterol absorption, stimulation of primary bile acid synthesis and its fecal losses were probably contributed from its dietary soluble fibers[18] and sterols.[19] Another mechanism involved probably through non-enzymatic lipid peroxidation by antioxidant properties of *N. sativa* making liver cells more efficient to remove LDL-C from blood by increasing LDL-C receptor densities in liver and binding to apolipoprotein, apo B.[20]

The changes on FBG observed in the present study were similar with a number of clinical studies in patients with diabetes type II. Incorporation of *N. sativa* as add on therapy at a dose of 2 g/day for 12 weeks improves significantly ($p<0.001$) the blood parameters of glycemia and diabetes control in patients with DM type II.[21] Moreover, fasting blood glucose and HbA1c levels were found to decrease significantly ($p = 0.006$) from 102.4 + 20.8 to 91.5 + n 12.5 mg/dL in *N. sativa* treated subjects as compared to control group at the end of two months treatment in a randomized control trial conducted in 70 healthy subjects attending general health check up at Bagiatallah Hospital, Iran.[22]

The hypoglycemic effect of *N. sativa* was mediated through multiple pharmacological actions. Study by Al-saif, 2008 and El- Dakhakkhny et al., 2002 reported that glucose lowering effects of *N. sativa* was due to improved insulin insensitivity and extra pancreatic actions of insulin in diabetic rats, respectively.[23,24] Fararh et al., 2005 demonstrated that hepatic glucose production from gluconeogenic precursors (alanine, glycerol and lactate) was significantly lowered in *N. sativa* treated hamsters indicating the hypoglycemic effect of *N. sativa* somehow partly mediated through decreased liver gluconeogenesis in menopausal women.[25] Kaleem et al., 2006 confirmed this anti-diabetic activity of *N. sativa* linking to its antioxidant effects. Thymoquinone, the active constituent of *N. sativa* has been demonstrated to attenuate oxidative stress in streptozotocin-induced diabetic rats through preserving pancreatic β- cell integrity leading to increased insulin levels.[26] *Nigella sativa* was also able to reduce glucose absorption from intestine as evidenced by aqueous extract of *N. sativa* (0.1 pg/ml to 100 ng/ ml) which exerted dose-dependent inhibition of sodium dependent glucose transport across isolated rat jejunum and controlled the activity of SGLT1, a major transporter of glucose in intestine.[27]

As suggested in the previous studies, the effect of *N. sativa* powder on metabolic parameters seem to be on multiple components and the synergistic action of its different constituents including thymoquinone and nigellamine, soluble fiber, sterols, flavanoids and high content of poly-unsaturated fatty acids.[28,29] A study evident the presence of phyto-sterols in amounts of 0.33 to 0.36% which further strengthens the protective effect of *N. sativa* interact with several metabolic pathways of human body.[30]

Conclusion

Nigella sativa has beneficial effects on fasting blood sugar and lipid profile in menopause women suggesting it as one such remedy that may prove beneficial in the future for the prevention and treatment of Mets. Even though there is positive correlation with the intakes of *N. sativa* on MetS but this finding is not enough to consider *N. sativa* as an alternative to drugs. However, it can be taken as complementary supplement in patients having mild or elevated risk of MetS which eventually leads to reduce dependency towards drugs.

Acknowledgements

This study was financially supported by the Research University Grant Scheme, RUGS (Vote No.: 91600), Universiti Putra Malaysia. We also would like to thank Sari Tani Desa SDN. BHD, Shah Alam for their contribution in sample capsulation. We also thank the administration and staffs of Pusat Kesihatan Universiti (PKU) and Institute Bioscience (IBS), Universiti Putra Malaysia for their assistance in respondent recruitment and sample analyses.

Conflict of Interest

The authors report no conflicts of interest.

References

1. Atsma F, Bartelink ML, Grobbee DE, Van Der Schouw YT. Postmenopausal status and early menopause as independent risk factors for cardiovascular disease: a meta-analysis. *Menopause* 2006;13(2):265-79.

2. Schneider JG, Tompkins C, Blumenthal RS, Mora S. The metabolic syndrome in women. *Cardiol Rev* 2006;14(6):286-91.

3. Wellons M, Ouyang P, Schreiner PJ, Herrington DM, Vaidya D. Early menopause predicts future coronary heart disease and stroke: the Multi-Ethnic Study of Atherosclerosis. *Menopause* 2012;19(10):1081-7.

4. Expert Panel on Detection E, Treatment of High Blood Cholesterol In A. Executive Summary of The Third Report of The National Cholesterol Education Program (NCEP) Expert Panel on Detection, Evaluation, And Treatment of High Blood Cholesterol In Adults (Adult Treatment Panel III). *JAMA* 2001;285(19):2486-97.

5. Goyal S, Baruah M, Devi R, Jain K. Study on Relation of Metabolic Syndrome with Menopause. *Ind J Clin Biochem* 2013;28(1):55-60.

6. Janssen I, Powell LH, Crawford S, Lasley B, Sutton-Tyrrell K. Menopause and the metabolic syndrome: the Study of Women's Health Across the Nation. *Arch Intern Med* 2008;168(14):1568-75.

7. Lin WY, Yang WS, Lee LT, Chen CY, Liu CS, Lin CC, et al. Insulin resistance, obesity, and metabolic syndrome among non-diabetic pre- and post-menopausal women in North Taiwan. *Int J Obes (Lond)* 2006;30(6):912-7.

8. Ainy E, Mirmiran P, Zahedi Asl S, Azizi F. Prevalence of metabolic syndrome during menopausal transition Tehranian women: Tehran Lipid and Glucose Study (TLGS). *Maturitas* 2007;58(2):150-5.

9. Kadir AA, Hamid HA, Hussain NHN. Metabolic syndrome among postmenopausal women: Prevalence of metabolic syndrome and its associated factors among postmenopausal women at Hospital Universiti Sains Malaysia. *Int J Coll Res Intern Med Public Health* 2012;4(6):1286-96.

10. Khoddami A, Ghazali HM, Yassoralipour A, Ramakrishnan Y, Ganjloo A. Physicochemical characteristics of Nigella Seed (Nigella sativa L.) oil as affected by different extraction Methods. *J Am Oil Chem Soc* 2011;88(4):533-40.

11. Salehisurmaghi MH. Nigella sativa. *Herbal Med Herbal Therapy* 2008;2:216-9.

12. Parhizkar S, Latif LA, Rahman SA, Dollah MA. Preventive effect of *Nigella sativa* on metabolic syndrome in menopause induced rats. *J Med Plants Res* 2011;5(8):1478-84.

13. Carr MC. The emergence of the metabolic syndrome with menopause. *J Clin Endocrinol Metab* 2003;88(6):2404-11.

14. Najmi A, Haque SF, Naseeruddin M, Khan RA. Effect of *Nigella Sativa* oil on various clinical and biochemical parameters of metabolic syndrome. *Int J Diabetes Metabolism* 2008;16(2):85-7.

15. Tasawar Z, Siraj Z, Ahmad N, Lashari MH. The effects of *Nigella sativa*(Kalonji) on lipid profile in patients with stable coronary artery disease in Multan Pakistan. *Pak J Nutr* 2011;10(2):162-7.

16. Sabzghabaee AM, Dianatkhah M, Sarrafzadegan N, Asgary S, Ghannadi A. Clinical evaluation of Nigella sativa seeds for the treatment of hyperlipidemia: a randomized, placebo controlled clinical trial. *Med Arh* 2012;66(3):198-200.

17. Bhatti IU, Ur Rehman F, Khan MA, Marwat SK. Effect of prophetic medicine kalonji (*Nigella sativa L.*) on lipid profile of human beings. An *in vivo* approach. *World Appl Sci J* 2009;6(8):1053-7.

18. Talati R, Baker WL, Pabilonia MS, White CM, Coleman CI. The effects of barley-derived soluble fiber on serum lipids. *Ann Fam Med* 2009;7(2):157-63.

19. Moruisi KG, Oosthuizen W, Opperman AM. Phytosterols/stanols lower cholesterol concentrations in familial hypercholesterolemic subjects: a systematic review with meta-analysis. *J Am Coll Nutr* 2006;25(1):41-8.

20. Al- Naqeeb G, Ismail M, Al- Zubairi AS. Fatty acid profile, α- tocopherol content and total antioxidant activity of oil extracted from N. sativa seeds. *Int J Pharmacol* 2009;5(4):244-50.

21. Bamosa AO, Kaatabi H, Lebdaa FM, Elq AM, Al-Sultanb A. Effect of Nigella sativa seeds on the glycemic control of patients with type 2 diabetes mellitus. *Indian J Physiol Pharmacol* 2010;54(4):344-54.

22. Mohtashami R, Amini M, Fallah Huseini H, Ghamarchehre M, Sadeqhi Z, Hajiagaee R, et al. Blood glucose lowering effects of *Nigella Sativa* L. seeds oil in healthy volunteers: A Randomized, Double-blind, placebo-controlled clinical trial. *J Med Plants* 2011;39(10):90-4.

23. Alsaif MA. Effect of *Nigella sativa* oil on impaired glucose tolerance and insulin insensitivity induced by high-fat-diet and turpentine-induced trauma. *Pak J Biol Sci* 2008;11(8):1093-9.

24. El-Dakhakhny M, Mady N, Lembert N, Ammon HP. The hypoglycemic effect of Nigella sativa oil is mediated by extrapancreatic actions. *Planta medica* 2002;68(5):465-6.

25. Fararh KM, Shimizu Y, Shiina T, Nikami H, Ghanem MM, Takewaki T. Thymoquinone reduces hepatic glucose production in diabetic hamsters. *Res Vet Sci* 2005;79(3):219-23.

26. Hamdy NM, Taha RA. Effects of Nigella sativa oil and thymoquinone on oxidative stress and neuropathy in streptozotocin-induced diabetic rats. *Pharmacology* 2009;84(3):127-34.

27. Meddah B, Ducroc R, El Abbes Faouzi M, Eto B, Mahraoui L, Benhaddou-Andaloussi A, et al. Nigella sativa inhibits intestinal glucose absorption and improves glucose tolerance in rats. *J Ethnopharmacol* 2009;121(3):419-24.

28. Ali BH, Blunden G. Pharmacological and toxicological properties of Nigella sativa. *Phytother Res* 2003;17(4):299-305.

29. Talati R, Baker WL, Pabilonia MS, White CM, Coleman CI. The effects of barley-derived soluble fiber on serum lipids. *Ann Fam Med* 2009;7(2):157-63.

30. Cheikh-Rouhoua S, Besbesa S, Lognayb G, Bleckerc C, Deroannec C, Attia H. Sterol composition of black cumin (*Nigella sativa* L.) and Aleppo pine (*Pinushalepensis Mill.*) seed oils. *J Food Compos Anal* 2008;21(2):162-8.

27

Selenium Effect on Oxidative Stress Factors in Septic Rats

Elmira Zolali[1,2], Hadi Hamishehkar[3,4]*, Nasrin Maleki-Dizaji[5], Naime Majidi Zolbanin[1], Hamed Ghavimi[3], Maryam Kouhsoltani[6], Parina Asgharian[1]

[1] Student Research Committee, Faculty of Pharmacy, Tabriz University of Medical Sciences, Tabriz, Iran.

[2] Biotechnology Research Center, Tabriz University of Medical Sciences, Tabriz, Iran.

[3] Drug Applied Research Center, Tabriz University of Medical Sciences, Tabriz, Iran.

[4] Clinical Pharmacy (Pharmacotherapy) Department, Faculty of Pharmacy, Tabriz University of Medical Sciences, Tabriz, Iran.

[5] Department of Pharmacology and Toxicology, Tabriz University of Medical Sciences, Tabriz, Iran.

[6] Department of Oral and Maxillofacial Pathology, Faculty of Dentistry, Tabriz University of Medical Sciences, Tabriz, Iran.

ARTICLE INFO

Keywords:
Sepsis
Selenium
CLP
Oxidative stress

ABSTRACT

Purpose: Severe oxidative stress is an important event that occurs in patients with sepsis. The body has extensive and multiple defense mechanisms against the reactive oxygen species (ROS) produced during inflammation and sepsis. One of these mechanisms includes a group of enzymes that utilize selenium as their cofactor. The purpose of this study is investigating of Selenium effect on oxidative stress factors in animal model of sepsis.

Methods: Sepsis was induced by caecal ligation and puncture (CLP) method. 30 Male Wistar rats were divided into following groups: sham group; CLP group; 100 μg/kg Selenium- treated CLP group. 12 hours after inducing sepsis animals were killed and lungs were removed. One of the lungs was frozen in liquid nitrogen and kept at $-70^{\circ C}$ for enzymatic activity analysis and the other was kept in formalin 10% until tissue section preparation performed for histopathological studies.

Results: The Myeloperoxidase (MPO) activity was decreased in Selenium- treated CLP group. Inflammation score of lung tissue was lowered in Selenium- treated CLP group, but it wasn't statically significant. Level of glutathione peroxidase (GPx) was higher in CLP and Selenium- treated CLP groups.

Conclusion: It seems that Selenium has protective effect on lung inflammation during acute lung injury. Also it may improve some stress oxidative profile during CLP model of sepsis.

Introduction

Sepsis is a systemic inflammatory syndrome occurring due to extraordinary immune system response to the microorganism or its toxin in bloodstream.[1] Sepsis is one of the most important public health concerns. Sepsis affects persons of all ages, and is the leading cause of morbidity and mortality in intensive care unit (ICU). When sepsis is associated with acute organ dysfunction, results from inflammation and activation of procoagulant response, it is called severe sepsis.[2]

In patients with severe sepsis, an early decrease in plasma selenium concentrations occurs that could be as a result of a defect in antioxidant defenses. Oxidative stress and free radicals might cause the development of multiple organ failure in patients with septic shock, so during severe oxidative stress like sepsis or septic shock, the requirement of selenium might be increased.[3] Selenium is a part of three major Se-containing proteins: selenoprotein-P, glutathione peroxidase (GPx), and

albumin. As a part of GPx, which is considered to be the most important antioxidant enzyme system preventing injury to cells, Selenium serves as a free radical scavenger and plays an important role in reducing oxidative damage.[4]

There is a good evidence that Selenium content is low in critically ill patients and patients with conditions of inflammation and high oxidative stress are at risk of its deficiency.[5] However, selenium can also be considered as a pro- oxidative agent, which may become toxic to cells and damage them. It is suggested that this toxicity is due to the pro-oxidant ability of selenium compounds to catalyze the oxidation of thiols and produce superoxide ($O2^-$), which causes depletion of intracellular glutathione, excessive oxidative stress, and organ damage.[6]

Therefore, to clarify the mechanism of selenium effect on sepsis and oxidative-stress pathway, we aimed to investigate the antioxidant effects of Selenium in animal

Corresponding author: Hadi Hamishehkar, Faculty of Pharmacy, Tabriz University of Medical Sciences, Tabriz, Iran.
Email: hamishehkar@tbzmed.ac.ir

model of sepsis on oxidative-stress biomarkers and evaluating histopathology properties of lung tissue.

Materials and Methods

Animals

The experiments were carried out on male Wistar rats weighing 270-300g and each group included ten rats. Animals were housed in standard polypropylene cages, four per cage, under a 12:12 h light/dark schedule at an ambient temperature of 23±2 °C. Animals had free access to food and water. All experiments were carried out under ethical guidelines for the care and use of laboratory animals (National Institutes of Health Publication No 85-23, revised 1985).

The rats were divided into three groups: (I) sham group, rats were subjected to laparotomy without any other manipulation; (II) CLP group, rats were subjected to CLP without any treatment; (III) 100 µg/kg Selenium- treated CLP group, rats received Selenium 0.5 hours after CLP. Selenium was administered i.p. The rats had free access to food and water after surgery, until they were killed.

Surgical procedure

Animal model of sepsis was induced through caecal ligation and one-hole puncture (CLP). Anaesthesia was induced through the intraperitoneal administration of ketamine (80–100 mg/kg) and xylazine (5–15 mg/kg). The abdomen was shaved and the peritoneum was opened. The caecum was ligated with a 4/0 silk ligature just distal to the ileocaecal valve. One puncture was made with an 18-gauge needle through the caecum, and the caecum was returned to the peritoneal cavity. The abdominal incision was then closed with a 4/0 sterile silk suture. The wound was treated by phenylbutazone to ensure analgesia.

The sham-operated group received laparotomy, but the caecum was not ligated or perforated. All the animals were given prewarmed normal saline (2ml/100g body weight) subcutaneously after surgery for fluid resuscitation.[7]

Specimen Collection

All three groups were anaesthetized after 12 h and lungs were removed quickly from all the rats and washed in ice-cold saline. Half the tissues were kept at -70°C for biochemical analyses, and the other half of the tissues were fixed in 10% formalin solution for histopathological analyses.

Measurement of Myeloperoxidase (MPO) activity

Myeloperoxidase (MPO) activity was measured according to the method of Bradley et al.[8] The lung tissues were chopped in 1 of 50 mM potassium phosphate buffer (pH=6), including 0.5% hexa-decyl-trimethyl-ammonium-bromide (HTAB) and homogenized for 3 min at 8500 rpm. The homogenates were sonicated for 10 seconds, frozen and thawed 3 times then centrifuged at 45000 rpm, in 4°C for 45 min.

The supernatant (100 µl) was added to 2.9 ml of phosphate buffer (50 mM; pH=6) including 0.167 mg/ml of O-dianisidine dihydrochloride and 0.0005% hydrogen peroxide. Five minutes later the reaction was stopped after addition 0.1 ml of 1.2 M hydrochloric acid and absorbance was measured spectrophotometrically at 400 nm. The concentrations were calculated by using calibration curve and expressed as units of MPO in mg weight of wet tissue (U/mg).

Measurement of Malondialdehyde (MDA)

Lipid per oxidation in the rat lung tissues was assayed by determination of the MDA levels according to the method of Olgen et al.[9] The tissues were homogenized in 1.15% KCl to achieve a 10% (W/V) homogenate, then were centrifuged and 1 ml of each supernatant was added to a mixture containing 3 ml of O-phosphorous acid (1%) and 1 ml of thiobarbituric acid (TBA; 0.67%) in an aqueous solution. The reaction mixture was heated for 60 min up to 90°C, and then was cooled in a room temperature. Then, 3 ml of n-butanol was added to each tube, and the tubes were shaken and then centrifuged. The absorbance of n-butanol phase was measured spectrophotometrically at 532 nm and the amount of thiobarbituric acid reactant substances (TBARS) was calculated from a calibration curve and reported as nmol MDA/ mg tissue.

Measurement of Superoxide Dismutase (SOD)

The rat lung tissues were homogenized in 1.15% KCl solution, 10% (w/v). The homogenates were centrifuged and the supernatants were used for SOD assay according to the method of Paoletti et al.[10] This method employs xanthine and xanthine oxidase to generate the superoxide radicals reacting with 2-(4-iodophenyl)-3-(4-nitrophenol)-5-phenyltetrazolium chloride (INT) to form a red formazan dye. The SOD activity was assayed by the degree of inhibition of the formazin production. The absorbance was measured at 505 nm; one unit of SOD was defined as the amount of the enzyme that caused a 50% inhibition of the INT reduction. Tissue SOD was measured by Randox commercial kit (Randox Laboratories Ltd., Crumlin, UK) and was reported as Unit/mg protein.

Measurement of Glutathione Peroxidase (GPx)

GPx activity was measured according to the method of Paglia and Valentine.[11] The rat lung tissues were homogenized in 1.15% KCl solution, 10% (w/v). The homogenates were centrifuged and the supernatants were used for GPx assay. GPx catalyzes the oxidation of glutathione by cumene hydroperoxide. In the presence of glutathione reductase and nicotinamide adenine dinucleotide phosphate-oxidase (NADPH), the oxidized glutathione is converted to the reduced form with a concomitant oxidation of NADPH to $NADP^+$. Tissue GPx was measured by Randox commercial kit at 340 nm and were reported as Unit/mg protein.

Data analysis

Data are expressed as the mean ± SD. One-way ANOVA test was used to find out differences in tissue extract oxidative stress levels in each measured time. P<0.05 was accepted as statistically significant differences.

Results

SOD activity, GPx levels, MDA levels and MPO enzymatic activity were evaluated in all lung tissues. There was no significant difference between groups in tissue SOD enzyme activity (P>0.05) (Figure 1).

The level of lung tissue MDA was significantly higher in the CLP group compared to sham group. MDA level has a relative decrease in Selenium- treated CLP group compared to CLP group but it was not significant (P>0.05) (Figure 1).

GPx activity was increased significantly in Selenium-treated CLP group compared to sham group (P<0.05) (Figure 1).

The activity of MPO in lung tissue was significantly higher in the CLP group. Treatment with Selenium significantly depressed the elevation in MPO activities (P<0.05) (Figure 1).

According to our analysis, there was a significant difference between sham group and CLP group, in terms of inflammation scores (P<0.05). Also histopathology studies showed decrease in lung tissue damage in Selenium- treated CLP group compared to CLP group, but it wasn't statistically significant (P>0.05) (Figure 2).

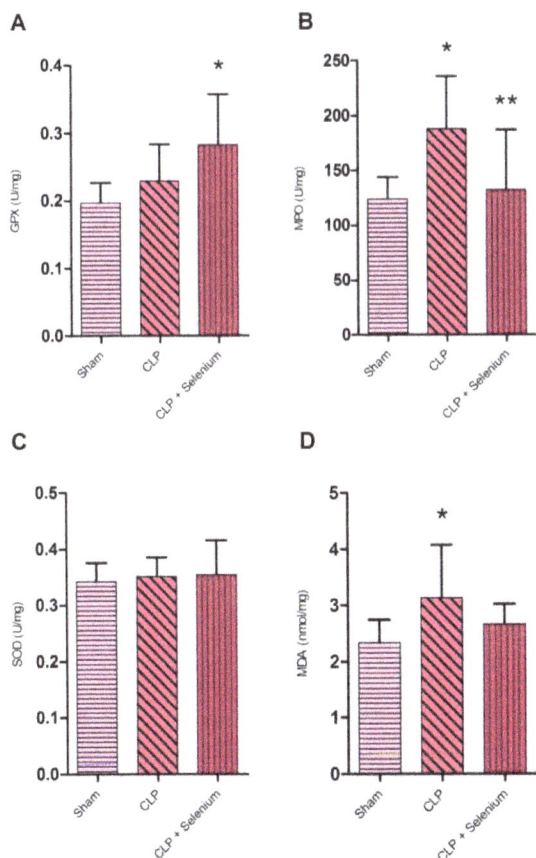

Figure 2. Lung tissue Inflammation scores measured 12 hours after caecal ligation and puncture (n = 6). *P<0.05 compared to sham group. Values are expressed as mean ± SD.

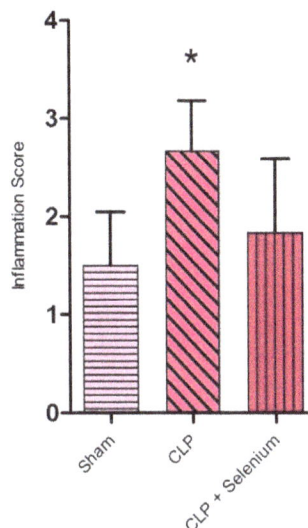

Figure 1. Lung tissue oxidative stress parameters measured 12 hours after caecal ligation and puncture (n= 10). (A) GPx level. (B) MPO activity. (C) SOD level. (D) MDA level. *P<0.05 compared to sham group. **P<0.05 compared to control group. Values are expressed as mean ± SD.

Discussion

Sepsis is an important health problem because it is complicated and difficult to treat and causes high mortality and morbidity; thus, it is important to diagnose and treat it as soon as possible. Microorganisms and their toxins cause the release of cytokines and the activation of inflammatory systems.[12] Oxidative stress is the imbalance between oxidants and antioxidants at the cellular level. This imbalance can cause oxidative damage which includes oxidative modification of cellular macromolecules, cell death, as well as structural tissue and organ damage.[13] Many antioxidants, such as selenium have been used to prevent defect of antioxidant defences in inflammatory and immune-related disease.

In septic patients, Selenium deficiency and defect of GPx detoxifying status has been proved, which correlates directly with high mortality rate.[5] Also it has been shown that Selenium replacement has improved the ability of immune system in oxidative stress conditions.[14] A study around the ability of Selenium to suppress respiratory problems showed that administration of selenium can decrease sepsis-induced change in lung tissue and improve GPx status to oppose oxidative stress.[12]

Considering recent studies of Selenium effects on systemic inflammatory response factors, we aimed to evaluate Selenium antioxidative effects on lung tissue parameters in septic rats to realize that whether it is able to improve outcome in septic patients or not. The

MPO activity is a marker of neutrophil accumulation in lung tissue that is affected strongly in sepsis.[15] In present study, decreasing level of MPO activity by treatment with Selenium may indicate that Selenium suppresses the severity of sepsis. Regarding to this result, lung inflammation following induction of sepsis was decreased in Selenium- treated CLP group. Obviously, lower neutrophil accumulation will result in lower tissue inflammation.

Superoxide anion (O_2^-) is the substrate of SOD that is converted to hydrogen peroxide (H_2O_2). SOD over activation in conditions like inflammation and sepsis, causes the accumulation of the H_2O_2 which could react with metal ions and generate hydroxyl radicals (OH^-) that is suggested to be the most dangerous radical.[16] Studies show an increase in SOD levels after sepsis as a feedback of ROS rise.[17] In this study SOD had no rise after 12 h after CLP in CLP group compared to sham group.

Our results showed that treatment with Selenium has improved GPx levels. GPx detoxifies H_2O_2 by reducing it to water. It also protects cytosolic organelles from oxidative damage by preventing lipid peroxidation.[15] Increasing in GPx level by prescription of Selenium may enable body to use antioxidative capacity in order to confront oxidative stress induced by invasive microorganism during sepsis.

Oxidized lipids and proteins play an important role in destruction and damaging cell membranes.[15] Secondary lipid peroxidation products have toxic effects and can prolong and potentiate the primary free-radical initiated oxidative damage.[18] Lipid peroxidation has been found in rats with sepsis, and MDA levels have been increased in patients with septic shock.[19] Lung tissue level of MDA was increased in septic rats compared to sham group. Also treatment with Selenium lowered MDA tissue levels but depression was not statistically significant. In conclusion, Selenium is seemed to partially overcome to lung manifestation of sepsis. However, more evidence is needed to prove its definite effect on process of sepsis.

Acknowledgments

The authors would like to acknowledge with gratitude Dr Nasrin Maleki and Dr Hamed Hamishehkar for their valuable comments. We also thank Amir M. Vatankhah for their helpful technical assistance (Drug Applied Research Center). This study was financially supported by grant no. 91/83 from the Drug Applied Research Center of Tabriz University of Medical Sciences.

Conflict of Interest

The authors report no conflicts of interest.

References

1. Kumar V, Sharma A. Is neuroimmunomodulation a future therapeutic approach for sepsis? Int Immunopharmacol 2010;10(1):9-17.

2. Bernard GR, Vincent JL, Laterre PF, Larosa SP, Dhainaut JF, Lopez-Rodriguez A, et al. Efficacy and safety of recombinant human activated protein C for severe sepsis. N Engl J Med 2001;344(10):699-709.

3. Macdonald J, Galley HF, Webster NR. Oxidative stress and gene expression in sepsis. Br J Anaesth 2003;90(2):221-32.

4. Carlos WG, Curtis Ramsey M, Fraiz J. Selenium in Early Sepsis: A Marker for Change? Advances in Sepsis 2008;6(3):99-102.

5. Strachan S, Wyncoll D. Selenium in critically ill patients. J Intensive Care Soc 2009;10:38-43.

6. Heyland DK. Selenium supplementation in critically ill patients: can too much of a good thing be a bad thing. Crit Care 2007;11(4):153.

7. Rittirsch D, Huber-Lang MS, Flierl MA, Ward PA. Immunodesign of experimental sepsis by cecal ligation and puncture. Nat Protoc 2008;4(1):31-6.

8. Bradley PP, Priebat DA, Christensen RD, Rothstein G. Measurement of cutaneous inflammation: estimation of neutrophil content with an enzyme marker. J Invest Dermatol 1982;78(3):206-9.

9. Olgen S, Coban T. Antioxidant evaluations of novel N-H and N-substituted indole esters. Biol Pharm Bull 2003;26(5):736-8.

10. Paoletti F, Aldinucci D, Mocali A, Caparrini A. A sensitive spectrophotometric method for the determination of superoxide dismutase activity in tissue extracts. Anal Biochem 1986;154(2):536-41.

11. Paglia DE, Valentine WN. Studies on the quantitative and qualitative characterization of erythrocyte glutathione peroxidase. J Lab Clin Med 1967;70(1):158-69.

12. Atli M, Erikoglu M, Kaynak A, Esen HH, Kurban S. The effects of selenium and vitamin E on lung tissue in rats with sepsis. Clin Invest Med 2012;35(2):E48-54.

13. Lykkesfeldt J, Svendsen O. Oxidants and antioxidants in disease: oxidative stress in farm animals. Vet J 2007;173(3):502-11.

14. Xu HB, Mei WD, Dong ZM, Liao BL. Study of the oxidative metabolic function and chemotaxis of neutrophils from patients with cancer influenced by selenium yeast. Biol Trace Elem Res 1990;25(3):201-9.

15. Ozturk E, Demirbilek S, Begec Z, Surucu M, Fadillioglu E, Kırımlıoglu H, et al. Does leflunomide attenuate the sepsis-induced acute lung injury? Pediatr Surg Int 2008;24(8):899-905.

16. Andrades M, Ritter C, Moreira JC, Dal-Pizzol F. Oxidative parameters differences during non-lethal and lethal sepsis development. J Surg Res 2005;125(1):68-72.

17. Warner BW, Hasselgren PO, James JH, Bialkowska H, Rigel DF, Ogle C, et al. Superoxide dismutase in rats with sepsis. Effect on survival rate and amino acid transport. Arch Surg 1987;122(10):1142-6.

18. Toklu HZ, Tunali Akbay T, Velioglu-Ogunc A, Ercan F, Gedik N, Keyer-Uysal M, et al. Silymarin, the antioxidant component of Silybum marianum, prevents sepsis-induced acute lung and brain injury. *J Surg Res* 2008;145(2):214-22.

19. Koksal G, Sayilgan C, Aydin S, Oz H, Uzun H. Correlation of plasma and tissue oxidative stresses in intra-abdominal sepsis. *J Surg Res* 2004;122(2):180-3.

28

Antinociceptive Effect of Some Biuret Derivatives on Formalin Test in Mice

Neda Adibpour[1,2]*, Ali Poornajjari[1], Mohammad Javad Khodayar[3,4], Saeed Rezaee[5,6]

[1] Department of Medicinal Chemistry, School of Pharmacy, Ahvaz Jundishapur University of Medical Sciences, Ahvaz, Iran.

[2] Department of Medicinal Chemistry, School of Pharmacy, Zanjan University of Medical Sciences, Zanjan, Iran. (current affiliation)

[3] Department of Pharmacology and Toxicology, School of Pharmacy, Ahvaz Jundishapur University of Medical Sciences, Ahvaz, Iran.

[4] Toxicology Research Center, Ahvaz Jundishapur University of Medical Sciences, Ahvaz, Iran.

[5] Department of Pharmaceutics, School of Pharmacy, Ahvaz Jundishapur University of Medical Sciences, Ahvaz, Iran.

[6] Department of Pharmaceutics, School of Pharmacy, Zanjan University of Medical Sciences, Zanjan, Iran. (current affiliation)

ARTICLE INFO

Keywords:
Biuret derivatives
Antinociceptive effect
Formalin test
Mice

ABSTRACT

Purpose: The current study was designed to investigate the antinociceptive effects of several biuret derivatives with N, N`-diphenyl, N-phenyl-N`-alkylphenyl, N,N`-bis alkylphenyl, 2-methylquinoline-4-yl, benzo[d]thiazol-2-ylthio and (1-phenyl-1H-tetrazol-5-yl)thio substituents on the formalin-evoked pain in mice.

Methods: Antinociceptive activity of the nine biurets derivatives were assessed at different doses in mice using formalin test and the results were compared with those of indomethacin(20 mg/kg) and vehicle of the compounds. Area under the pain score curve against time (AUEC) up to 60 minutes was used as the measure of pain behavior.

Results: A rather good analgesic effect was seen for most of the tested biuret derivatives. Significant reduction in median $AUEC_{0-5 minutes}$ was observed at the doses of 50 and 25 mg/kg for biurets with either benzyl and 2-methylquinoline-4-yl (C8) or phenylethyl and benzo[d]thiazol-2-ylthio(C9) moieties, respectively(p-value<0.0044). Antinociceptive activities of compound C7 (with bis phenylropyl substituent), C8 and C9 during the late phase of formaldehyde-induced pain were comparable to that of indomethacin.

Conclusion: Unlike indomethacin, the tested biuret compounds are able to induce antinociception in both phases of formalin test and could be considered comparable to indomethacin at the selected doses.

Introduction

Various pharmacological activities have been reported for biuret derivatives with the general structure shown in Figure 1. McColl reported synthesis of some phenyl biurets and assessed their effects on gastric acid secretion and prevention of peptic ulcer.[1] p-Toluenesulfonyl-biurets and alkyl p-toluenesulfonylthiocarbamates described by Kriesel et al showed hypoglycemic activity.[2] Fouaddel and her colleagues reported synthesis N,N`-diphenyl, N-phenyl-N`-alkylphenyl, and N,N`-bis alkylphenyl biurets and analogous compounds by replacing one phenyl group with 2-methylquinoline-4-yl, benzo[d]thiazol-2-ylthio and (1-phenyl-1H-tetrazol-5-yl)thio moieties and cytotoxicity of them against T47D breast cancer cell line.[3]

During an in silico study by Adibpour et al, it has been shown that biuret derivatives could inhibit pteridine reductase 1 of different strains of leishmania and could be considered as potential antileishmaniasis agents.[4] This effect was further confirmed by Khademvatan and his

coworkers. They found that some of N,N`-diphenyl, N-phenyl-N`-alkylphenyl, and N,N`-bis alkylphenyl biurets were more active against Leishmania major and Leishmania infantumpromastigotes in comparison to glucantime.[5]

In an attempt to find new anti-inflammatory and analgesic agents, Kajitani and his co-workers were prepared several arylbiurets and tested them as anti-inflammatory and analgesic agents.[6] Their results showed that the analgesic activities of 1.3-dimethyl-5-phenylbiuret and 5-(4-chlorophenyl)1, 1, 3, trimethylphenyl biuret were higher than that of aminopyrine. Following their investigation, this study was conducted to assess the antinociceptive activity of several N,N`-diphenyl, N-phenyl-N`-alkylphenyl, and N,N`-bis alkylphenyl biurets and analogous 2-methylquinoline-4-yl, benzo[d]thiazol-2-ylthio and (1-phenyl-1H-tetrazol-5-yl)thio derivatives using pain model of formalin in mice.

*Corresponding author: Neda Adibpour, Department of Medicinal Chemistry, School of Pharmacy, Zanjan University of Medical Sciences, Zanjan, Iran. Email: n.adibpour@zums.ac.ir

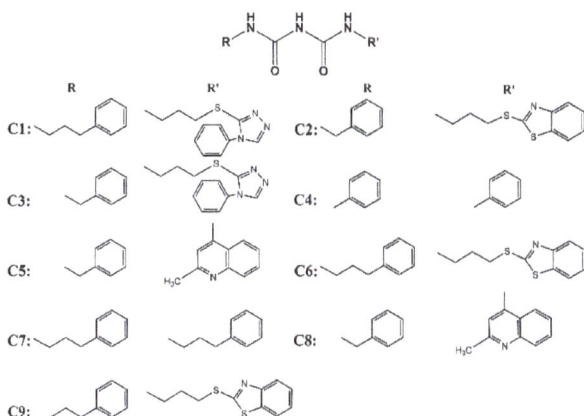

Figure 1. Biuret derivatives

Materials and Methods

Chemicals

Biuret derivatives (C1-C9 in Figure 1) were synthesized and purified as previously reported.[3] Indomethacin was a gift from Darou Pakhsh Pharmaceutical Manufacturing Company, Tehran, Iran. Formalin and dimethyl sulfoxide (DMSO) were purchased from Merck, Germany.

Animal experiments and drug administration

Adult male NMRI mice weighing 24-29 gram were obtained from experimental animal house of Ahvaz Jundishapur University of Medical Sciences and maintained on a 12 hours light/dark cycle with free access to food and water, except during the time of experiments. Mice were randomly divided into groups of 4-5 for test and each animal was used only once. All the ethical issues were considered based on the Ahvaz Medical University Ethical Protocols (AMUEP) on animal experiments. Antinociceptive activity of biuret derivatives were assessed using formalin test and compared with vehicle and indomethacine. Biurets were first dissolved in DMSO and then diluted in saline. Indomethacin was prepared in the minimum amount of alkali solution. Different doses of tested compounds and indomethacin (20 mg/kg) were freshly prepared and injected intraperitoneally in a volume of 10 mL/kg. Fifteen minutes after drug injection, 20 µL of 2.5% formalin was injected intraplantar into the left hind paw using a microsyringe with a 29-gauge needle. Mice were immediately returned to the observation box to monitor pain scores. The animals were placed individually in a Plexiglas box and all observations were carried out by a trained investigator blind to the experimental treatment of the animals. A mirror was placed at 45° angle under the observation box to allow the experimenter an unimpeded view of the injected paw. Animal behavior was continuously scored in 15-second intervals for a total of 60 minutes[7-9] and pain behavior was calculated as the area under the pain score curve (AUEC) of pain score-time curve between 0 and 5 minutes and also from 5 up to 60 minutes post drug administration by using of trapezoidal rule.[10]

Statistical analysis

Comparison of median $AUEC_{0-5 \text{ minutes}}$ and $AUEC_{5-60 \text{ minutes}}$ between different groups of mice were done using Kruskal-Walis followed by Connover-Inman post hoc tests. Differences between medians were considered statistically significant at p-values of less than 0.05.

Results

Descriptive statistics summary of $AUEC_{0-5 \text{ minutes}}$ and $AUEC_{5-60 \text{ minutes}}$ for different groups of mice receiving either the tested biuret derivatives, indomethacin or vehicle are presented in Tables 1 and 2. No significant difference was detected between median of AUEC values in mice receiving indomethacin as compared to those of vehicle group during the early phase of formaldehyde-induced pain as could be seen from notched box plot of $AUEC_{0-5 \text{ minutes}}$ in Figure 2. Median $AUEC_{0-5 \text{ minutes}}$ in all groups of mice received different doses of biurets were lower than those of animals in vehicle and indomethacin groups. However, these differences could be only considered statistically significant for compounds C3 and C7-C9 at the dose of 100 mg/kg in comparison to both indomethacin and vehicle (p-value<0.0125). For C9 and C8, significant reduction in median $AUEC_{0-5 \text{ minutes}}$ also observed at lower doses of biurets i.e. 25 and 50 mg/kg, respectively (p-value<0.0044). Figure 3 shows notched box plot of $AUEC_{0-5 \text{ minutes}}$ values for compounds C7-C9 at different levels of administered dose. These compounds showed the greatest antinociceptive activity at early phase of the formaldehyde-induced pain (Table 1). Increasing the dose of compounds C7-C9 lead to increase in antinociceptive activity (decreasing of median $AUEC_{0-5 \text{ minutes}}$) , however, this increase was not always statistically significant.

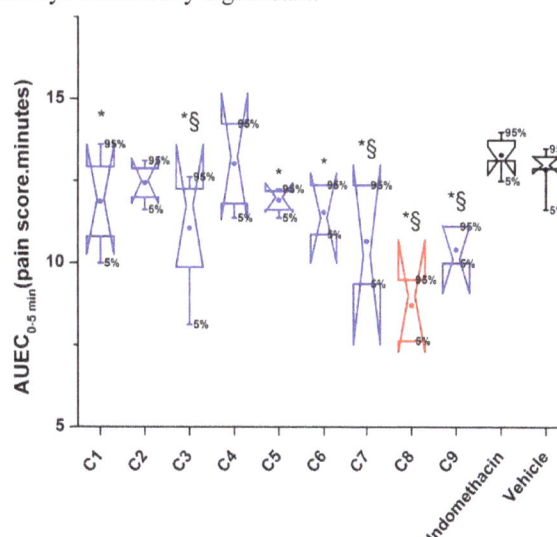

Figure 2. Notched box plot of area under the pain score-time profile up to 5 minutes post administration ($AUEC_{0-5 \text{ minutes}}$) at the biuret dose of 100 mg/kg and 20 mg/kg of indomethacin. Solid circles represent the mean of the values in each group. Boxes and whiskers show the interquartile range and 5 and 95 percentiles, respectively. 95% confidence intervals around the medians are illustrated by the notches. Significant difference of median $AUEC_{0-5 \text{ minutes}}$ with indomethacin and vehicle groups are depicted by (*) and (§), respectively. Plots of the groups that their median AUECs were not statistically significant are shown in the same color.

Advanced Research in Pharmacology

Table 1. Descriptive statistics summary of area under the pain score-time curve between 0 and 5 minutes ($AUEC_{0-5\ minutes}$) in different groups of mice receiving either biuret derivatives at various doses, indomethacin(5 mg/kg) or vehicle.

-	N[a]	Mean	SD[b]	1st Quartile	Median	3rd Quartile	5th Percentile	5th Percentile	Rank Sum[c]
C1-100 mg/Kg	4	11.9	1.5	10.8	11.9	12.9	10.0	13.6	205
C1-200 mg/Kg	4	10.6	2.9	9.1	11.9	12.1	6.3	12.4	164.5
C2-100 mg/Kg	4	12.4	0.6	12.0	12.5	12.9	11.6	13.1	262.5
C2-200 mg/Kg	4	10.3	1.8	8.3	11.3	11.5	8.3	11.5	74.5
C2-50 mg/Kg	4	12.3	1.4	11.3	12.1	13.3	10.9	14.0	230
C3-100 mg/Kg	4	11.1	2.0	9.9	11.8	12.3	8.1	12.6	169
C3-200 mg/Kg	4	11.5	1.0	10.7	11.6	12.3	10.3	12.4	172
C4-100 mg/Kg	4	13.0	1.5	11.8	13.3	14.3	11.4	14.3	279.5
C4-200 mg/Kg	4	10.6	2.5	9.2	11.4	12.0	7.0	12.6	145.5
C5-100 mg/Kg	4	11.9	0.4	11.6	12.0	12.2	11.4	12.3	201
C5-200 mg/Kg	4	9.8	2.2	8.0	10.2	11.5	7.0	11.6	86
C6-100 mg/Kg	4	11.5	0.8	10.9	11.4	12.4	10.9	12.4	126.5
C6-200 mg/Kg	4	10.3	1.1	9.7	9.9	10.9	9.5	12.0	94
C7-100 mg/Kg	4	10.7	1.5	9.4	10.3	12.4	9.4	12.4	96
C7-25 mg/Kg	4	12.6	1.1	11.9	12.2	13.3	11.9	14.3	260.5
C7-50 mg/Kg	4	12.7	0.9	12.3	12.4	13.2	12.1	14.0	279
C8-100 mg/Kg	4	8.7	1.0	7.6	9.0	9.5	7.6	9.5	22
C8-25 mg/Kg	4	12.4	1.0	11.9	12.0	13.0	11.9	13.9	241
C8-50 mg/Kg	4	10.7	1.0	10.1	10.5	11.4	9.8	12.1	115.5
C9-100 mg/Kg	4	10.4	0.6	10.0	10.1	11.1	10.0	11.1	64.5
C9-10 mg/Kg	4	11.6	1.6	10.3	11.6	12.9	9.9	13.1	193
C9-25 mg/Kg	4	11.0	1.0	10.4	11.2	11.6	9.6	11.9	119
Indomethacin	5	13.3	0.6	13.1	13.1	13.8	12.5	14.0	407
Vehicle	5	12.9	0.7	12.9	13.0	13.3	11.6	13.5	363.5

[a] Number of mice in the treatment group , [b] Standard deviation , [c] Kruskal-Wallis sum of the ranks in each groups of mice

Table 2. Descriptive statistics summary of area under the pain score-time curve between 5 and 60 minutes ($AUEC_{5-60 minutes}$) in different groups of mice receiving either biuret derivatives at various doses, indomethacin(5 mg/kg) or vehicle .

-	N[a]	Mean	SD[b]	1st Quartile	Median	3rd Quartile	5th Percentile	95th Percentile	Rank Sum[c]
C1-100 mg/Kg	4	84.4	15.1	73.0	84.6	95.8	66.4	102.1	337.0
C1-200 mg/Kg	4	25.8	9.2	18.3	26.4	33.3	15.1	35.3	116.0
C2-100 mg/Kg	4	22.6	6.9	16.9	22.0	28.3	15.8	30.5	105.0
C2-200 mg/Kg	3	16.6	6.2	11.1	15.4	23.3	11.1	23.3	58.5
C2-50 mg/Kg	4	79.0	15.0	67.6	75.5	90.4	65.9	99.0	320.0
C3-100 mg/Kg	4	66.4	7.3	60.9	64.3	71.8	60.8	76.3	279.0
C3-200 mg/Kg	4	23.4	22.2	4.6	23.0	42.3	1.1	46.5	103.0
C4-100 mg/Kg	4	82.1	8.3	76.4	82.8	87.7	71.3	91.4	345.0
C4-200 mg/Kg	4	21.7	15.2	12.1	19.0	31.3	6.1	42.5	100.5
C5-100 mg/Kg	4	66.2	5.9	61.3	67.1	71.1	59.0	71.5	278.0
C5-200 mg/Kg	4	39.0	14.2	29.1	35.9	48.9	25.6	58.5	166.5
C6-100 mg/Kg	3	66.4	0.6	66.0	66.1	67.1	66.0	67.1	206.5
C6-200 mg/Kg	4	31.1	18.3	17.6	36.2	44.6	6.0	46.0	134.0
C7-100 mg/Kg	3	7.9	7.4	1.1	6.8	15.8	1.1	15.8	28.0
C7-25 mg/Kg	4	52.2	16.0	39.4	49.3	65.0	38.0	72.3	225.5
C7-50 mg/Kg	4	27.6	9.0	20.9	26.3	34.3	18.5	39.3	128.0
C8-100 mg/Kg	3	6.3	5.6	0.0	8.4	10.6	0.0	10.6	25.0
C8-25 mg/Kg	4	58.8	13.5	48.9	62.3	68.6	40.3	70.1	248.5
C8-50 mg/Kg	4	19.3	13.2	8.0	18.0	30.5	7.8	33.3	86.0
C9-100 mg/Kg	3	14.4	4.7	9.0	16.6	17.6	9.0	17.6	53.0
C9-10 mg/Kg	4	65.3	1.1	64.4	65.2	66.1	64.0	66.6	262.0
C9-25 mg/Kg	4	22.1	16.3	8.1	23.0	36.0	5.0	37.3	97.0
Indomethacin	5	52.7	3.4	50.9	54.5	54.5	47.6	55.9	265.0
Vehicle	5	73.8	5.7	70.8	73.6	75.0	67.3	82.5	404.0

[a] Number of mice in the treatment group , [b] Standard deviation , [c] Kruskal-Wallis sum of the ranks in each groups of mice

As it could be seen from Figure 3 and Table 2, in the late phase of formalin-induced pain (up to 60 minutes post drug administration), difference of median $AUEC_{5-60\ minutes}$ values between indomethacin and vehicle groups was significant (p-value=0.0006). A rather good analgesic activity was seen by compounds C2 and C7-C9 at the dose of 100 mg/kg in comparison to indomethacin (Figure 4). However, these compounds did not show any statistically significant difference of median $AUEC_{5-60\ minutes}$ at this level of dose. Compounds C7-C9 had comparable analgesic activity to indomethacin at the dose of 25 mg/kg (Figure 5). Increasing the dose of compounds C7-C9 to the values greater than 25 mg/kg did not result in significant reduction of median $AUEC_{5-60\ minutes}$.

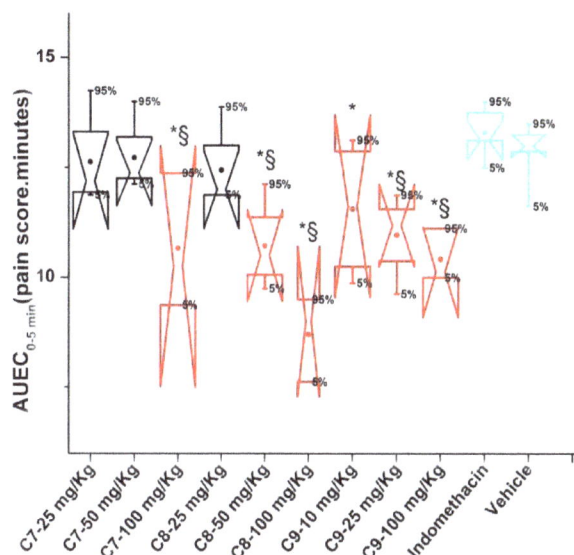

Figure 3. Notched box plot of area under the pain score-time profile up to 5 minutes post administration ($AUEC_{0-5\ minutes}$) at different doses of compounds C7-C9 and 20 mg/kg of indomethacin. Solid circles represent the mean of the values in each group. Boxes and whiskers show the interquartile range and 5 and 95 percentiles, respectively. 95% confidence intervals around the medians are illustrated by the notches. Significant difference of median $AUEC_{0-5\ minutes}$ with indomethacin and vehicle groups are depicted by (*) and (§), respectively. Plots of the groups that their median AUECs were not statistically significant are shown in the same color.

Discussion

Among the several models of persistent nociception, formalin test has been well established as a valid model for screening of anti-inflammatory and antinociceptive agents.[11,12] A number of analogies have been specified between formalin-evoked pain and human persistent clinical pain.[13] Intraplantar injection of formalin evokes signs of nociception (flinching and licking of the injected paw) with early (phase 1), followed by a quiescent period characterized by fewer pain behaviours, and late-hyperalgesic (phase 2) components that last for approximately 1 hr.[7,8] The early phase or neurogenic nociception results direct activation of peripheral nociceptors whereas the late phase due to inflammatory nociception that reflect induction of a spinal state of facilitation, central sensitization, development of

inflammation and enlargement of receptive fields and also the concurrent presence of low-level input from both large and small afferents.[11,13]

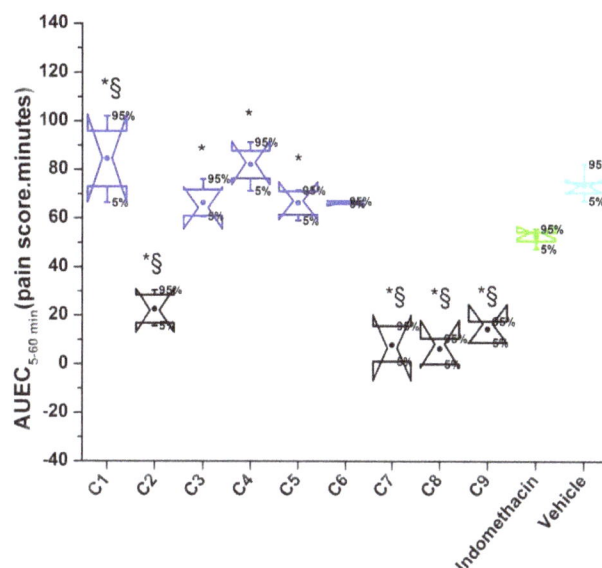

Figure 4. Notched box plot of area under the pain score-time profile between 5 and 60 minutes post administration ($AUEC_{5-60\ minutes}$) at the biuret dose of 100 mg/kg and 20 mg/kg of indomethacin. Solid circles represent the mean of the values in each group. Boxes and whiskers show the interquartile range and 5 and 95 percentiles, respectively. 95% confidence intervals around the medians are illustrated by the notches. Significant difference of median $AUEC_{0-5\ minutes}$ with indomethacin and vehicle groups are depicted by (*) and (§), respectively. Plots of the groups that their median AUECs were not statistically significant are shown in the same color.

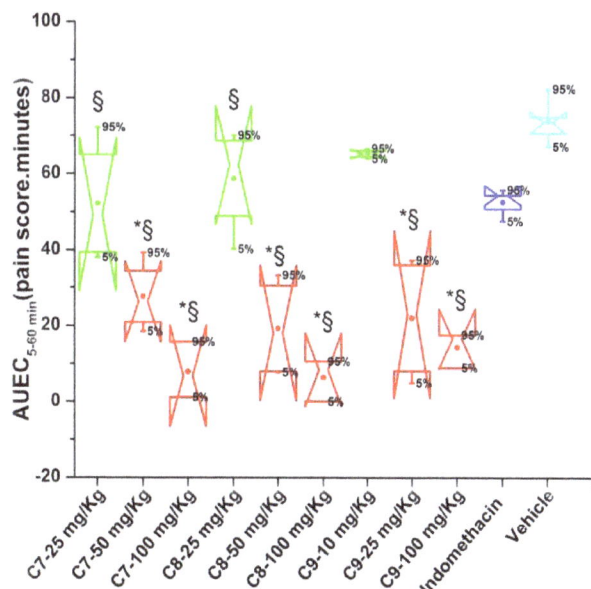

Figure 5. Notched box plot of area under the pain score-time profile between 5 and 60 minutes post administration ($AUEC_{5-60\ minutes}$) at different doses of compounds C7-C9 and 20 mg/kg of indomethacin. Solid circles represent the mean of the values in each group. Boxes and whiskers show the interquartile range and 5 and 95 percentiles, respectively. 95% confidence intervals around the medians are illustrated by the notches. Significant difference of median $AUEC_{0-5\ minutes}$ with indomethacin and vehicle groups are depicted by (*) and (§), respectively. Plots of the groups that their median AUECs were not statistically significant are shown in the same color.

Several aryl biurets like 1,3-dimethyl-5-phenylbiuret, l-ethyl-3-methyl-5-phenylbiuret and 1,1,3-trimethyl-5-phenyl biuret were found to have more potent anti-inflammatory activity than pheylbutazone using carrageenan-induced paw edema in rat. It has also be shown that 1.3-dimethyl-5-phenylbiuret and 5-(4-chlorophenyl) 1,1,3-trimethylpheyl biuret showed higher analgesic activity than that of aminopyrine in acetic acid stretching test.[6]

Unlike indomethacin, the biuret derivatives under investigation in the current study showed antinociceptive activity in both phases of formaldehyde-induced pain in mice. The highest activity was seen by biuret derivative with phenylethyl and benzo[d]thiazol-2-ylthio moieties (C9). Compounds C7 and C8 with phenylpropyl, benzyl and 2-methylquinoline-4-yl substituents also showed good activities in comparison to indomethacin. However, difference between median AUECs were not significant at doses higher than 25 mg/kg in both phases of pain. Almost all the biuret compounds, showed a rather good analgesic activities at the dose of 100 mg/kg. It seems that the more lipophilic show higher analgesic activity.

Conclusion

In conclusion, our findings may suggest that biuret compounds, unlike indomethacin are able to induce antinociception in both phases of formalin test and could be considered comparable to indomethacin at the selected doses. However, further investigations are necessary to elucidate their safety and efficacy.

Acknowledgments

This paper was extracted from Pharm.D thesis of Ali Poornajjari that submitted in School of Pharmacy of Ahvaz Jundishapur University of Medical Sciences and financially supported by grant no. u-91203 from Vice Chancellor of Research of this university.

Conflict of Interest

There is no conflict of interest to be reported.

References

1. Mccoll JD, Chubb FL, Lee CF, Hajdu A, Komlossy J. Synthesis and Pharmacological Properties of Phenyl-Substituted Biurets. *J Med Chem* 1963;6:584-7.
2. Kriesel DC, Menzie J. Synthesis and pharmacological evaluation of some tosylbiurets and tosylthiocarbamates as potential hypoglycemic agents. *J Pharm Sci* 1968;57(10):1791-3.
3. Fouladdel S, Khalaj A, Adibpour N, Azizi E. Synthesis and cytotoxicity of some biurets against human breast cancer T47D cell line. *Bioorg Med Chem Lett* 2010;20(19):5772-5.
4. Adibpour N, Rahim F, Rezaeei S, Khalaj A, Ebrahimi A. In silico designing selective inhibitor of drugs, medicinal plants compounds and experimental ligands for pteridine reductase targeting visceral leishmaniasis. *Afr J Microbiol Res* 2012;6(5):917-26.
5. Khademvatan S, Adibpour N, Eskandari A, Rezaee S, Hashemitabar M, Rahim F. In silico and in vitro comparative activity of novel experimental derivatives against Leishmania major and Leishmania infantum promastigotes. *Exp Parasitol* 2013;135(2):208-16.
6. Kajitani M, Yamazaki T, Yamada S, Tanaka M, Ogawa K, Honna T, et al. Syntheses, antiinflammatory, and analgesic activities of arylbiurets. *Arch Pharm (Weinheim)* 1990;323(6):355-9.
7. Abbott FV, Franklin KB, Westbrook RF. The formalin test: scoring properties of the first and second phases of the pain response in rats. *Pain* 1995;60(1):91-102.
8. Dubuisson D, Dennis SG. The formalin test: a quantitative study of the analgesic effects of morphine, meperidine, and brain stem stimulation in rats and cats. *Pain* 1977;4(2):161-74.
9. Tjolsen A, Berge OG, Hunskaar S, Rosland JH, Hole K. The formalin test: an evaluation of the method. *Pain* 1992;51(1):5-17.
10. Khodayar MJ, Shafaghi B, Naderi N, Zarrindast MR. Antinociceptive effect of spinally administered cannabinergic and 2-adrenoceptor drugs on the formalin test in rat: possible interactions. *J Psychopharmacol* 2006;20(1):67-74.
11. Coderre TJ, Melzack R. The contribution of excitatory amino acids to central sensitization and persistent nociception after formalin-induced tissue injury. *J Neurosci* 1992;12(9):3665-70.
12. Diaz A, Dickenson AH. Blockade of spinal N- and P-type, but not L-type, calcium channels inhibits the excitability of rat dorsal horn neurones produced by subcutaneous formalin inflammation. *Pain* 1997;69(1-2):93-100.
13. Yaksh TL, Hua XY, Kalcheva I, Nozaki-Taguchi N, Marsala M. The spinal biology in humans and animals of pain states generated by persistent small afferent input. *Proc Natl Acad Sci U S A* 1999;96(14):7680-6.

29

Nucleostemin Depletion Induces Post-G1 Arrest Apoptosis in Chronic Myelogenous Leukemia K562 Cells

Negin Seyed-Gogani[1], Marveh Rahmati[2], Nosratollah Zarghami[2,3], Iraj Asvadi-Kermani[3], Mohammad Ali Hoseinpour-Feyzi[1], Mohammad Amin Moosavi[1,3,4]*

[1] Department of Zoology, Faculty of Natural Science, University of Tabriz, Tabriz, Iran.

[2] Department of Biochemistry, Faculty of Medicine, Tabriz University of Medical Science, Tabriz, Iran.

[3] Hematology and Oncology Research Center, Tabriz University of Medical Science, Tabriz, Iran.

[4] National Institute of Genetic Engineering and Biotechnology, Tehran, Iran.

ARTICLE INFO

Keywords:
Apoptosis
Cell cycle
Chronic myelogenous leukemia
K562
Nucleostemin
RNA interference

ABSTRACT

Purpose: Despite significant improvements in treatment of chronic myelogenous leukemia (CML), the emergence of leukemic stem cell (LSC) concept questioned efficacy of current therapeutical protocols. Remaining issue on CML includes finding and targeting of the key genes responsible for self-renewal and proliferation of LSCs. Nucleostemin (NS) is a new protein localized in the nucleolus of most stem cells and tumor cells which regulates their self-renewal and cell cycle progression. The aim of this study was to investigate effects of *NS* knocking down in K562 cell line as an in vitro model of CML.

Methods: *NS* gene silencing was performed using a specific small interfering RNA (NS-siRNA). The gene expression level of *NS* was evaluated by RT-PCR. The viability and growth rate of K562 cells were determined by trypan blue exclusion test. Cell cycle distribution of the cells was analyzed by flow cytometry.

Results: Our results showed that *NS* knocking down inhibited proliferation and viability of K562 cells in a time-dependent manner. Cell cycle studies revealed that *NS* depletion resulted in G_1 cell cycle arrest at short times of transfection (24 h) followed with apoptosis at longer times (48 and 72 h), suggest that post-G1 arrest apoptosis is occurred in K562 cells.

Conclusion: Overall, these results point to essential role of *NS* in K562 cells, thus, this gene might be considered as a promising target for treatment of CML.

Introduction

Chronic myelogenous leukemia (CML) is a clonal pluripotent hematopoietic stem cell disorder caused by indefinite proliferation of leukemic stem cells (LSCs).[1] Reciprocal translocation between the *abl* gene (on chromosome 9) and the *bcr* gene (on chromosome 22) causes formation of *Bcr-Abl* oncogene.[1,2] The fusion product of *Bcr-Abl* is an oncogenic protein displays up-regulated tyrosine kinase activity.[2] At present, CML therapies mostly included chemotherapy, differentiation therapy, α-interferon treatment, Bcr-Abl tyrosine kinase inhibitors and bone marrow transplantation.[3,4] Although, recent tyrosine kinase inhibitors improved therapeutical options in CML patients, some adverse effects such as drug resistance and late relapse were observe in clinical trials.[5] It has been suggested that current therapeutic approaches would not completely eliminate all LSC in CML patients and relapse of disease was observed. In fact, unlimited self-renewal capacity and impaired differentiation property of LSCs allow continuously proliferation and prevent terminal differentiation and apoptosis that normally occur in blood cells.[6,7] Obviously, elucidation of the mechanisms involved in LSC proliferation, differentiation and apoptosis enumerates first-line investigations for improving CML therapeutic strategies.

In 2002, Tsai and McKay discovered that a novel gene called *Nucleostemin* (*NS*), apparently expressed in rat embryonic and adult central nervous system stem cells.[8] The protein coded by *NS* gene was found in the nucleoli of undifferentiated cells, such as adult and embryonic stem cells, neural stem cells and human bone marrow stem cells but not in differentiated counterpart cells, indicating that *NS* is silenced during normal cells differentiation.[9,10] Interestingly, recent reports suggest that *NS* gene is also abundantly expressed in several human cancer cell lines such as SGC-7901 (gastric), Hela (cervical), 5637

---

*Corresponding author: Mohammad Amin Moosavi, Nanobiomaterial and Tissue Engineering Research Center, National Institute of Genetic Engineering and Biotechnology, P.O Box: 14965/161, Tehran, Iran. Email: a-moosavi@nigeb.ac.ir

(bladder), PC-3 (prostate), and HL-60 (acute myelocytic leukemia).[11-15] In parallel with significant of this gene in cancer, several knocking down experiments using RNA interference (RNAi) showed that inhibition of *NS* gene expression markedly inhibited proliferation and cell cycle progression of cancerous cells followed with induction of differentiation and/or apoptosis.[11-15] Recently, a high expression level of NS has been reported in leukemia patients, particularly CML.[15] Consistent with this, RNAi-mediated *NS* knocking down inhibited proliferation and induced differentiation and apoptosis in HL-60 human acute myeloblastic leukemia.[16] However, importance of *NS* in other types of leukemia, especially CML, needs to be addressed.

This study was designed to investigate functional importance and therapeutic potential of *NS* gene expression and effects of *NS* knockdown on cell cycle and apoptosis in K562 cells. Our result showed that RNA interference (RNAi)-mediated *NS* silencing induced G_1 cell cycle arrest followed with apoptosis in K562 leukemia cells.

Materials and Methods
Cell culture
The human K562 cell line was cultured in RPMI 1640 medium supplemented with heat-inactivated fetal bovine serum (10% v/v), streptomycin (100µg/ml) and penicillin (100 U/ml) at 37 °C in a humidified atmosphere of 5% CO_2.

siRNA design and synthesis
NS specific double-stranded small interfering RNA (NS-siRNA) was designed by siRNA target finder program at the Ambion website: (http://www.ambion.com/techlib/misc/ siRNA_finder.html). The NS-siRNA and irrelevant scrambeled siRNA (IR-siRNA) oligonucleotides were synthesized by Eurofin MWG Operon (Germany). A siRNA labeled by fluorescein at 3' end of antisense strand was used to determine efficiency of cellular transfection. The sense and antisense sequence of NS-siRNA and IR-siRNA were as followed:
NS-siRNA Sense: 5'-GAACUAAAACAGCAGCAGAdTdT-3' and Antisense: 5'-UCUGCUGCUGUUUUAGUUCdTdT-3'
IR-siRNA (Sense: 5'-CACCGCCTCTCATCGTCGTC-3', Antisense: AAUCAGACGUGGACCAGAAGAdTdT)

K562 cells transfection
The day before transfection, cells were diluted at a density of 3×10^5/ml in culture medium containing FBS (10%) and antibiotics in cell culture flask. After 24 h, 2×10^5 cells/ well were seeded in 24-well plates (SpL Life sciences, South Korea) with 100 µl culture medium containing FBS (10%) and antibiotics. For cell transfection, 200 nM siRNA associated with 6 µl HiPerfect (Qiagen, USA) transfection reagent and 100 µl serum free medium mixed and vortexed. This mixture was incubated for 10 min at room temperature and then added

to cells. After 6 h, 400 µl culture medium containing FBS (12.5%) and antibiotics were added to the cells.

RNA extraction and reverse transcriptase polymerase chain reaction (RT-PCR)
Total RNA was isolated from transfected cells as well as untransfected cells 12-72 h after transfection, using RNX plus™ (Cinagen, Tehran) according to the manufacturer's protocol. Total RNA (1 µg) converted to cDNA in a final volume of 20 µl by oligo dT and RevertAid™ M-MuLV reverse transcriptase (Fermentase, UK). PCR reactions were carried out using Taq DNA polymerase. The sequences of primers for all isoforms of NS (NM014366, NM206825, NM206826) were: Reverse: 5 '-AAAGCCATTCGGGTTGGAGT-3', Forward: 5'-ACCACAGCAGTTTGGCAGCAC-3'. *β2microglobulin (β2m)* gene was used as a control for adjusting the relative amounts of total RNA between the samples. *β2m* forward primer and reverse primer were 5'- CTA CTC TCT CTT TCT GGC CTG-3' and 5'- GAC AAG TCT GAA TGC TCC AC-3', respectively. PCR for *NS* gene included an initial denaturation step at 94 °C for 2 min, followed by 35 amplification cycles consisting of denaturation at 94 °C for 30 s, annealing at 60 °C for 40 s, extension at 72 °C for 1 min and final extension at 72 °C for 5 min (418 bp). PCR for *β2m* gene included an initial denaturation step at 94 °C for 5 min, followed by 30 amplification cycles consisting of denaturation at 94 °C for 30 s, annealing at 57 °C for 30 s, extension at 72 °C for 1 min and final extension at 72 °C for 5 min (191 bp). The amplified product was identified by electrophoresis on 1.5% agarose gel. *NS* and *β2m* primers were synthesized by Eurofin MWG Operon (Germany).

Growth inhibition and viability
To study proliferation and viability, the transfected and untransfected cells were seeded at a density of 2×10^4 cells/well in 24-well plates. After different times of transfection, viable and dead cells were counted by trypan blue exclusion assay and percent of growth inhibition and cytotoxixicty were determined as mentioned previously.[17] The transfected cells were stained with 0.4% trypan blue at a dilution of 1:1, and counted using a neubauer hemocytometer slide under an inverted light microscopy (Olympus, Japan). Morphological studies of cells were also performed by inverted light microscopy (Olympus, Japan).

Cell cycle analyses
DNA contents of cells were analyzed using flow cytometry as described previously.[18] Control and transfected cells were harvested and washed twice with PBS (Phosphate Buffer Saline), fixed in 70% ethanol and kept at −20 °C until analysis. Then the cells were stained with 20 µg/ml PI containing 20 µg/ml RNase (DNase free) for 2 h. The stained cells were analyzed by flow cytometry (Partec Pas, Germany). The population of G_0/G_1, S, G_2/M and sub-G_1 cells was determined using Mulicycle Cell

Cycle Software. The results are expressed as percentage of the cells in each phase.

Fluorescent microscopic study of apoptosis

Control and transfected cells were washed in cold PBS and adjusted to a cell density of 5×10^4 cell/20µl of PBS and gently mixed with a mixture of AO (1 µg/ml) and EtBr (1 µg/ml) solution (1 : 1, v/v). The suspension was placed on a microscopic slide and viewed under a fluorescent microscopy (Nikon E-1000, Japan).

Statistical analyses

All data represent the mean ±SEM of three independent experiments. Significant differences between groups were evaluated by multiple mean comparisons via one-way ANOVA test, SPSS 14.0 and Microsoft Excel 210. $P<0.05$ were considered statistically significant.

Results

Expression of NS was efficiently inhibited by NS-siRNA in K562 cells

Based on our preliminary data about high expression level of *NS* in leukemia cell lines, we examined different RNAi techniques for silencing of this gene in K562 cells.[19] One of the designed siRNAs, called NS-siRNA, could efficiently inhibit NS expression in K562 cells (Figure 1). As depicted in Figure 1, NS-siRNA at 200 nM was efficiently delivered into K562 cells (Figure 1A) and significantly inhibited *NS* expression in a time-dependent manner (Figure 1B). In fact, no significant reduction in *NS* expression was observed after 6-12 h NS-siRNA transfection of K562 cells, whereas *NS* mRNA level were significantly inhibited between 16 h and 48 h of transfection (Figure 1B and C). The inhibition rate of *NS* expression in comparison with corresponding *β2m* internal control after 16 h, 24 h and 48 h were about 20%, 24% and 55%, respectively (Figure 1C).

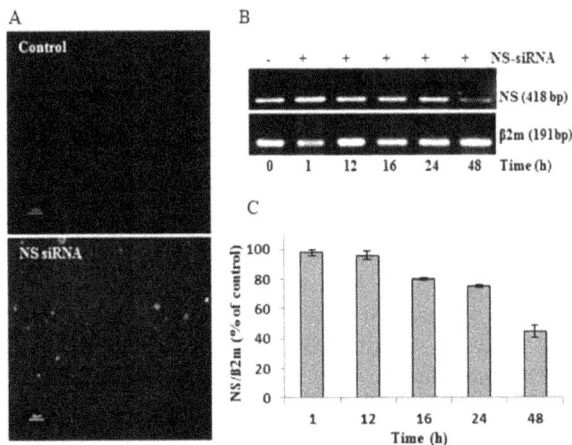

Figure 1. Knockdown of *NS* expression by siRNA in K562 cell line. (A) NS-siRNA delivery into K562 cells. After 24 h of transfection with fluorescein-labeled NS-siRNA, K562 cells were harvested and analyzed by fluorescent microscopy. (B) RT-PCR study of *NS* gene expression level in K562 cells. Following transfection with 200 nM IR- and NS-siRNAs, K562 cells were collected and mRNA levels of NS were dtermined by semi quantitative RT-PCR. (C) Analyzing of NS mRNA level in K562 cells. The densitometry analysis of *NS* mRNA over *β2m* mRNA data was studied by UVItec software. Each value represents the mean±SEM of three independent experiments and *P*<0.05 (*) were considered statistically significant.

Knockdown of NS inhibits growth and viability of K562 cells

To evaluate biological consequence of *NS* silencing, the growth rate and viability of K562 cells were studied for various time intervals (Figure 2). No significant growth inhibitory effects were observed 12 h after transfection, while growth was inhibited by 28.8%, 33.7% and 36.4% after 24 h, 48 h and 72 h, respectively (Figure 2A). In comparison with control or IR-siRNA transfected cells, the viability of NS depleted cells was also reduced but with different kinetics (Figure 2B). Indeed, no significant cell death was observed after 12-24 h of NS depletion, while viability of K562 cells was significantly reduced by 17.6% and 34.9% after 48 h and 72h, respectively. These findings together with the growth results (Figure2A) suggest that growth inhibition is prominent effects of NS-siRNA at short times while cell death is appeared at long times (48-72 h).

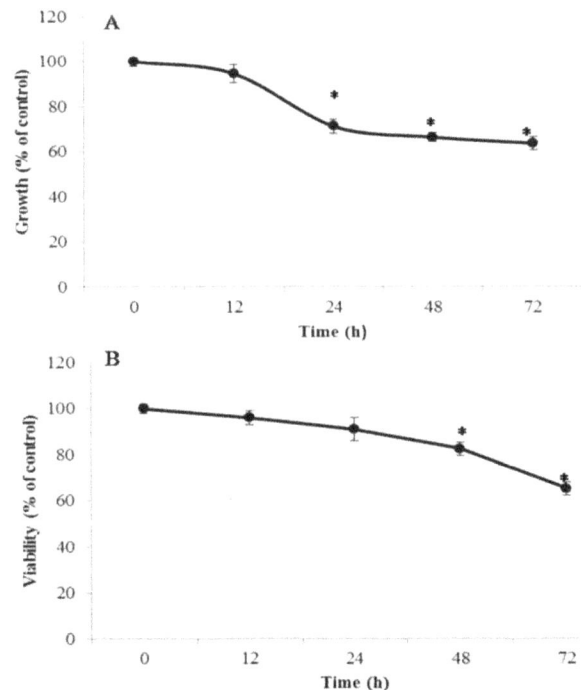

Figure 2. Effects of NS-siRNA on growth and viability of K562 cells. Following transfection with 200 nM IR- and NS-siRNAs, K562 cells were collected and number of viable cells (white cells), and dead cells (blue cells) were estimated . Growth inhibition (a) and viability (b) were studied using trypan blue test , respectively. Each value represents the mean±SEM of three independent experiments. *P*<0.05 (*) were considered statistically significant.

Knockdown of NS leads to profound morphological changes in K562 cells

The morphology of K562 cells after NS-siRNA transfection was shown in Figure 3. Aggregation of K562 cells and decrees in cell confluency was typically observed in *NS* depleted K562 cells. However, some cell death criteria such as cell shrinking and cell debris were observed after 48-72 h of NS-siRNA transfection.

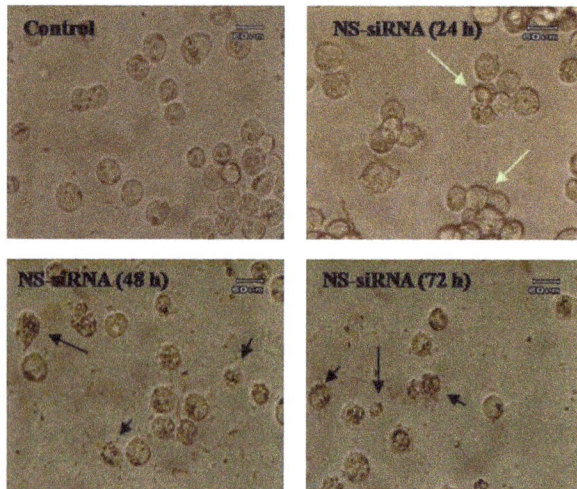

Figure 3. Morphological changes of K562 leukemia cells after transfection with NS- siRNA. The cells were transfected by 200 nM NS-siRNA for 24-72 h, and then morphological changes were studied using light microscopy (magnification 40x). After 24 h, cell aggregation (white arrow) were observed in NS-siRNA transfected K562 cells whereas after longer times (48-72 h) cell shrinking (long black arrows) and apoptotic bodies (short black arrows) were clearly observed.

Knockdown of NS induces apoptosis in K562 cells

To determine mode of cell death in NS-siRNA transfection cells, we studied apoptosis and necrosis by AO/EtBr double staining of the cells (Figure 4). The results clearly showed that *NS* siRNA transfected cells underwent apoptosis after 48 h. The apoptotic criteria, including nuclear fragmentation chromatin condensation, and apoptotic bodies were clearly observed. In these figure, viable cells were equally green whereas early apoptotic cells had bright green blots in their nuclei indicating chromatin condensation and nuclear fragmentation. Late apoptotic cells, however, stained orange and showed condense and fragmented nuclei. Necrotic cells were uniformly orange.

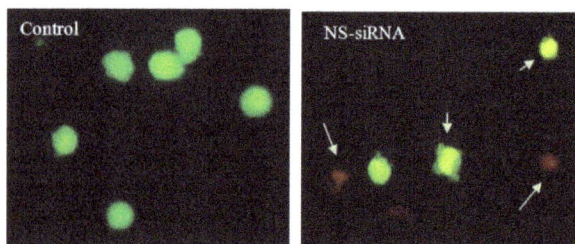

Figure 4. Apoptotic effects of NS-siRNA in K562 cells. Frothy eight hours after transfection of K562 cells with 200 nM IR- and NS-siRNAs, the cells were collected.
Control (IR-siRNA) and NS-siRNA transfected K562 cells were double stained with AO/EtBr and studied by fluorescent microscopy (magnification, 40x).Viable cells are equally green, early apoptotic cells are green and contained bright green dots in their nuclei (short arrows) and late apoptotic cells are orange (long arrows).

Knockdown of NS induces G_0/G_1 cell cycle arrest in K562 cells

Evidence suggests that the cell fate decision is made within G1 phase of cell cycle. Therefore, the cell cycle

distribution of NS-siRNA transfected K562 cells was also studied in this work (Figure 5). When compared with control cells, NS-siRNA transfected cells showed a significant increase in G_0/G_1 phase of cell cycle population with concurrent decrease in S and G_2M phase after 24 h of transfection. As might be expect, a sub-G_1 peak (apoptotic cells) was apparent after longer times of transfection. For example, After 24 h, the G_0/G_1 cell cycle population of NS-siRNA transfected cells (59%) was higher than control cells (45%). Moreover, the sub- G_1cell population (apoptotic cells) was increased from from 18-36% 48 -72 h of transfection, respectively.

Discussion

Several reports have suggested that *NS* is a marker of stem cells that is involved in controlling self-renewal, cell cycle progression and proliferation in both stem cells and cancerous cells.[10,20] As we took this matter into consideration that *NS* plays a critical role in cell proliferation, consequently, we examined *NS* expression and its function in K562 cell line as a model of CML stem cells. K562 cell line has been established from the pleural extravasation of a patient with CML in blast crisis which behaves as pluripotent hematopoietic stem cells. In addition to abnormal *Bcr-Abl* gene, K562 cells have also mutated p53 gene.[16] These combined mutations make the cells a suitable and worldwide *in vitro* model to study effects of new chemotherapy drugs and CML stem cells targeted therapies.[16] With our knowledge, functional importance of NS in CML has not been studied until now. Our results indicated that *NS* mRNA was highly expressed in K562 cells. This finding is aligned with previous studies based on *NS* over-expression in several human cancer cell lines.[11-15] In our study, role of NS in cell cycle progress and apoptosis of K562 cells was determined by a *NS* specific siRNA as a genomic nanoparticle. These oligos led to a significant decrease in the *NS* mRNA expression (Figure 1). The results showed that *NS* knocking down inhibited growth of K562 cells 24 h after transfection. Apoptosis began after 48 h and increased to its highest level after 72 h. Therefore, NS depletion in K562 cells resulted in growth inhibition at short times and apoptosis at longer times. These results are in full agreement with cell cycle results where an accumulation in G_1 phase population was observed after 24 h of NS-siRNA transfection. After this time point, however, the cells population at G_1 phase decreased and a sub-G_1 peak was appeared, suggest that post-G_1 arrest apoptosis is exact mode of action of NS-siRNA in K562 cells. Most literature reports suggest that NS depletion inhibited proliferation and induced cell cycle arrest in cancer cell lines.[13,14,21,22] For instance, *NS* specific siRNA in bladder cancer cells led to G_1 cell cycle arrest in prostate PC-3 cells and bladder cancer 5637cells.[13,14] However, NS may also induce G_2/M cell cycle arrest as the case of bladder cancer SW1710 cells.[13] Apparently, the role of NS in regulation of G_1 phase of cell cycle in K562 cells are in full agreement with most of these literature reports.

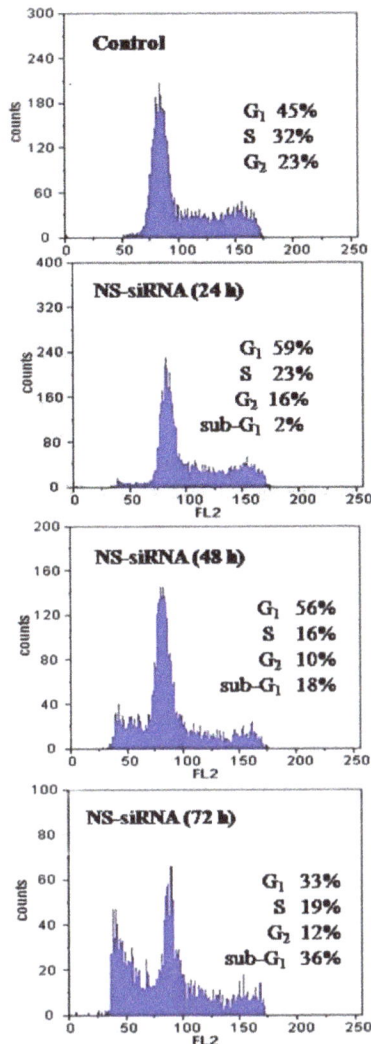

Figure 5. Effects of NS-siRNA on cell cycle distribution of K562 cells. Following NS –siRNA transfection, the K562 cells were collected at different time intervals (24-72 h) and their DNA contents were analyzed by flow cytometry as mentioned in materials and methods. The results are from a typical experiment.

Although, several reports point to apoptotic effects of NS depletion in different cancerous cells, induction of apoptosis following G_1 cell cycle arrest is a novel finding of this paper. In fact, it has been previously reported that *NS* depletion induced a rapid apoptosis response in HeLa cells, PC-3 cells, human bladder (5637) cells and HL-60 cells.[12-14,16] In our experiments, however, we observed a delayed apoptosis response in K562 cells. This may be related to different levels of NS depletion and protein contents of the cells used in distinct experiments.

Several studies have provided evidence that the p53 signaling pathway is involved in cell-cycle arrest induced by the NS depletion. The knockdown of NS enhanced the interaction between the p53-binding protein MDM2 and the ribosomal protein L5 or L11, preventing MDM2 from inducing ubiquitylation-based p53 degradation.[8,21] However, NS depletion induced cell-cycle arrest and decreased cell proliferation in rat

bone marrow stromal stem cells and several cancerous cells in a p53-independent manner.[22] Considering this fact that K562 cells and three other cancerous cell lines HL-60, PC-3 and 5637 cells have no functional p53 protein, it can be concluded other proteins might be involved in NS effects.[14] It is possible that NS induces apoptosis via interaction with other molecules than p53. Consistent with this conclusion, it has been reported that NS depletion inhibited ribosome biogenesis in a p53-depndent manner.[23] Further works are in progress to address this question.

Conclusion

Attain to potent growth inhibitory and apoptotic effects of NS-siRNA in human myeloid leukemia K562 cells, the silencing of this gene can be a considered as a therapiutic target for treatment of leukemia.

Acknowledgments

The authors appreciate the financial support of this investigation by the research grants of the Hematology and Oncology Research Center of Tabriz University of Medical Science, and National Institute of Genetic engineering and Biotechnology.

Conflict of Interest

The authors declare that they have no conflict of interest.

References

1. Wong S, Witte ON. The BCR-ABL story: bench to bedside and back. *Annu Rev Immunol* 2004;22:247-306.
2. Tefferi A, Dewald GW, Litzow ML, Cortes J, Mauro MJ, Talpaz M, et al. Chronic myeloid leukemia: current application of cytogenetics and molecular testing for diagnosis and treatment. *Mayo Clin Proc* 2005;80(3):390-402.
3. Deininger MW, Goldman JM, Melo JV. The molecular biology of chronic myeloid leukemia. *Blood* 2000;96(10):3343-56.
4. Druker BJ, Sawyers CL, Kantarjian H, Resta DJ, Reese SF, Ford JM, et al. Activity of a specific inhibitor of the BCR-ABL tyrosine kinase in the blast crisis of chronic myeloid leukemia and acute lymphoblastic leukemia with the Philadelphia chromosome. *N Engl J Med* 2001;344(14):1038-42.
5. Thiesing JT, Ohno-Jones S, Kolibaba KS, Druker BJ. Efficacy of STI571, an abl tyrosine kinase inhibitor, in conjunction with other antileukemic agents against bcr-abl-positive cells. *Blood* 2000;96(9):3195-9.
6. Sell S. Leukemia: stem cells, maturation arrest, and differentiation therapy. *Stem cell reviews* 2005;1(3):197-205.
7. Normile D. Cell proliferation. Common control for cancer, stem cells. *Science* 2002;298(5600):1869.

8. Tsai RY, Mckay RD. A nucleolar mechanism controlling cell proliferation in stem cells and cancer cells. *Genes Dev* 2002;16(23):2991-3003.

9. Nomura J, Maruyama M, Katano M, Kato H, Zhang J, Masui S, et al. Differential requirement for nucleostemin in embryonic stem cell and neural stem cell viability. *Stem Cells* 2009;27(5):1066-76.

10. Kafienah W, Mistry S, Williams C, Hollander AP. Nucleostemin is a marker of proliferating stromal stem cells in adult human bone marrow. *Stem Cells* 2006;24(4):1113-20.

11. Liu SJ, Cai ZW, Liu YJ, Dong MY, Sun LQ, Hu GF, et al. Role of nucleostemin in growth regulation of gastric cancer, liver cancer and other malignancies. *World J Gastroenterol* 2004;10(9):1246-9.

12. Sijin L, Ziwei C, Yajun L, Meiyu D, Hongwei Z, Guofa H, et al. The effect of knocking-down nucleostemin gene expression on the in vitro proliferation and in vivo tumorigenesis of HeLa cells. *J Exp Clin Cancer Res* 2004;23(3):529-38.

13. Nikpour P, Mowla SJ, Jafarnejad SM, Fischer U, Schulz WA. Differential effects of Nucleostemin suppression on cell cycle arrest and apoptosis in the bladder cancer cell lines 5637 and SW1710. *Cell Prolif* 2009;42(6):762-9.

14. Liu RL, Zhang ZH, Zhao WM, Wang M, Qi SY, Li J, et al. Expression of nucleostemin in prostate cancer and its effect on the proliferation of PC-3 cells. *Chin Med J (Engl)* 2008;121(4):299-304.

15. Yue B, Sun L, Zhao X, Chen Y, Wang Q, Liu S, et al. Expression of nucleostemin gene in human acute leukemic cells. *Life Sci J* 2006;3:12-6.

16. Yue B, Lu J, Wang Y, Yu L, Wang Q, Liu S, et al. Effects of nucleostemin gene silencing on morphology and cytochemistry of HL-60 cells. *Life Sci J* 2008;5(2):9-14.

17. Moosavi MA, Yazdanparast R, Lotfi A. ERK1/2 inactivation and p38 MAPK-dependent caspase activation during guanosine 5'-triphosphate-mediated terminal erythroid differentiation of K562 cells. *Int J Biochem Cell Biol* 2007;39(9):1685-97.

18. Moosavi MA, Yazdanparast R. Distinct MAPK signaling pathways, p21 up-regulation and caspase-mediated p21 cleavage establishes the fate of U937 cells exposed to 3-hydrogenkwadaphnin: differentiation versus apoptosis. *Toxicol Appl Pharmacol* 2008;230(1):86-96.

19. Moosavi MA, Googani N, Asadi M, Asvadi kermani I. Knocking-down nucleostemin gene expression inhibits proliferation and induces apoptosis in human leukemia K562 cells. *Clin Biochem* 2011;44(13):S61.

20. Ma H, Pederson T. Nucleostemin: a multiplex regulator of cell-cycle progression. *Trends Cell Biol* 2008;18(12):575-9.

21. Ma H, Pederson T. Depletion of the nucleolar protein nucleostemin causes G1 cell cycle arrest via the p53 pathway. *Mol Biol Cell* 2007;18(7):2630-5.

22. Jafarnejad SM, Mowla SJ, Matin MM. Knocking-down the expression of nucleostemin significantly decreases rate of proliferation of rat bone marrow stromal stem cells in an apparently p53-independent manner. *Cell Prolif* 2008;41(1):28-35.

23. Lubbert M, Miller CW, Crawford L, Koeffler HP. p53 in chronic myelogenous leukemia. Study of mechanisms of differential expression. *J Exp Med* 1988;167(3):873-86.

Evolutionary Origin and Conserved Structural Building Blocks of Riboswitches and Ribosomal RNAs: Riboswitches as Probable Target Sites for Aminoglycosides Interaction

Elnaz Mehdizadeh Aghdam[1], Abolfazl Barzegar[2,3]*, Mohammad Saeid Hejazi[1,3]*

[1] *Drug Applied Research Center and Department of Pharmaceutical Biotechnology, Faculty of Pharmacy, Tabriz University of Medical Sciences, Tabriz, Iran.*

[2] *Research Institute for Fundamental Sciences (RIFS), University of Tabriz, Tabriz, Iran.*

[3] *The School of Advanced Biomedical Sciences (SABS), Tabriz University of Medical Sciences, Tabriz, Iran.*

ARTICLE INFO

Keywords:
Riboswitch
Ribosomal RNA
Structural similarity
Motif
Docking

ABSTRACT

Purpose: Riboswitches, as noncoding RNA sequences, control gene expression through direct ligand binding. Sporadic reports on the structural relation of riboswitches with ribosomal RNAs (rRNA), raises an interest in possible similarity between riboswitches and rRNAs evolutionary origins. Since aminoglycoside antibiotics affect microbial cells through binding to functional sites of the bacterial rRNA, finding any conformational and functional relation between riboswitches/rRNAs is utmost important in both of medicinal and basic research.

Methods: Analysis of the riboswitches structures were carried out using bioinformatics and computational tools. The possible functional similarity of riboswitches with rRNAs was evaluated based on the affinity of paromomycin antibiotic (targeting "A site" of 16S rRNA) to riboswitches via docking method.

Results: There was high structural similarity between riboswitches and rRNAs, but not any particular sequence based similarity between them was found. The building blocks including "hairpin loop containing UUU", "peptidyl transferase center conserved hairpin A loop"," helix 45" and "S2 (G8) hairpin" as high identical rRNA motifs were detected in all kinds of riboswitches. Surprisingly, binding energies of paromomycin with different riboswitches are considerably better than the binding energy of paromomycin with "16S rRNA A site". Therefore the high affinity of paromomycin to bind riboswitches in comparison with rRNA "A site" suggests a new insight about riboswitches as possible targets for aminoglycoside antibiotics.

Conclusion: These findings are considered as a possible supporting evidence for evolutionary origin of riboswitches/rRNAs and also their role in the exertion of antibiotics effects to design new drugs based on the concomitant effects via rRNA/riboswitches.

Introduction

Today, it is evident that RNAs are not just intermediates between DNA and proteins. Their catalytic and regulating characteristics have been more verified since more than a decade ago. It has been revealed that there are RNA-based mechanisms which regulate gene expression in response to internal or external signals.[1-3] Accordingly, mRNA structure plays an essential role in this process and determines the fate of the mRNA.[4-7] As ribosome binds mRNA before transcription is completed, most regulatory regions are located within the 5' untranslated region (UTR) of mRNAs. These regulatory regions contain either *cis*

acting binding sites or *trans*-acting regulators (non-coding RNAs).

Riboswitches, usually found within the 5'UTR of mRNAs, are *cis* acting RNA elements. They can adopt various conformations in response to environmental signals, including stalled ribosomes, uncharged tRNAs, elevated temperatures or small molecule ligands.[8] These metabolite sensors, which were identified a decade ago,[9] regulate the genes involved in the uptake and use of related metabolites without proteins interpretation.[1,9]

An ever-increasing number and variety of riboswitches are being identified in bacteria, as well as some

*Corresponding authors: Mohammad Saeid Hejazi and Abolfazl Barzegar, The School of Advanced Biomedical Sciences (SABS), Tabriz University of Medical Sciences, Tabriz, Iran. Email: saeidhejazi@tbzmed.ac.ir,
Email: barzegar@tabrizu.ac.ir

eukaryotes. For example, as much as 2% of all *Bacillus subtilis* genes are regulated by riboswitches that bind to metabolites such as flavin mononucleotide (FMN), thiamin pyrophosphate (TPP), S-adenosylmethionine (SAM), lysine, and purines. Riboswitches generally consist of two parts: the aptamer region, a conserved sequence which binds the ligand, and the so-called expression platform, which regulates gene expression through alternative RNA structures that affect transcription or translation.[10,11] Upon binding of the ligand, the riboswitch changes the conformation which forms or disrupts transcriptional terminators or antiterminators, respectively. Therefore, in order to find out their mechanistic details, 2D and 3D structure of riboswitches' aptamers[12] and their binding characteristics[13] were extensively analyzed experimentally or computationally.[14-16] On the other hand, other possible interactions are suggested to introduce some molecules as new drugs which exert their effects via riboswitches.[17,18]

RNA structure is basically expressed at the sequence or primary structure level, the secondary and tertiary levels. Initially, RNA motifs were identified at the sequence level as generally existing short sequences in functional RNAs, such as transfer RNA (tRNA) or ribosomal RNA (rRNA).[19] Base-pairing or secondary structure constitutes both the canonically base-paired regions (helices) and non-paired regions (loops). Structural studies and comparative sequence analyses have suggested that biological RNAs are composed primarily of conserved structural building blocks or motifs[20] of secondary and tertiary structures. Forms and functions of RNAs in the biological systems which connected to their three-dimensional (3D) structures lead RNA molecules to perform specific roles. However, there are some similarities between various motifs in RNAs types with diverse functionalities.

Barrick and Breaker in 2007 detected some motifs in riboswitches, which are close in relation to rRNA structures.[21] In 2008, an artificial riboswitch for the aminoglycoside antibiotic, neomycin B, was engineered[22] which partially resembles the ribosomal A-site, the natural target for aminoglycoside antibiotics.[23] Based on the previous studies we aimed to investigate relation between rRNAs and riboswitches structures and their subsequent functions such as binding to specific antibiotics. In this path, in current study we attempted to survey structural similarity including primary, 2D, 3D and motifs as well as functional similarity among rRNAs and riboswitch elements through bioinformatics and computational tools.

Materials and Methods
Databases and Programs
Riboswitches data were collected from Rfam database[24] and structure information was acquied through PDB database (www.pdb.org). Sequences mostly gained from NCBI based on Rfam sequences information.

Multiple sequence alignment was carried out via ClustalW implemented in Mega5 program. Needle (http://www.ebi.ac.uk/Tools/psa/emboss_needle/nucleo tide.html) and Water (http://www.ebi.ac.uk/Tools/psa/emboss_water/nucleot ide.html) servers were applied in order to accomplish optimal pairwise global and local alignment, respectively.[25] Also, functional and structural alignments were done by means of SARA server (http://structure.biofold.org/sara/)[26] and R3D Align (http://rna.bgsu.edu/R3DAlign) servers,[27] respectively. Eventually, the interactions of an antibiotic with RNA structures were carried out via Autodock version 4.2 program.

Functional and structural riboswitch alignments
Ten riboswitch classes which have not only the most representatives in microorganisms,[28] but also have available PDB structures, were selected. Their PDB codes which represent preferably unbound state of riboswitches were extracted first from Rfam (http://rfam.sanger.ac.uk/) and then PDB (http://www.rcsb.org/pdb/home/home.do). They included TPP (PDB code: 2gdi), FMN (PDB code: 2yie), SAM-I (PDB code: 3iqn), lysine (PDB code: 3d0x), glycine (PDB code: 3ox0), purine (PDB code: 4fe5), c-di-GMP-I (PDB code: 3iwn), c-di-GMP-II (PDB code: 3q3z), preQ1(PDB code: 3fu2), THF (PDB code: 3suy) riboswitches. Each code was analyzed via SARA server (http://structure.biofold.org/sara/) to perform structure based function alignment. Default parameters are -7.00 for opening gap, -0.60 for extension gap and 3 consecutive vectors (4 atoms) for length of the Unit-Vector used to generate the comparison matrix. The results were sorted based on PSS (percentages of secondary structure identity) and top rRNA structures were selected and their sequences were acquired.

Sequences alignment
All rRNA sequences which have high similarity with a definite riboswitch sequence were aligned applying ClustalW[29] implemented in Mega5[30] with the default parameters for multiple alignment stages as 15 and 6.66 for gap opening and gap extension penalties, respectively. If necessary, minor adjustments were manually made to the alignments. Also, global and local pairwise alignments of same rRNAs with the riboswitches sequences were conducted through Needle and Water server programs. All the parameters were set by default as 10 and 0.5 for gap opening and gap extension penalties, respectively.

Motifs categorization
The category (more than 50 percent secondary structure identity) for each type of riboswitches was used to organize similar rRNA motifs. Afterward, motifs were sorted out based on the number of similar riboswitches types. Also, average of PSS (percentages of secondary

structure identity) level for each type of motifs was determined. In addition, according to results, types of riboswitches are organized based on each kind of motif they could possess.

Docking
Preparation of the macromolecules
All crystal structures of 10 riboswitches (PDB IDs: 2gdi, 2yie, 3iqn, 3d0x, 3ox0, 4fe5, 3iwn, 3q3z, 3fu2, 3suy) and 16S-rRNA A-site (PDB ID: 1j7t) were selected. Water and ligand molecules were eliminated by the software program ViewerPro Version 5.0. Also non-polar hydrogens and Gasteiger charges were added during the preparation of the macromolecule input file using the AutoDockTools package.

Preparation of the ligand
Complex between paromomycin and the 16S-rRNA A-site (PDB code: 1j7t) was used to provide the three-dimensional (3D) structure of paromomycin by removing other atoms using ViewerPro Version 5. Gasteiger charges were added to the obtained structure of the ligand and the rotatable bonds were set to 9 by using AutoDock Tools.

Preparation of the grid files
The complex crystal structure of paromomycin antibiotic and 16S-rRNA A-site motif (PDB code: 1j7t) was selected as a control sample for assessments of the results. In order to find out the similar and conserved building blocks of the riboswitches with the rRNA, the 3D structure of 16S-rRNA A-site and 10 different riboswitches were structurally aligned via R3D Align. The aligned part of each riboswitch with "A site" motif of 16S rRNAs was considered to generate Grid maps. The interaction of the antibiotic ligand (paromomycin) and 16S-rRNA A-site as well as the homologue parts in different riboswitches were analyzed. Grid maps were generated by AutoGrid 4.2 based on the superimposed area of each riboswitch with 16S-rRNA A-site. The numbers of points in the grid boxes were 60×56×80; 84×86×82; 72×86×86; 76×68×100; 100×100×100; 98×88×88; 108×80×90; 76×98×100; 100×74×86; 98×74×88; 72×86×86 for 1j7t, 3iwn, 3q3z, 3ox0, 3d0x, 3fu2, 4fe5, 3iqn, 3suy, 2gdi and 2yie, respectively, with a grid spacing of 0.375A°.

Preparation of the docking files
Molecular docking was carried out by the molecular docking software, AutoDock Version 4.2 based on the Lamarckian genetic algorithm.[31] For each complex, 100 independent docking runs were conducted containing a population of 150 randomly positioned individuals. The maximum number of energy-evaluation retries and generations were 2500000 and 27000, respectively. Also, crossover rate of 0.8 and a mutation rate of 0.02 were set up. The docking results were clustered on the results of docking by using a root mean square (RMS) tolerance of 2.0 A°. During docking, macromolecules

were set rigid, whereas all the torsional bonds of ligands were set free. The docking results were clustered according to a root-mean-square deviation (RMSD) tolerance of 0.2 nm.

The structure of 16S-rRNA A-site (PDB code: 1j7t) was taken as the control for docking. First, the ligand (paromomycin) was removed from the complex. Then, the ligand-free structure of 16S-rRNA A-site was docked with ligand for 100 independent runs. At last, binding energies obtained from docking of riboswitches with paromomycin were compared to control binding energy.

Statistical Analyses
Where needed, results were evaluated by excel (version 2007) and SPSS (version 16). Statistical analyses were performed using one-way analysis of variance (ANOVA). Statistical assessment of difference between mean values was performed by least significance difference (LSD) test at $p<0.05$ using SPSS (16 version) software.

Results and Discussion
Structural riboswitch alignments
Recent interest in non-coding RNA transcripts has culminated in a rapid increase of deposited RNA structures in the PDB database. However, functional classification and characterization of the RNA structure have not completely been addressed. There are many bioinformatics tools to investigate 2D and 3D structural alignments of DNA and RNA structures.[32-34] SARA (Structure Alignment of Ribonucleic Acids) web server (http://sgu.bioinfo.cipf.es/services/SARA)[26] is a promising program for aligning RNA 3D structures via PDB files based on unit-vector root mean square (URMS). Herein, PDB codes of a total of 10 riboswitch types were analyzed by SARA server and all rRNA PDB codes were collected. For all PDB codes in each group of data achieved from SARA server, primary, secondary and tertiary similarity percentages were calculated. Also they were sorted by average natural logarithm of PID (Percentage of sequence identity), PSS (percentages of secondary structure identity) and PSI (percentages of tertiary structure identity). For instance, among similar rRNA PDB codes for lysine riboswitch, the highest 2D similarity belongs to "helix 45" (PDB code: 1wts-chain A) which shares 28.6, 100 and 92.9 % primary, secondary and tertiary identity with this type of riboswitch, respectively. According to Figure 1, there is a correlation between tertiary structure identity (based on PSI) and secondary structure identity (based on PSS) with approximate coefficient of determination (R^2) of 0.8. As a result, the observed correlation between the similarity of 2D and 3D structures demonstrate that both 2D and 3D structures could be utilized for similarity studies in current study. Besides, those concerned with RNA-ligand interactions, generally give greater weight to secondary structure similarity, as ligand binding sites

typically consist of a single type of secondary structure.[35] As a result and due to interaction analysis in the subsequent stages of this study, secondary structure could be more useful and debatable in our study. Hence, in the following steps, sorting in order of PSS (based on secondary structure identity) was performed.

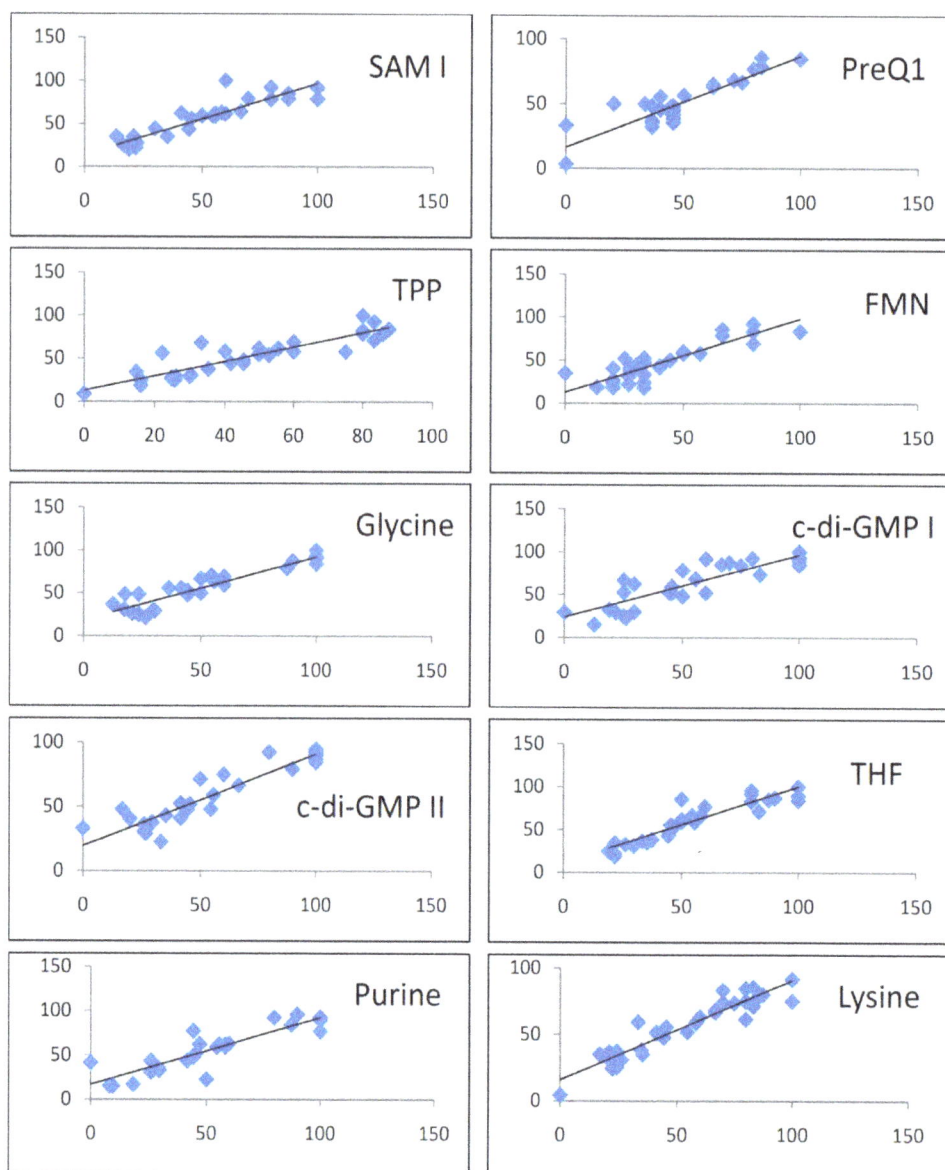

Figure 1. Correlation of secondary structure identity and 3D structure of rRNAs with the mentioned riboswitches. Vertical and horizontal axes are percentage of secondary structure similarity (PSS) and tertiary structure identity (PSI) of rRNAs with the associated riboswitches, respectively. There is high correlation between PSS and PSI of rRNAs with 10 different types of riboswitches ($R^2 \sim 0.8$).

Motifs categorization

The Structural Classification of RNA (SCOR) is a database designed to provide a comprehensive perspective and understanding of RNA motif structures, functions, tertiary interactions and their relationships (http://scor.berkeley.edu/). It is an inclusive, manually created source of RNA structural motifs which applies automated tools and literature descriptions to assist in the classification of RNA secondary and tertiary structure motifs such as Kink turns, S-turns, GNRA loops.[36,37]

All of the rRNA motifs having more than 50 percent secondary structure identity (PSS) with similar riboswitches were exploited to categorize in similar

groups. In addition, averages of PSS for each type of motifs were calculated. Figure 2 illustrates rRNA motifs against the number of similar riboswitches. As it is shown these rRNA motifs are in common with different kinds of riboswitches structures. Also, there is a remarkable high amount of secondary structure identity between shown rRNA motifs and riboswitches. Table 1 shows the rRNA motifs/ riboswitches correlation with more details. Accordingly, glycine and THF riboswitches are similar to the most number of detected rRNA motifs (18 motifs). However, apart from "18S rRNA A site" and "helix 21", all of the mentioned ribosomal RNA motifs are similar among different 10 types of riboswitches. In this issue, 4 motifs including hairpin loop containing UUU, peptidyl transferase center conserved hairpin A loop, helix 45 and S2 (G8) hairpin are common in all kinds of riboswitches (see Table 1 and Figure 2). It means these motifs are highly similar among different types of riboswitches. Already, Winkler *et al.* figured out that the GA motif is a highly conserved structure in both TPP and SAM riboswitches and 23S rRNAs. In addition, it was observed that UA_handle motif , is common within both ribosomal RNAs and riboswitches.[38] Hence, our findings revealed that not only the mentioned GA and UA_handle motifs but also several other important and highly conserved rRNA motifs such as hairpin UUU, A loop, helix 45 and S2 (G8) hairpin and GNRA tetraloop are found in riboswitches with high similarity. GNRA motif provides tertiary contacts which are important for group I introns, hammerhead ribozymes, and the ribosome.[39-41] It is believed that GNRA has high selectivity and specificity in binding to different kinds

of compounds;[42-44] a common characteristics for riboswitches. GNRA tetaraloop is a common motif in some riboswitches including glycine, purine, FMN, THF, c-di-GMP I (see Figure 2 and Table 1). The structural similarity of this motif with rRNAs is more than 75 percent. Consequently, the findings proposed that the common motifs in riboswitches structures should have common functional properties in similar rRNAs such as binding ligand molecules. The ligand binding characteristics of 10 riboswitches and RNAs which share similar motifs with them were considered as well (see section 3.3). Considering these findings, common evolutionary aspects of riboswitches and rRNAs are confirmed. As a result the resemblance of rRNA building blocks and riboswitches domains may be resulted either from connecting evolution or the dependent byproducts of historical events such as local segment duplication and recombination mechanisms that cause elevation of structural complexity of natural functional molecules.

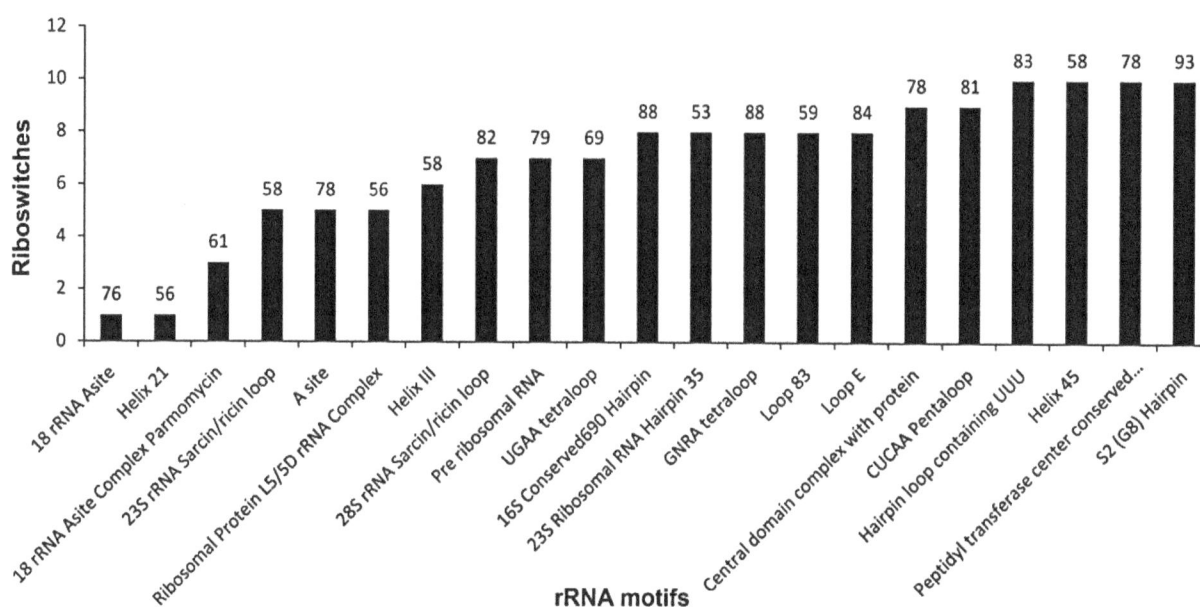

Figure 2. Correlation of ribosomal RNA motifs with 10 different types of riboswitches. Vertical axis demonstrates the number of similar riboswitches types which share at least 50% secondary structure identity (PSS>50%) with the shown rRNA motifs (average of PSS for each motif is shown above on the relative column). Please note that 4 motifs including "Hairpin loop containing UUU", "Helix 45", "Peptidyl transferase center conserved hairpin A loop", and "S2 (G8) Hairpin" are similar with all 10 types of riboswitches having 83, 58, 78, 93% PSS, respectively.

Sequences alignment
Multiple sequence alignment is a way of arranging the sequences of DNA, RNA, or protein molecules to similar regions that may be a consequence of functional, structural, or evolutionary origin. Multiple alignments are often used in identifying conserved sequences across a group of sequences hypothesized to be evolutionarily related. Herein, multiple sequence alignment of the riboswitches and similar rRNAs with more than 50 percent secondary structure identity (PSS, discussed above) was carried out. Although, all of the sequences were structurally similar to each other

(PSS>50%) there were not any particular sequence similarity results using different programs (ClustalW2 and M-Coffee, data not shown). In order to do the alignment more precisely, pairwise alignment of each rRNA with the riboswitches was accomplished by Needle and Water servers as global and local alignment tools, respectively. Figure 3 illustrates the results achieved for each pairwise global alignment between every rRNAs and associated riboswitches. Each one of 10 riboswitches sequences was aligned with related rRNAs and an average for every kind of riboswitches was represented in Mean ± SEM (Standard Error of the

Mean). As it was shown, global identity percentage is considerably lower than 25% identity. More importantly, based on local alignment there is no unique region in rRNA sequences aligned with the similar riboswitches (Table S1). As a result, no common assembly of nucleotides was recognized in the alignments by different programs. Despite this fact that aptamer domains of riboswitches are highly conserved sequences,[1,9] no particular conserved element was observed in their similar rRNAs. In agreement with our findings, it is commonly established that functionally important RNA sequences could be less conserved than their structures[45] where maintaining the structure is more important than maintaining the sequence.[46] For instance, a study on human and mouse genome sequences suggested that there are corresponding non-coding RNA sequences regions between human and mouse with common RNA structures which are not alignable in primary sequence.[46] Therefore, in spite of the structurally similarity of riboswitches and rRNAs, no particular conserved primary sequence element observed in their similar rRNAs using pairwise/multiple alignment approach.

Table 1. Types of riboswitches which share more than 50% secondary structure identity with ribosomal RNA motifs. The type of riboswitch which include a motif is checked under its name.

Motif*	Riboswitch									
	Glycine	Lysine	Purine	THF	FMN	TPP	preQ1	SAM	c-di-GMP I	c-di-MP II
16S Conserved 690 Hairpin	✓	✓	-	✓	✓	✓	✓	-	✓	✓
18 rRNA A site	✓	-	-	-	-	-	-	-	-	-
18 rRNA A site Complex Parmomycin	✓	-	-	-	-	-	-	✓	✓	-
23S rRNA Sarcin/ricin loop	✓	✓	✓	✓	-	-	-	-	✓	-
23S Ribosomal RNA Hairpin 35	✓	✓	✓	✓	-	✓	-	✓	✓	✓
28S rRNA Sarcin/ricin loop	✓	✓	✓	✓	-	✓	-	✓	✓	-
A site	✓	✓	-	✓	-	-	-	✓	-	✓
Central domain complex with protein	-	✓	✓	✓	✓	✓	✓	✓	✓	✓
CUCAA Pentaloop	✓	✓	✓	✓	-	✓	✓	✓	✓	✓
GNRA tetraloop	✓	-	✓	✓	✓	✓	-	✓	✓	✓
Hairpin loop containing UUU	✓	✓	✓	✓	✓	✓	✓	✓	✓	✓
Helix 21	-	-	-	-	-	✓	-	-	-	-
Helix 45	✓	✓	✓	✓	✓	✓	✓	✓	✓	✓
Helix III	✓	-	✓	✓	-	-	-	✓	✓	✓
Loop 83	✓	✓	✓	✓	✓	-	-	✓	✓	✓
Loop E	-	-	✓	✓	✓	✓	✓	✓	✓	✓
Peptidyl transferase center conserved hairpin A loop	✓	✓	✓	✓	✓	✓	✓	✓	✓	✓
Pre ribosomal RNA	✓	✓	✓	✓	-	✓	-	✓	-	✓
Ribosomal Protein L5/5D rRNA Complex	✓	✓	-	✓	-	✓	-	-	✓	-
S2 (G8) Hairpin	✓	✓	✓	✓	✓	✓	✓	✓	✓	✓
UGAA tetraloop	✓	-	✓	✓	✓	✓	✓	✓	-	-
16S Conserved 690 Hairpin	✓	✓	-	✓	✓	✓	✓	-	✓	✓
Total number	18	14	15	18	10	15	9	16	16	14

*The name of each motif is extracted from SCOR (Structural Classification of RNA, http://scor.berkeley.edu/).

Functional properties of riboswitches-rRNAs motifs

Ligand binding is one of the main functions of RNAs for structural stabilization, as well as producing signals. RNA ligand binding is important for ribozymes, riboswitches and splicing functions, along with mediating RNA-protein and RNA-RNA intermolecular interactions.[47] The first ribosomal RNA identified as a small molecule target was 16S RNA component of the prokaryotic ribosome.[48] Various antibiotics, such as aminoglycosides, affect bacterial cells through binding to functional sites of the bacterial rRNA which leads to miscoding during the translation process. Since similarity between riboswitches and different rRNA motifs were revealed in previous parts of current study, a question was raised that "could binding characteristics of these structures be similar too?" Therefore, the binding affinity of riboswitches for paromomycin as a functional characteristic of these structures was evaluated for a common motif in riboswitches-rRNA structures using molecular docking approach via Autodock 4.2. Paromomycin is a member of aminoglycosides antibiotics family that has high functional affinity for "A site" motif of 16S rRNAs.[49-51] The aligned part of each riboswitch with "A site" motif of 16S rRNAs (1j7t) was considered to evaluate the possibility of functional antibiotic binding affinity. Table 2 illustrated the binding energy of docked ligand with riboswitches and 16S rRNA structures. According to the docking results, except for c-di-GMP I riboswitch, there is a high functional affinity of paromomycin to the riboswitches in comparison with 16S rRNA. Statistical analysis showed that apart from c-di-GMP I, p value for all kinds of riboswitches relative to "16S rRNA A site" is less than 0.01. As a result, there is a remarkable significant upshift was occurred in binding energy of different riboswitches types with paromomycin. The range of appropriate binding energies for riboswitches is from -13 to -22 kcal/mol whereas it is -11.7 kcal/mol for "16S rRNA A site" (see Table 2). Seven riboswitches including lysine, THF, SAM, c-di-GMP II, purine, glycine and TPP riboswitches have 1.5-~2 times higher affinity for paromomycin than "A site" motif. Among them, lysine, THF, SAM and c-di-GMP II have more than 50% of secondary structure similarity with "A site" motif (Table 1). However, despite having less similarity of purine and TPP riboswitches with "A site" motif, they have also considerable low binding energy with paromomycin. But only c-di-GMP I riboswitch showed completely different functional behavior of quite not suitable interaction with the desired ligand. It could be possibly due to nucleotide types in defined binding site which cause weak electrostatic interaction with paromomycin. According to Table 2, maximum and minimum binding energy of each type of riboswitches

demonstrates that the most involved intermolecular energy (van der Waals, H bonding, desolvation and electrostatic energy) in mentioned interactions is electrostatic energy.

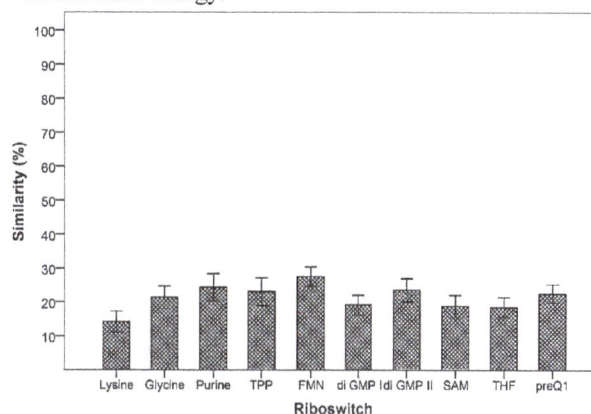

Figure 3. Average of global pairwise alignment similarity percentage of rRNA sequences with structurally-based similar riboswitches via Needle program [25]. The sequences of all structurally similar rRNAs (PSS>50%.) were aligned with related riboswitch and the similarity percentages were represented in Mean ± SEM for all types of riboswitches (it should be noted that the average number of rRNAs for the analysis were more than 30 strings for each type of riboswitches). Global identity percentages in the range of 14% to 26% denote no sequence correlation between riboswitch and structurally similar rRNAs (For complete data see Table S1).

Table 2. Binding energy of paromomycin interactions with different types of riboswitches and "16S rRNA A site" as receptors. Binding energy of each interaction is divided to van der Waals energy, hydrogen bonding energy, desolvation energy and electrostatic energy.

Receptors*	Mean binding energy ± SD (kcal/mol)	Max binding energy(kcal/mol)			Min binding energy(kcal/mol)		
		vdW + Hbond + desolv Energy	Electrostatic Energy	Total binding energy	vdW + Hbond + desolv Energy	Electrostatic Energy	Total binding energy
Lysine (3d0x)	-22.75 ± 1.12	-6.87	-20.91	-25.1	-5.5	-17.4	-20.22
THF (3suy)	-20.29 ± 1.47	-5.5	-19.99	-22.8	-3.35	-16.49	-17.15
SAM (3iqn)	-19.05 ± 0.77	-8.32	-15.6	-21.24	-3.66	-16.66	-17.64
c-di-GMP II (3q3z)	-19.3295 ± 0.61	-5.62	-17.96	-20.9	-3.95	-16.48	-17.75
Purine (4fe5)	-19.17 ± 0.62	-6.02	-17.25	-20.59	-4.81	-15.58	-17.7
Glycine (3ox0)	-18.97 ± 0.90	-6.04	-17.48	-20.83	-2.52	-17.06	-16.89
TPP (2gdi)	-18.52 ± 0.94	-6.32	-16.92	-20.56	-3.1	-15.88	-16.3
preQ (3fu2)	-15.12 ± 1.64	-5.67	-15.33	-18.32	-3.39	-11.47	-12.17
FMN (2yie)	-13.07 ± 0.93	-5.16	-12.74	-15.21	-3.68	-9.65	-10.65
c-di-GMP I (3iwn)	0.53 ± 0.76	-7.04	2.89	-25.1	-3.47	2.98	2.2
A site (1j7t)**	-11.75 ± 0.79	-5.29	-10.93	-13.54	-3.54	-9.23	-10.08
*Receptors indicated riboswitches with their PDB codes. ** "A site" refers to "16S rRNA A site" set as a control.							

Figure 4 shows RMSD (Root Mean Square Deviation) against binding energy for all kinds of riboswitches and "16S rRNA A site". Accordingly, the steadiness of all graphs showed that most conformations in studied structures have similar behavior to interact with receptors. Consequently, it verified the docking results and similar condition of docking in all of the riboswitches and 16S rRNA A site. Figure 5

illustrates the schematic interaction of paromomycin with "A site" and the riboswitches types. As paromomycin and "A site" interaction, the ligand binds to minor groove of riboswitches too. However, this kind of binding is not observed in c-di-GMP I riboswitch which may be the reason for not suitable interaction. Apart from c-di-GMP I riboswitch, paromomycin is covered in all types of riboswitches which may reduce the access of the molecule with around environment.

These findings support a report which introduced an engineered riboswitch for the aminoglycoside antibiotic neomycin B.[22] The resulting neomycin B responsive RNA-element partially resembles the ribosomal A-site, the natural target for aminoglycoside antibiotics.[23] Furthermore, recently Jia et al. discovered an aminoglycoside-binding riboswitch that is related to induction of aminoglycosides antibiotic resistance.[52]

The targeting of RNA with small molecules is the complementary or even basic of targeting of proteins. Through this phenomenon, riboswitches demonstrate regulatory mechanisms in which proteins do not take part. Furthermore, the importance of RNA-binding

small molecules such as antibiotics is undeniable. All clinically approved drugs which exert their effects by binding to RNA are totally recognized as rRNA-targeting molecules.[35] Accordingly, it could be discussed that some of resulted motifs in this study could be alternative binding sites for antibiotics and related small molecules in riboswitches. As though, if further studies on other motifs and antibiotics verify these findings, there is another mechanism for antibiotics effects or resistance apart from rRNA binding signaling in bacteria. It means these kinds of small molecules may bind to same motifs in riboswitches to generate their impact leading to bacteria's death or growth repression. However, this suggestion needs more computational and experimental confirming findings.

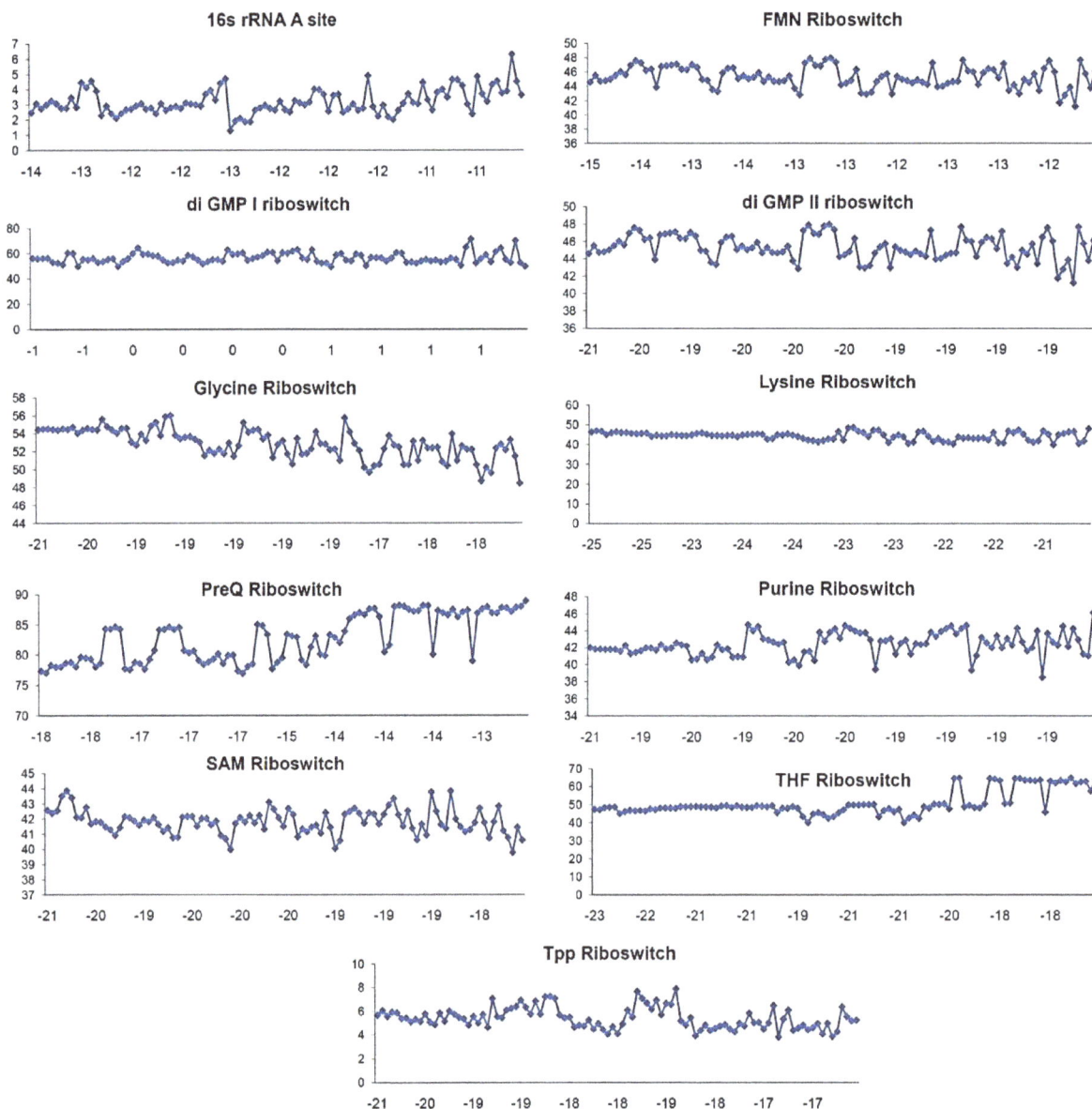

Figure 4. RMSD vs. binding energy for 10 types of riboswitches and "16S rRNA A site" based on Autodock results. Vertical and horizontal axes represented RMSD and binding energy of each docked conformations.

Evolutionary Origin and Conserved Structural Building Blocks of Riboswitches and Ribosomal...

183

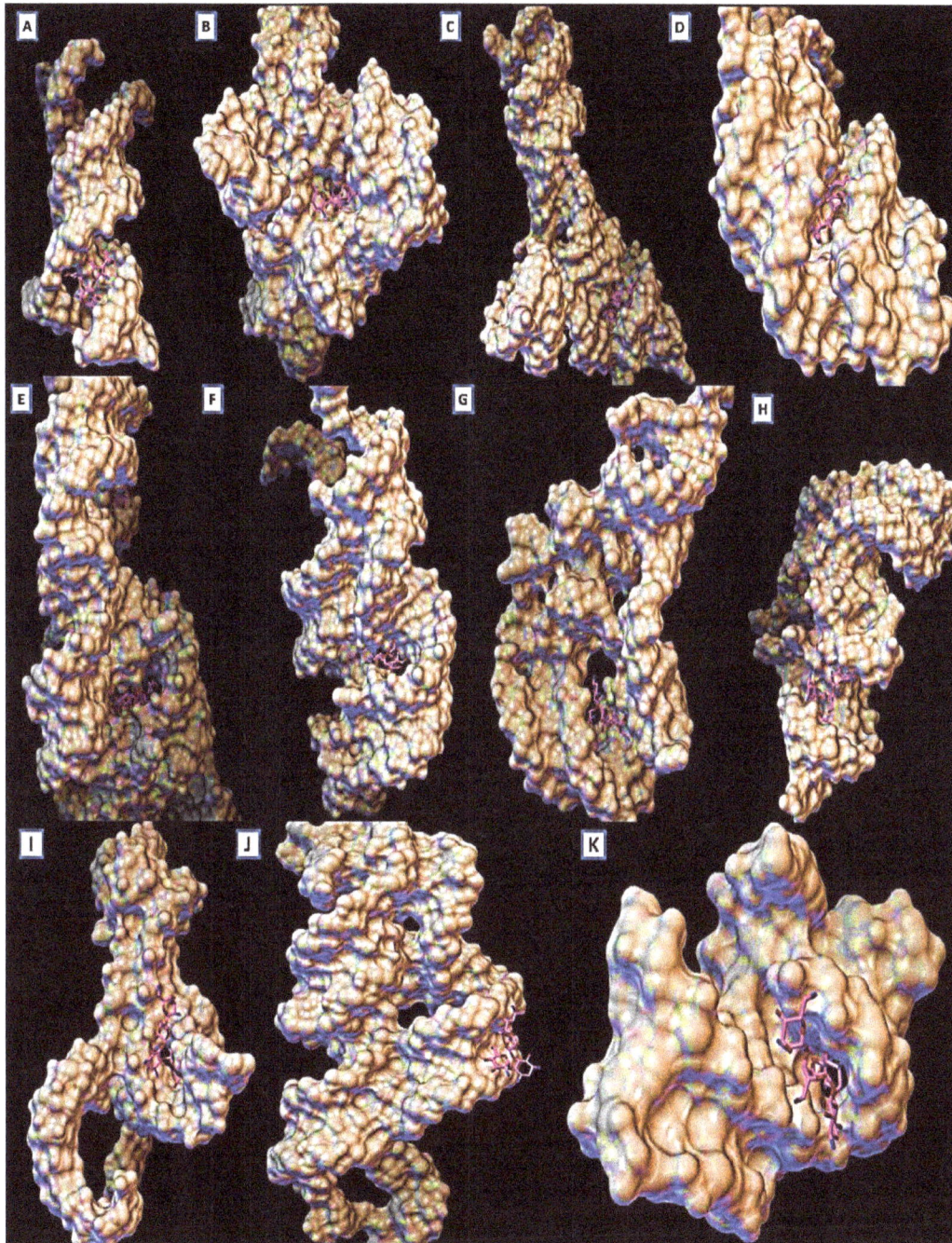

Figure 5. Docking conformations of paromomycin and RNAs. The ligand Paromomycin was shown stick-line and all of receptors were presented charge-space including (**A**) "16S rRNA A site" (1j7t), (**B**) SAM riboswitch (3iqn), (**C**) Glycine riboswitch (3ox0), (**D**) Purine riboswitch (4fe5), (**E**) Lysine riboswitch (3d0x), (**F**) THF riboswitch (3suy), (**G**) c-di-GMP II riboswitch (3q3z), (**H**) TPP riboswitch (2gdi), (**I**) FMN riboswitch (2yie), (**J**) c-di-GMP I riboswitch (3iwn), (**K**) preQ riboswitch (3fu2). The conformation with lowest binding energy was selected for each structure.

Conclusion

In this study, the relation between ribosomal RNAs and riboswitches in terms of structural and functional similarity was evaluated. Our findings indicated these two types of RNAs are structurally similar (secondary and tertiary based level) rather than in primary sequences. Accordingly, similar secondary structure motifs with high identity as Hairpin loop containing UUU, Peptidyl transferase center conserved hairpin A loop, Helix 45 and S2 (G8) Hairpin were detected between riboswitches and rRNAs. Consequently, investigation on the connection between binding sites of aminoglycosides in rRNAs and riboswitches using docking method revealed that riboswitches bind more tightly than "16S rRNA A site" to paromomycin. Considering other studies suggesting any kind of structural, functional or evolutionary similarity of ribosomal RNAs and riboswitches, these results could verify that these two apparent diverse types of RNAs show strong correspondence to each other.

Conflict of Interest

The authors declare that they have no conflict of interest.

References

1. Montange RK, Batey RT. Riboswitches: emerging themes in RNA structure and function. *Annu Rev Biophys* 2008;37:117-33.
2. Toledo-Arana A, Repoila F, Cossart P. Small noncoding RNAs controlling pathogenesis. *Curr Opin Microbiol* 2007;10(2):182-8.
3. Waters LS, Storz G. Regulatory RNAs in bacteria. *Cell* 2009;136(4):615-28.
4. Serganov A, Patel DJ. Amino acid recognition and gene regulation by riboswitches. *Biochim Biophys Acta* 2009;1789(9-10):592-611.
5. Serganov A. The long and the short of riboswitches. *Curr Opin Struct Biol* 2009;19(3):251-9.
6. Geissmann T, Marzi S, Romby P. The role of mRNA structure in translational control in bacteria. *RNA Biol* 2009;6(2):153-60.
7. Cruz JA, Westhof E. The dynamic landscapes of RNA architecture. *Cell* 2009;136(4):604-9.
8. Grundy FJ, Henkin TM. From ribosome to riboswitch: Control of gene expression in bacteria by RNA structural rearrangements. *Crit Rev Biochem Mol Biol* 2006;41(6):329-38.
9. Nahvi A, Sudarsan N, Ebert MS, Zou X, Brown KL, Breaker RR. Genetic control by a metabolite binding mRNA. *Chem Biol* 2002;9(9):1043.
10. Nudler E, Mironov AS. The riboswitch control of bacterial metabolism. *Trends Biochem Sci* 2004;29(1):11-7.
11. Mandal M, Breaker RR. Gene regulation by riboswitches. *Nat Rev Mol Cell Biol* 2004;5(6):451-63.
12. Petrone PM, Dewhurst J, Tommasi R, Whitehead L, Pomerantz AK. Atomic-scale characterization of conformational changes in the preQ(1) riboswitch aptamer upon ligand binding. *J Mol Graph Model* 2011;30:179-85.
13. Ling B, Wang Z, Zhang R, Meng X, Liu Y, Zhang C, et al. Theoretical studies on the interaction of modified pyrimidines and purines with purine riboswitch. *J Mol Graph Model* 2009;28(1):37-45.
14. Vicens Q, Mondragon E, Batey RT. Molecular sensing by the aptamer domain of the FMN riboswitch: A general model for ligand binding by conformational selection. *Nucleic Acids Res* 2011;39(19):8586-98.
15. Kelley JM, Hamelberg D. Atomistic basis for the on-off signaling mechanism in SAM-II riboswitch. *Nucleic Acids Res* 2010;38(4):1392-400.
16. Gong Z, Zhao Y, Chen C, Xiao Y. Computational study of unfolding and regulation mechanism of preQ1 riboswitches. *PLoS One* 2012;7(9):e45239.
17. Mulhbacher J, Brouillette E, Allard M, Fortier LC, Malouin F, Lafontaine DA. Novel riboswitch ligand analogs as selective inhibitors of guanine-related

metabolic pathways. *PLoS Pathog* 2010;6(4):e1000865.
18. Daldrop P, Reyes FE, Robinson DA, Hammond CM, Lilley DM, Batey RT, et al. Novel ligands for a purine riboswitch discovered by RNA-ligand docking. *Chem Biol* 2011;18(3):324-35.
19. Woese CR, Winker S, Gutell RR. Architecture of ribosomal RNA: Constraints on the sequence of "tetra-loops". *Proc Natl Acad Sci U S A* 1990;87(21):8467-71.
20. Leontis NB, Westhof E. Analysis of RNA motifs. *Curr Opin Struct Biol* 2003;13(3):300-8.
21. Barrick JE, Breaker RR. The distributions, mechanisms, and structures of metabolite-binding riboswitches. *Genome Biol* 2007;8(11):R239.
22. Weigand JE, Sanchez M, Gunnesch EB, Zeiher S, Schroeder R, Suess B. Screening for engineered neomycin riboswitches that control translation initiation. *RNA* 2008;14(1):89-97.
23. Duchardt-Ferner E, Weigand JE, Ohlenschlager O, Schmidtke SR, Suess B, Wohnert J. Highly modular structure and ligand binding by conformational capture in a minimalistic riboswitch. *Angew Chem Int Ed Engl* 2010;49(35):6216-9.
24. Burge SW, Daub J, Eberhardt R, Tate J, Barquist L, Nawrocki EP, et al. Rfam 11.0: 10 years of RNA families. *Nucleic Acids Res* 2013;41(D1):D226-32.
25. Rice P, Longden I, Bleasby A. EMBOSS: the European Molecular Biology Open Software Suite. *Trends Genet* 2000;16(6):276-7.
26. Capriotti E, Marti-Renom MA. Sara: A server for function annotation of RNA structures. *Nucleic Acids Res* 2009;37(Web Server issue):W260-5.
27. Rahrig RR, Leontis NB, Zirbel CL. R3d align: Global pairwise alignment of RNA 3D structures using local superpositions. *Bioinformatics* 2010;26(21):2689-97.
28. Breaker RR. Riboswitches and the RNA world. *Cold Spring Harb Perspect Biol* 2012;4(2).
29. Thompson JD, Higgins DG, Gibson TJ. Clustal W: Improving the sensitivity of progressive multiple sequence alignment through sequence weighting, position-specific gap penalties and weight matrix choice. *Nucleic Acids Res* 1994;22(22):4673-80.
30. Tamura K, Peterson D, Peterson N, Stecher G, Nei M, Kumar S. Mega5: Molecular evolutionary genetics analysis using maximum likelihood, evolutionary distance, and maximum parsimony methods. *Mol Biol Evol* 2011;28(10):2731-9.
31. Morris GM, Goodsell DS, Halliday RS, Huey R, Hart WE, Belew RK, et al. Automated docking using a Lamarckian genetic algorithm and an empirical binding free energy function. *J Comput Biol* 1998;19(14):1639-62.
32. Chang YF, Huang YL, Lu CL. SARSA: A web tool for structural alignment of RNA using a structural alphabet. *Nucleic Acids Res* 2008;36(Web Server issue):W19-24.

33. Dror O, Nussinov R, Wolfson H. Arts: Alignment of RNA tertiary structures. *Bioinformatics* 2005;21 (Suppl 2):ii47-53.

34. Ferre F, Ponty Y, Lorenz WA, Clote P. DIAL: A web server for the pairwise alignment of two RNA three-dimensional structures using nucleotide, dihedral angle and base-pairing similarities. *Nucleic Acids Res* 2007;35(Web Server issue):W659-68.

35. Thomas JR, Hergenrother PJ. Targeting RNA with small molecules. *Chem Rev* 2008;108(4):1171-224.

36. Klosterman PS, Hendrix DK, Tamura M, Holbrook SR, Brenner SE. Three-dimensional motifs from the SCOR, structural classification of RNA database: Extruded strands, base triples, tetraloops and U-turns. *Nucleic Acids Res* 2004;32(8):2342-52.

37. Tamura M, Hendrix DK, Klosterman PS, Schimmelman NR, Brenner SE, Holbrook SR. SCOR: Structural classification of RNA, version 2.0. *Nucleic Acids Res* 2004;32(Database issue):D182-4.

38. Jaeger L, Verzemnieks EJ, Geary C. The UA_handle: A versatile submotif in stable RNA architectures. *Nucleic Acids Res* 2009;37(1):215-30.

39. Nissen P, Ippolito JA, Ban N, Moore PB, Steitz TA. RNA tertiary interactions in the large ribosomal subunit: The A-minor motif. *Proc Natl Acad Sci U S A* 2001;98(9):4899-903.

40. Cate JH, Gooding AR, Podell E, Zhou K, Golden BL, Kundrot CE, et al. Crystal structure of a group I ribozyme domain: Principles of RNA packing. *Science* 1996;273(5282):1678-85.

41. Scott WG, Finch JT, Klug A. The crystal structure of an all-RNA hammerhead ribozyme: A proposed mechanism for RNA catalytic cleavage. *Cell* 1995;81(7):991-1002.

42. Yan Z, Baranger AM. Binding of an aminoacridine derivative to a GAAA RNA tetraloop. *Bioorg Med Chem Lett* 2004;14(23):5889-93.

43. Yan Z, Rao Ramisetty S, Bolton PH, Baranger AM. Selective recognition of RNA helices containing dangling ends by a quinoline derivative. *Chembiochem* 2007;8(14):1658-61.

44. Yan Z, Sikri S, Beveridge DL, Baranger AM. Identification of an aminoacridine derivative that binds to RNA tetraloops. *J Med Chem* 2007;50(17):4096-104.

45. Chursov A, Walter MC, Schmidt T, Mironov A, Shneider A, Frishman D. Sequence-structure relationships in yeast mRNAs. *Nucleic Acids Res* 2012;40(3):956-62.

46. Torarinsson E, Sawera M, Havgaard JH, Fredholm M, Gorodkin J. Thousands of corresponding human and mouse genomic regions unalignable in primary sequence contain common RNA structure. *Genome Res* 2006;16(7):885-9.

47. Hendrix DK, Brenner SE, Holbrook SR. RNA structural motifs: Building blocks of a modular biomolecule. *Q Rev Biophys* 2005;38(3):221-43.

48. Moazed D, Noller HF. Interaction of antibiotics with functional sites in 16S ribosomal RNA. *Nature* 1987;327(6121):389-94.

49. Francois B, Szychowski J, Adhikari SS, Pachamuthu K, Swayze EE, Griffey RH, et al. Antibacterial aminoglycosides with a modified mode of binding to the ribosomal-RNA decoding site. *Angew Chem Int Ed Engl* 2004;43(48):6735-8.

50. Vicens Q, Westhof E. Crystal structure of paromomycin docked into the eubacterial ribosomal decoding A site. *Structure* 2001;9(8):647-58.

51. Fourmy D, Recht MI, Blanchard SC, Puglisi JD. Structure of the A site of *Escherichia coli* 16S ribosomal RNA complexed with an aminoglycoside antibiotic. *Science* 1996;274(5291):1367-71.

52. Jia X, Zhang J, Sun W, He W, Jiang H, Chen D, et al. Riboswitch control of aminoglycoside antibiotic resistance. *Cell* 2013;152(1-2):68-81.

Construction of pPIC9 Recombinant Vector Containing Human Stem Cell Factor

Behrooz Farhadi[1], Mahmoud Shekari khaniani[2], Sima Mansoori Derakhshan[2]*

[1] Department of Biochemistry, Faculty of Medicine, Tabriz University of Medical Sciences Tabriz, Iran.

[2] Department of Medical Genetics, Faculty of Medicine, Tabriz University of Medical Sciences Tabriz, Iran.

ARTICLE INFO

Keywords:
Human SCF
Cloning
Expression
Pichia pastoris

ABSTRACT

Purpose: Various cytokine regulates hematopoesis; they promote number of stages in stem cells biology such as proliferation, differentiation and endurance. Biological effects of SCF, as a hematopoietic cytokine; is triggered by binding to its ligand c-kit. Potential therapeutic applications of SCF include hematopoietic stem cell mobilization, exvivo stem/progenitor cell expansion, gene therapy, and immunotherapy. In this study we tried to construct of pPIC9 recombinant vector containing human SCF. *Methods:* hSCF cDNA was amplified by PCR and both hSCF cDNA and pPIC9 as yeast expression vector (shuttle vector) digested by *EcoR I* and *Xho I* restriction enzymes. Subsequent the digestion reaction, ligation reaction was carried out. In order to verifying of pPIC9 recombinant vector containing hSCF, PCR and sequence analysis was performed. *Results:* The construction of recombinant expression vector of pPIC9 containing hSCF cDNA was confirmed by sequencing method successfully. *Conclusion:* rhSCF/pPIC9 vector can be transformed into the *Picha pastoris* yeast as a eukaryotic host in order to produce human SCF at industrial scale.

Introduction

HEMATOPOIESIS is regulated by several cytokines that endorse the survival, proliferation, and differentiation of hematopoietic stem cells and progenitor cells.[1] Stem Cell Factor (SCF) plays an important role in hematopoiesis, spermatogenesis, and melanogenesis. Biological effects of SCF; as a hematopoietic cytokine; is triggered by binding to its ligand c-kit.[2-4] The SCF gene is located on the Sl locus in mice[4] and on chromosome 12q22-12q24 in humans.[5-6] SCF can exist both as a transmembrane protein and a soluble protein[7] (Figure 1, described in detail below). The both forms of SCF are produced by alternative splicing of the same RNA transcript and depending on inclusion or exclusion of exon 6, the proteolytic cleavage site can remain or not.[8-9]

Translation of mRNA including exon 6 contains proteolytic cleavage site and leads to production of the soluble form of human SCF (SCF248). Whereas the transmembrane form of SCF (SCF220) is produced by alternative spliced mRNA translation which excludes exone 6 that the cleavage occurs after Ala165. Gly residue which is replace with amino acids 149-177 in SCF220.

The soluble form of SCF is glycosylated and circulates as a dimer. The SCF's soluble form has noticeable secondary structure which includes a helices and β sheets regions.[10-13] The molecular weight of the *soluble form of SCF is about 18.5 kDa. SCF contains four Cys residues which construct the two intramolecular* bonds

Cys4-Cys89 and Cys43-Cys138.[14-15] Deletion of the area containing Cys138 in carboxyterminal region reduces biologic activity of the soluble SCF. This concept recommends that the Cys43- Cys138 disulfide bond might be essential for its full biologic activity.[16] Subsequent studies show that both intramolecular disulfide pairs are important to retain SCF entire biologic activity.[17]

HUMAN SCF

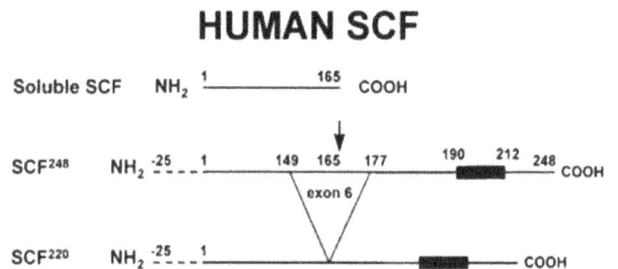

Figure 1. Soluble and transmembrane forms of human stem cell factor are shown. The arrow points to the primary proteolytic cleavage site of SCF248 in exon 6. The transmembrane form of SCF, SCF220 lacks the primary proteolytic cleavage site in exon 6. Dotted lines show the 25 amino acid signal sequence and dark box indicates the hydrophobic transmembrane domain.

SCF has a great role in acceleration of hematopoietic stem cells entry into the cell cycle.[18] Colony forming unit- spleen CFU-S survival *in vitro* needs the presence of SCF, and when SCF accompanies with IL-3 *in vitro*, the production of CFU-S increases significantly along a two-week period.[19]

The mast cell deficiency in W/Wv and Sl/Sld mice indicated that SCF might be necessary for mast cell production. Mast cells survival, proliferation, and maturation are promoted by SCF in vitro. In vitro proliferation and differentiation of pro-mastocyte, the earliest committed mast cell progenitor, occurs in the presence of both SCF and IL-3.[20]

In according to mast cell studies,[7,21-23] hematopoietic cell lines studies[24,25] and of normal hematopoietic cells studies,[25] we can conclude that SCF can regulate the adhesive properties of hematopoietic cells.

CD34[+] marrow cells adherence to fibronectin is enhanced by SCF Exposure, and hematopoietic progenitor cells adhesion to stromal cells decreases in W/Wv mice.[26]

Sensitivity to radiotherapy changes in the presence of SCF. Sl and W mutations increases radiosensitivity in mice[27] it might be due to the capability of SCF to suppress apoptosis and promote cell cycle progression.[4,28]

According to the properties of SCF, this protein can be used in clinical applications. Thus production of human Stem Cell Factor as a recombinant protein is a necessity in our country. We tried to construct recombinant shuttle vector of pPIC9 contains human stem cell factor gene. This vector can be used for transformation into *pichia pastoris* yeast. The Figure 2 shows the map of pPIC9.

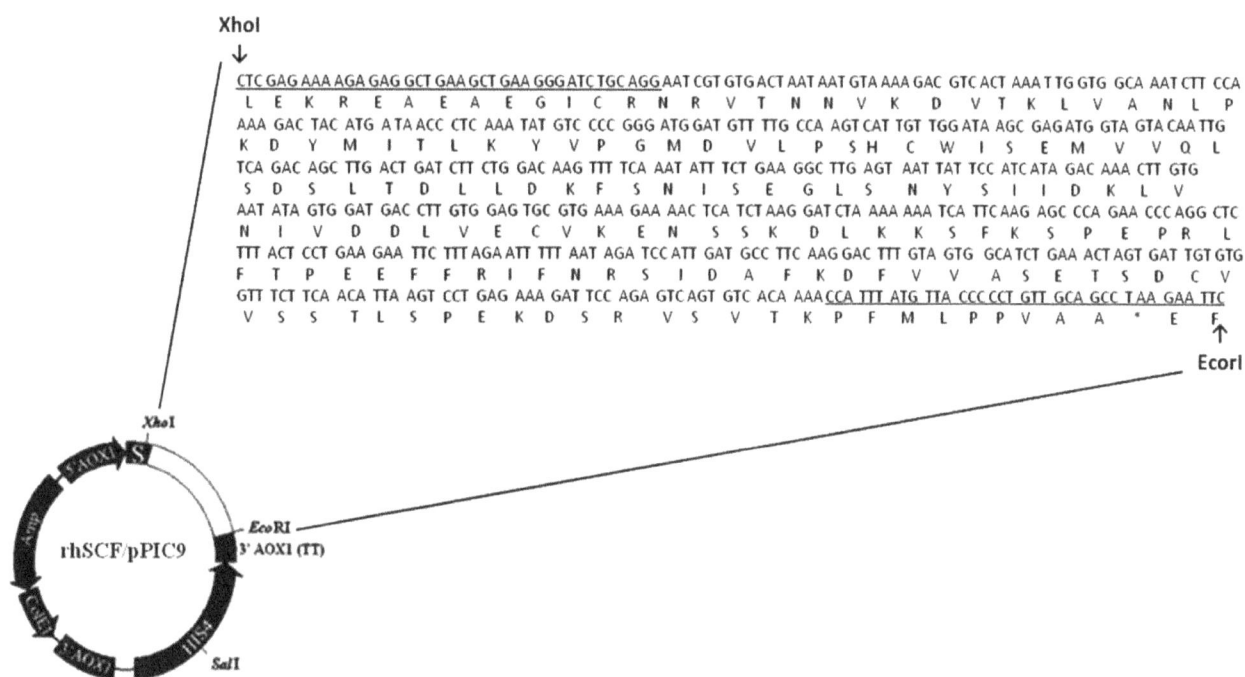

Figure 2. Expression vector used for production of recombinant *hSCF* in *Pichia pastoris*. The *hSCF* cDNA nucleotide sequence in shown in details and sequences belong to primers which used in specific amplification of cDNA. Sequences found in the vector: 5' AOX1-alcohol oxidase promoter, 3'AOX1(TT)- Transcriptional termination sequence,using 3' AOX1– sequences for direct integration into the yeast genome, HIS4 –histidiol dehydrogenase codifying gene, S-secretion signal sequence, ColE1-Escherichia coli replication origin, Amp –ampicillin resistance gene in Escherichia coli.

Materials and Methods
PCR Amplification of hSCF cDNA
The SCF cDNA sequence (protein coding nucleotides) was amplified by PCR, using specific primers), corresponding to the N- and C-terminal amino acid sequence of SCF. The human SCF cDNA sequence was derived from NCBI gene bank (Homo sapiens KIT ligand (KITLG), transcript variant b, mRNA. ACCESSION # NM_000899). Recognition sites sequence of XhoI and EcoR I restriction enzymes were added to 5' ends of reverse and forward primers to introduce Xho I site at the 5' and EcoR I site (Italics and bold) at the 3' end of the PCR products. We included the sequence between Xho I site and SnaBI site (underlined) in the 5' site of the SCF-fwd primer after the XhoI recognition site sequence. These 24 nucleotides between Xho I site and SnaBI site which encodes the KEX2 and STE13 cleavage sites must be recreated in order for efficient cleavage of the fusion protein to occur. Meanwhile the stop codon (TAA) was included after the EcoR I site in reverse primer. The sequences of the primers were 5'-ATCTCGAGAAAAGAGAGGCTGAAGCTGAAGG GATCTGCAGG-3' and 5' AATGAATTCTTAGGCTGCAACAGGGGGTAACA TAAATGG-3'.

A 498 bp fragment including whole coding sequence of SCF gene was amplified with these primers by PCR in a final volume 50μl. The final concentration of materials for PCR was as follows: Primers: 0.4μM, dNTP: 200µM and Mg2+: 1.5mM. PFU polymerase was used for amplification. Reaction was performed at an initial denaturation at 94 °C *for 3 min followed by 30 cycles amplification, each cycle including denaturation for 30 sec, annealing at 68 °C for 1 min and extension at 72 °C* for 1 min with an extra final 10 min incubation at 72 °C to complete all extensions.

Cloning of hSCF cDNA into pPIC9 Expression Vector

pPIC9 Vector and PCR product were double digested by *Xho1/EcoR1* enzymes at 37 °C over night (Fermentas) separately. Final volume of reaction was 40 µl and tango buffer was used as buffer in the reaction. Following electrophoresis of digested products, extraction of digested vector and insert from gel agarose was performed using QIAGENE kit. Ligation was performed with T4 DNA Ligase enzyme and 100ng of vector with the ratio 1:3 of insert to vector. Following ligation, transformation to the DH5-α strain was performed by CaCl2 method. Transformant cells were plated on LB Agar containing Ampicilin (50µl/ml) and incubated overnight at 37 °C. Recombinant plasmids were extracted from several clones by miniprep kit (Fermentas).

Verifying of Recombinant Vector by PCR and Sequencing

PCR was performed at the same conditions on extracted plasmids with SCF-Fwd and SCF-Rev primers. PCR product were analysed by sequencing.

Results

The SCF cDNA was amplified by PCR. A single band of the expected size (498 bp) corresponding to human SCF cDNA was detected by agarose gel electrophoresis (Figure 3).

Double digestion of pPIC9 vector was performed with *Xho1/EcoR1* restriction enzymes. Digested products were resolved on agarose gel using electrophoresis and gel picture is presented in Figure 4. Following double digestion of vector by Xho1/EcoR, a small fragment of pPIC9 vector including 40 bp is separated which was electrophorsed out of gel and not observed on the gel. The bound A belongs to undigested vector and bounds B and C belong to digested vectors (Figure 4).

Following *Xho I/EcoR I* digestion and purification of both vector and PCR product, the PCR product was ligated into the corresponding *EcoR* I and *Xho* I sites within the multi-cloning site (MCS) of pPIC9 plasmid. Subsequent the ligation reaction, bacterial transformation and Amp selection on LB agar plates, a few numbers of clones were obtained. A total of 10 bacterial clones were screened by PCR using the SCF-Fwd and SCF-Rev primers. These primers yielded cloned PCR products containing the 498 bp PCR product representing SCF cDNA (Figure 5).

Sequence analysis of the 498 bp cloned PCR products confirmed SCF cDNA (Figure 6).

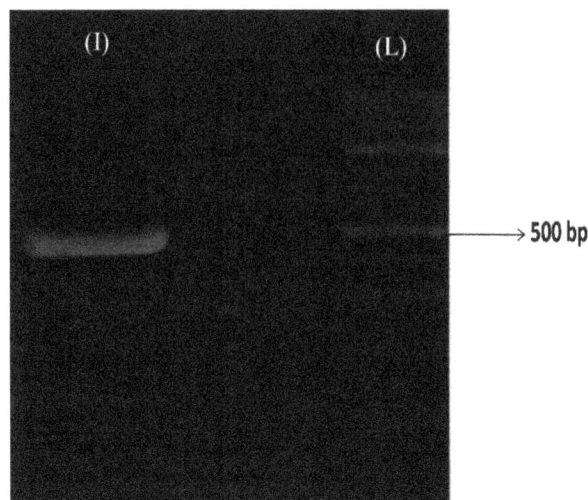

Figure 3. Agarose gel electrophoresis of PCR products of SCF cDNA. Lane of (I) corresponds to PCR Product of human SCF cDNA. Lane (L) corresponds to 100bp Ladder (Fermentas).

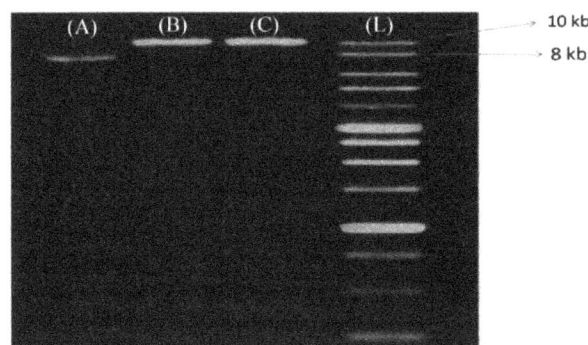

Figure 4. Double digestion of pPIC9 vector by Xho1/EcoR. bound A correspond to undigested vector. bound s B and C correspond to double digested pPIC9 vector. Lane L correspond to 10 Kbp ladder.

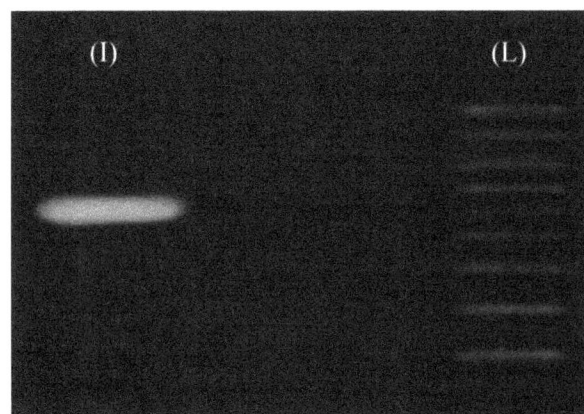

Figure 5. PCR screening of cloned SCF cDNA PCR products. The clones on Ampicillin plates were picked and screened by PCR. Lane L corresponds to 100 bp ladder (Fermentas). Bound I represent bacterial clone containing the SCF cDNA PCR product.

(A)

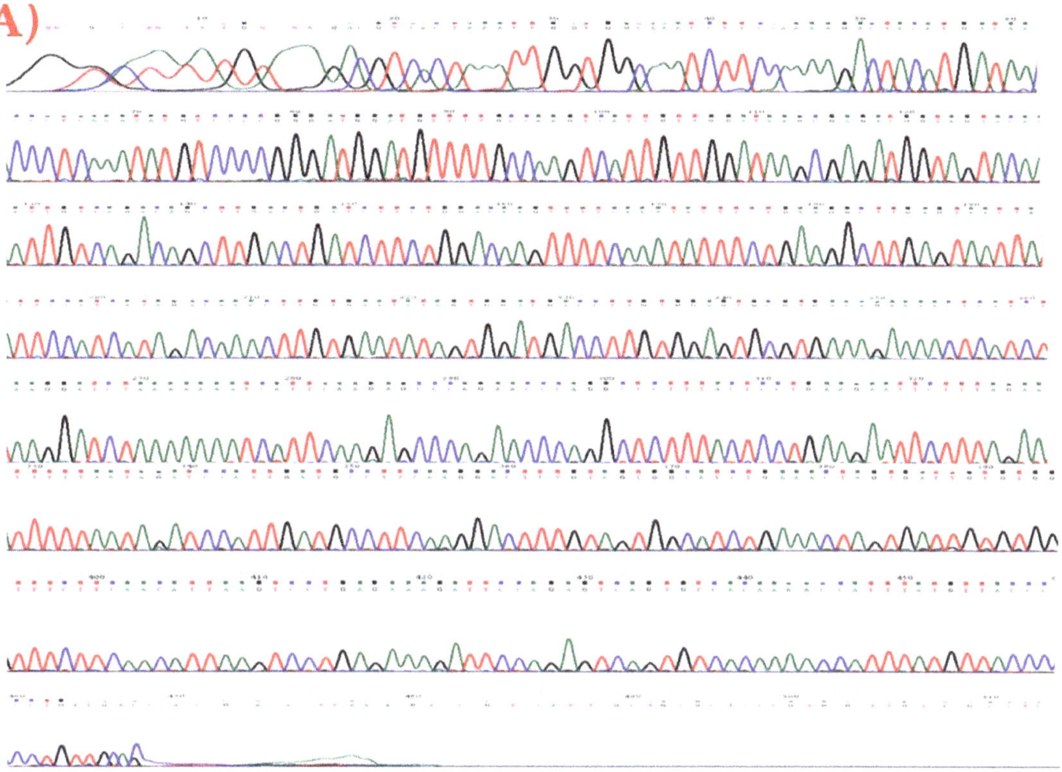

(B)

ref|NM_000899.4| U E G M Homo sapiens KIT ligand (KITLG), transcript variant b, mRNA
Length=5460
Score = 835 bits (452), Expect = 0.0
Identities = 452/452 (100%), Gaps = 0/452 (0%)
Strand=Plus/Plus

Query 15   AGACGTCACTAAATTGGTGGCAAATCTTCCAAAAGACTACATGATAACCCTCAAATATGT 74
            |||||||||||||||||||||||||||||||||||||||||||||||||||||||||||||
Sbjct 309 AGACGTCACTAAATTGGTGGCAAATCTTCCAAAAGACTACATGATAACCCTCAAATATGT 368

Query 75   CCCCGGGATGGATGTTTTGCCAAGTCATTGTTGGATAAGCGAGATGGTAGTACAATTGTC 134
            |||||||||||||||||||||||||||||||||||||||||||||||||||||||||||||
Sbjct 369 CCCCGGGATGGATGTTTTGCCAAGTCATTGTTGGATAAGCGAGATGGTAGTACAATTGTC 428

Query 135 AGACAGCTTGACTGATCTTCTGGACAAGTTTTCAAATATTTCTGAAGGCTTGAGTAATTA 194
            |||||||||||||||||||||||||||||||||||||||||||||||||||||||||||||
Sbjct 429 AGACAGCTTGACTGATCTTCTGGACAAGTTTTCAAATATTTCTGAAGGCTTGAGTAATTA 488

Query 195 TTCCATCATAGACAAACTTGTGAATATAGTGGATGACCTTGTGGAGTGCGTGAAAGAAAA 254
            |||||||||||||||||||||||||||||||||||||||||||||||||||||||||||||
Sbjct 489 TTCCATCATAGACAAACTTGTGAATATAGTGGATGACCTTGTGGAGTGCGTGAAAGAAAA 548

Query 255 CTCATCTAAGGATCTAAAAAAAATCATTCAAGAGCCCAGAACCCAGGCTCTTTACTCCTGA 314
            |||||||||||||||||||||||||||||||||||||||||||||||||||||||||||||
Sbjct 549 CTCATCTAAGGATCTAAAAAAAATCATTCAAGAGCCCAGAACCCAGGCTCTTTACTCCTGA 608

Query 315 AGAATTCTTTAGAATTTTTAATAGATCCATTGATGCCTTCAAGGACTTTGTAGTGGCATC 374
            |||||||||||||||||||||||||||||||||||||||||||||||||||||||||||||
Sbjct 609 AGAATTCTTTAGAATTTTTAATAGATCCATTGATGCCTTCAAGGACTTTGTAGTGGCATC 668

Query 375 TGAAACTAGTGATTGTGTGGTTTCTTCAACATTAAGTCCTGAGAAAGATTCCAGAGTCAG 434
            |||||||||||||||||||||||||||||||||||||||||||||||||||||||||||||
Sbjct 669 TGAAACTAGTGATTGTGTGGTTTCTTCAACATTAAGTCCTGAGAAAGATTCCAGAGTCAG 728

Query 435 TGTCACAAAACCATTTATGTTACCCCCTGTTG 466
            ||||||||||||||||||||||||||||||||
Sbjct 729 TGTCACAAAACCATTTATGTTACCCCCTGTTG 760

Figure 6. Sequencing analysis of recombinant vector. A) Chromatogram of sequencing result related to SCF cDNA. B) Blast analysis of the sequencing result. The results reveal that 498 bp bond which obtained from PCR reaction which belongs to human SCF.

This approach allowed heterologous gene insertion between the 5' AOX1 promoter sequence and the transcription termination sequence. The resultant plasmid (rhSCF/pPIC9), shown in Figure 1, was transformed into Escherichia coli, enabling rhSCF expression plasmid propagation.

Discussion

The survival, differentiation, and mobilization of numerous cell types (myeloid, erythroid, megakaryocytic, lymphoid, germ cell, and melanocyte progenitors) are promoted by SCF.[29,30]

SCF is widely used in stem cell research area and purchasing this recombinant protein is costly and time-consuming in Iran. Considering the cost and problem in accessibility of this product, clears the importance of indigenizing production of rhSCF.

The occurrence of multiple disulfide bridges in the native SCF protein (5) prompted us to use the *Pichia pastoris* eukaryotic expression system, since it is known that disulfide bridge formation of eukaryotic proteins expressed in prokaryotes is often erratic, leading to improper folding and tertiary structure destabilization.

For expression of SCF gene under the transcriptional control of AOX1 promoter, a 498 bp *XhoI/EcoR I* fragment composed of a 498-bp region beginning immediately 5' of methionine initiator ATG of SCF was generated by PCR.

In designing primers for cloning SCF coding gene in pPIC9 vector, we attempted to clone the SCF ORF under control of AOX1 promoter with α-factor secretion signal sequence in downstream of the AOX1 promoter. Recent evidences suggest that the a-factor secretion signal sequence might be modified to include KEX2-like processing sites for efficient cleavage to occur.[31] Choosing *Xho I* restriction site in the 5'-end allowed in-frame cloning into the a-factor secretion signal of pPIC9 expression vector and a sequence encoding the KEX2 and STE13 cleavage sites comprising 24 nucleotides was placed ahead of the mature SCF cDNA. The reverse primer was designed based on the C-terminal amino acid sequence of SCF, a stop codon, and an EcoRI restriction site in the 3'-end.

Using these primers, the 498-bp fragment encoding hSCF was cloned in pPIC9 inframe to the α-factor secretion signal, downstream of the alcohol oxidase promoter. The resultant plasmid (rhSCF/pPIC9) was transformed into E. coli DH5α, purified, and analyzed by sequencing, confirming the presence of rhSCF/pPIC9 expression plasmid.

Acknowledgements

Authors are highly thankful to stem cell research center for financial support.

Conflict of Interest

The authors report no conflicts of interest.

References

1. Metcalf D. Hematopoietic regulators: redundancy or subtlety? *Blood* 1993;82(12):3515-23.
2. Williams DE, Eisenman J, Baird A, Rauch C, Ness KV, March CJ, et al. Identification of a ligand for the c-kit protooncogene. *Cell* 1990;63(1):167-74.
3. Flanagan JG, Leder P. The kit ligand: a cell surface molecule altered in steel mutant fibroblasts. *Cell* 1990;63(1):185-94.
4. Zsebo KM, Williams DA, Geissler EN, Broudy VC, Martin, FH, Atkins HL, et al. Stem cell factor is encoded at the Sl locus of the mouse and is the ligand for the c-kit tyrosine kinase receptor. *Cell* 1990;63:213.
5. Anderson DM, Williams DE, Tushinski R, Gimpel S, Eisenman J, Cannizzaro LA, et al. Alternate splicing of mRNAs encoding human mast cell growth factor and localization of the gene to chromosome 12q22-q24. *Cell Growth Differ* 1991;2(8):373-8.
6. Geissler EN, Liao M, Brook JD, Martin FH, Zsebo KM, Housman DE, et al. Stem cell factor (SCF), a novel hematopoietic growth factor and ligand for c-kit tyrosine kinase receptor, map on human chromosome 12 between 12q14.3 and 12qter. *Somat Cell Mol Genet* 1991;17(2):207-14.
7. Flanagan JG, Chan DC, Leder P. Transmembrane form of the kit ligand growth factor is determined by alternative splicing and is missing in the Sld mutant. *Cell* 1991;64(5):1025-35.
8. Huang EJ, Nocka KH, Buck J, Besmer P. Differential expression and processing of two cell associated forms of the kit-ligand. KL-1 and KL-2. *Mol Biol Cell* 1992;3(3):349-62.
9. Anderson DM, Lyman SD, Baird A, Wignall JM, Eisenman J, Rauch C, et al. Molecular cloning of mast cell growth factor, a hematopoietin that is active in both membrane bound and soluble forms. *Cell* 1990;63(1):235-43.
10. Toksoz D, Zsebo KM, Smith KA, Hu S, Brankow D, Suggs SV, et al. Support of human hematopoiesis in long-term bone marrow cultures by murine stromal cells selectively expressing the membrane-bound and secreted forms of the human homolog of the steel gene product, stem cell factor. *Proc Natl Acad Sci USA* 1992;89(16):7350-4.
11. Huang EJ, Manova K, Packer AI, Sanchez S, Bachvarova RF, Besmer P. The murine steel panda mutation affects kit ligand expression and growth of early ovarian follicles. *Dev Biol* 1993;157(1):100-9.
12. Huang E, Nocka K, Beier DR, Chu TY, Buck J, Lahm HW, et al. The hematopoietic growth factor KL is encoded by the Sl locus and is the ligand of the c-kit receptor, the gene product of the W locus. *Cell* 1990;63(1):225-33.
13. Lu HS, Clogston CL, Wypych J, Fausset PR, Lauren S, Mendiaz EA, et al. Amino acid sequence and posttranslational modification of stem cell factor isolated from Buffalorat liver cell-conditioned medium. *J Biol Chem* 1991;266(13):8102-7.
14. Zsebo KM, Wypych J, McNiece IK, Lu HS, Smith KA, Karkare SB, et al. Identification, purification, and biological characterization of hematopoietic

stem cell factor from buffalo rat liver-conditioned medium. *Cell* 1990;63(1):195-201.

15. Langley KE, Wypych J, Mendiaz EA, Clogston CL, Parker VP, Farrar DH, et al. Purification and characterization of soluble forms of human and rat stem cell factor recombinantly expressed by Escherichia coli and by Chinese hamster ovary cells. *Arch Biochem Biophys* 1992;295(1):21-8

16. Nishikawa M, Tojo A, Ikebuchi K, Katayama K, Fujii N, Ozawa K, et al. Deletion mutagenesis of stem cell factor defines the c-terminal sequences essential for its biological activity. *Biochem Biophys Res Commun* 1992;188(1):292-7.

17. Jones MD, Narhi LO, Chang WC, Lu HS. Refolding and oxidation of recombinant human stem cell factor produced in Escherichia coli. *J Biol Chem* 1996;271(19):11301-8.

18. Leary AG, Zeng HQ, Clark SC, Ogawa M. Growth factor requirements for survival in G0 and entry into the cell cycle of primitive human hemopoietic progenitors. *Proc Natl Acad Sci USA* 1992;89(9):4013-7.

19. De Vries P, Brasel KA, Eisenman JR, Alpert AR, Williams DE. The effect of recombinant mast cell growth factor on purified murine hematopoietic stem cells. *J Exp Med* 1991;173(5):1205-11.

20. Rodewald HR, Dessing M, Dvorak AM, Galli SJ. Identification of a committed precursor for the mast cell lineage. *Science* 1996;271(5250):818-22.

21. Dastych J, Metcalfe DD. Stem cell factor induces mast cell adhesion to fibronectin. *J Immunol* 1994;152(1):213-9.

22. Kinashi T, Springer TA. Steel factor and c-kit regulate cell matrix adhesion. *Blood* 1994;83(4):1033-8.

23. Kaneko Y, Takenawa J, Yoshida O, Fujita K, Sugimoto K, Nakayama H, et al. Adhesion of mouse mast cells to fibroblasts: adverse effects of

steel (Sl) mutation. *J Cell Physiol* 1991;147(2):224-30.

24. Kovach NL, Lin N, Yednock T, Harlan JM, Broudy VC. Stem cell factor modulates avidity of a4b1 and a5b1 integrins expressed on hematopoietic cell lines. *Blood* 1995;85(1):159-67.

25. Levesque JP, Leavesley DI, Niutta S, Vadas M, Simmons PJ. Cytokines increase human hemopoietic cell adhesiveness by activation of very late antigen (VLA)-4 and VLA-5 integrins. *J Exp Med* 1995;181(5):1805-15.

26. Kodama H, Nose M, Niida S, Nishikawa S, Nishikawa S. Involvement of the c-kit receptor in the adhesion of hematopoietic stem cells to stromal cells. *Exp Hematol* 1994;22(10):979-84.

27. Russell ES, Bernstein SE, McFarland EC, Modeen WR. The cellular basis of differential radiosensitivity of normal and geneti cally anemic mice. *Radiat Res* 1963;20:677-94.

28. Geissler EN, McFarland EC, Russell ES. Analysis of pleiotropism at the dominant white-spotting (W) locus of the house mouse: A description of ten new W alleles. *Genetics* 1981;97(2):337-61.

29. Bashamboo A, Taylor AH, Samuel K, Panthier JJ, Whetton AD, Forrester LM. The survival of differentiating embryonic stem cells is dependent on the SCF-KIT pathway. *J Cell Sci* 2006;119(Pt 15):3039-46.

30. Ashman LK. The biology of stem cell factor and its receptor C-kit. *Int J Biochem Cell Biol* 1999;31(10):1037-51.

31. Laroche Y, Storme V, De Meutter J, Messens J, Lauwereys M. High-level secretion and very efficient isotopic labeling of tick anticoagulant peptide (TAP) expressed in the methylotrophic yeast, Pichia pastoris. *Biotechnol (N Y)* 1994;12(11):1119-24.

Permissions

All chapters in this book were first published in APB, by Tabriz University of Medical Sciences; hereby published with permission under the Creative Commons Attribution License or equivalent. Every chapter published in this book has been scrutinized by our experts. Their significance has been extensively debated. The topics covered herein carry significant findings which will fuel the growth of the discipline. They may even be implemented as practical applications or may be referred to as a beginning point for another development.

The contributors of this book come from diverse backgrounds, making this book a truly international effort. This book will bring forth new frontiers with its revolutionizing research information and detailed analysis of the nascent developments around the world.

We would like to thank all the contributing authors for lending their expertise to make the book truly unique. They have played a crucial role in the development of this book. Without their invaluable contributions this book wouldn't have been possible. They have made vital efforts to compile up to date information on the varied aspects of this subject to make this book a valuable addition to the collection of many professionals and students.

This book was conceptualized with the vision of imparting up-to-date information and advanced data in this field. To ensure the same, a matchless editorial board was set up. Every individual on the board went through rigorous rounds of assessment to prove their worth. After which they invested a large part of their time researching and compiling the most relevant data for our readers.

The editorial board has been involved in producing this book since its inception. They have spent rigorous hours researching and exploring the diverse topics which have resulted in the successful publishing of this book. They have passed on their knowledge of decades through this book. To expedite this challenging task, the publisher supported the team at every step. A small team of assistant editors was also appointed to further simplify the editing procedure and attain best results for the readers.

Apart from the editorial board, the designing team has also invested a significant amount of their time in understanding the subject and creating the most relevant covers. They scrutinized every image to scout for the most suitable representation of the subject and create an appropriate cover for the book.

The publishing team has been an ardent support to the editorial, designing and production team. Their endless efforts to recruit the best for this project, has resulted in the accomplishment of this book. They are a veteran in the field of academics and their pool of knowledge is as vast as their experience in printing. Their expertise and guidance has proved useful at every step. Their uncompromising quality standards have made this book an exceptional effort. Their encouragement from time to time has been an inspiration for everyone.

The publisher and the editorial board hope that this book will prove to be a valuable piece of knowledge for researchers, students, practitioners and scholars across the globe.

List of Contributors

Saeed Ghanbarzadeh
Drug Applied Research Center and Faculty of Pharmacy, Tabriz University of Medical Sciences, Tabriz, Iran
Student Research Committee, Tabriz University of Medical Sciences, Tabriz, Iran

Hadi Valizadeh
Research Center for Pharmaceutical Nanotechnology and Faculty of Pharmacy, Tabriz University of Medical Sciences, Tabriz, Iran

Parvin Zakeri-Milani
Liver and Gastrointestinal Diseases Research Center and Faculty of Pharmacy, Tabriz University of Medical Sciences, Tabriz, Iran

Behrooz Farhadi
Department of Biochemistry, Faculty of Medicine, Tabriz University of Medical Sciences Tabriz, Iran

Mahmoud Shekari khaniani and Sima Mansoori Derakhshan
Department of Medical Genetics, Faculty of Medicine, Tabriz University of Medical Sciences Tabriz, Iran

Hossein Babaei and Mohammad Ali Eghbal
Drug Applied Research Center, Tabriz University of Medical Sciences, Tabriz, Iran
Pharmacology and toxicology department, School of pharmacy, Tabriz University of Medical Sciences, Tabriz, Iran

Reza Heidari
Drug Applied Research Center, Tabriz University of Medical Sciences, Tabriz, Iran
Pharmacology and toxicology department, School of pharmacy, Tabriz University of Medical Sciences, Tabriz, Iran
Students' Research Committee, Tabriz University of Medical Sciences, Tabriz, Iran

Hamdolah Sharifi
Department of Pharmacology and Toxicology, Faculty of Pharmacy, Tabriz University of Medical Sciences. Tabriz, Iran

Alireza Mohajjel Nayebi and Safar Farajnia
Drug Applied Research Center, Tabriz University of Medical Science, Tabriz, Iran

Mahnaz Talebi, Sasan Andalib and Hormoz Ayromlou
Neurosciences Research Center, Tabriz University of Medical Sciences, Tabriz, Iran

Shohreh Bakhti and Alireza Aghili
School of Medicine, Tabriz University of Medical Sciences, Tabriz, Iran

Ashraf Talebi
School of Pharmacy, Tabriz University of Medical Sciences, Tabriz, Iran

Reza Ghotaslou and Morteza Milani
Liver and Gastroenterology Diseases Research Center, Tabriz University of Medical Sciences, Tabriz, Iran

Mohammad Taghi Akhi, Mohammad Reza Nahaei and Mohammad Meshkini
Department of Microbiology, School of Medicine, Tabriz University of Medical Sciences, Tabriz, Iran

Alka Hasani
Department of Microbiology, School of Medicine, Tabriz University of Medical Sciences, Tabriz, Iran
Infectious Diseases and Tropical Medicine Research Centre, Tabriz University of Medical Sciences, Tabriz, Iran

Mohammad Saeid Hejazi
Department of Pharmaceutical Biotechnology, School of Pharmacy, Tabriz University of Medical Sciences, Tabriz, Iran

Saadat Parhizkar
Medicinal Plants Research Centre, Yasuj University of Medical Sciences (YUMS), Yasuj, Iran

Maryam Jamielah Yusoff and Mohammad Aziz Dollah
Biomedical Department, Faculty of Medicine and Health Sciences,University Putra Malaysia, Malaysia

Saeideh Razi Soofiyani and Behzad Baradaran
Drug Applied Research Center, Tabriz University of Medical Sciences, Tabriz, Iran
Immonuology Research Center, Tabriz University of Medical Sciences, Tabriz, Iran

Tohid Kazemi and Leila Mohammadnejad
Immonuology Research Center, Tabriz University of Medical Sciences, Tabriz, Iran

Farzaneh Lotfipour
Faculty of Pharmacy, Tabriz University of Medical Sciences, Tabriz, Iran

Zohreh Ataie, Mina Ghahramanian Golzar, Hadi Ebrahimi and Fariba Mirzaie
Neuroscience Research Centre (NSRC), Tabriz University of Medical Sciences, Tabriz, Iran

Shirin Babri and Gisou Mohaddes
Neuroscience Research Centre (NSRC), Tabriz University of Medical Sciences, Tabriz, Iran
Neuroscience Research Centre, Shahid Beheshti Universiy of Medical Sciences, Tehran, Iran

Maliki Reddy Dastagiri Reddy, Yadati Narasimha Spoorthy and Lakshmana Rao Krishna Rao Ravindranath
Sri Krishnadevaraya University, Anantapur, A.P., India

Aluru Raghavendra Guru Prasad
ICFAI Foundation for Higher Education, Hyderabad, A.P., India

Saadat Parhizkar
Medicinal Plants Research Centre, Yasuj University of Medical Sciences (YUMS),Yasuj, Iran

Latiffah A Latiff
Community Health Department, Faculty of Medicine and Health Sciences, University Putra Malaysia (UPM), Malaysia

Zohreh Babaloo, Jafar Majidi and Behzad Baradaran
Immunology Research Center, Tabriz University of Medical Sciences, Tabriz, Iran

Elnaz Mosaferi
Immunology Research Center, Tabriz University of Medical Sciences, Tabriz, Iran
Tabriz International University of Medical Sciences, Tabriz, Iran

Mozhdeh Mohammadian
Hematology and Oncology Research Center, Tabriz University of Medical Sciences, Tabriz, Iran

Amir Monfaredan
Department of Hematology, Faculty of Medicine, Tabriz Branch of Islamic Azad University, Tabriz, Iran

Laleh Payahoo, Alireza Ostadrahimi, Yaser Khaje Bishak, Nazila Farrin and Sepide Mahluji
Nutrition Research Center, Faculty of Health and Nutrition, Tabriz University of Medical Science, Tabriz, Iran

Majid Mobasseri
Department of Internal Medicine, Tabriz University of Medical Science, Tabriz, Iran

Mohammad Asghari Jafarabadi
Tabriz Health Management Research Center, Faculty of Health and Nutrition, Tabriz University of Medical Science, Tabriz, Iran

Shirin Babri and Saeideh Hasani Azami
Neuroscience Research Center, Tabriz University of Medical Sciences, Tabriz, Iran

Gisou Mohaddes
Drug Applied Research Center, Tabriz University of Medical Sciences, Tabriz, Iran

Paniz Sajjadi
Department of Pharmaceutics, School of Pharmacy, Ahvaz Jundishapur University of Medical Sciences, Ahvaz, Iran

Mohammad Javad Khodayar
Department of Pharmacology and Toxicology, School of Pharmacy, Ahvaz Jundishapur University of Medical Sciences, Ahvaz, Iran

Behzad Sharif Makhmalzadeh and Saeed Rezaee
Nanotechnology Research Center, Ahvaz Jundishapur University of Medical Sciences, Ahvaz, Iran

Nosratollah Zarghami
Drug Applied Research Center, Tabriz University of Medical Sciences, Tabriz, Iran

Fatemeh Kazemi-Lomedasht
Drug Applied Research Center, Tabriz University of Medical Sciences, Tabriz, Iran
Pasteur Institute of Iran, Tehran, Iran

Abbas Rami
Pasteur Institute of Iran, Tehran, Iran

Reza Heidari, Hossein Babaei and Mohammad Ali Eghbal
Drug Applied Research Center, Tabriz University of Medical Sciences, Tabriz, Iran
Pharmacology and Toxicology Department, Faculty of Pharmacy, Tabriz University of Medical Sciences, Tabriz, Iran

Leila Roshangar
Anatomical Sciences Department, Faculty of Medicine, Tabriz University of Medical Sciences, Tabriz, Iran

Behzad Baradaran
Immunology Research Center, Tabriz University of Medical Sciences, Tabriz, Iran

Hadi Karami
Immunology Research Center, Tabriz University of Medical Sciences, Tabriz, Iran
Department of Biochemistry, Faculty of Medicine, Tabriz University of Medical Sciences, Tabriz, Iran

Ali Esfahani
Hematology and Oncology Research Center, Shahid Ghazi Hospital, Tabriz University of Medical Sciences, Tabriz, Iran

Masoud Sakhinia
Faculty of Medicine, University of Liverpool, Liverpool, United Kingdom

Ebrahim Sakhinia
Department of Genetics, Faculty of Medicine, Tabriz University of Medical Sciences, Tabriz, Iran
Tuberculosis and Lung Disease Reseach Center, Tabriz University of Medical Sciences, Tabriz, Iran

Laleh Pejman, Hasan Omrani and Zahra Mirzamohammadi
Department of Physiology, Faculty of Medicine, Tabriz University of Medical Sciences, Tabriz, Iran

Amir Ali Shahbazfar
Department of Pathology, Faculty of Veterinary Medicine, Tabriz University, Tabriz, Iran

Majid Khalili and Rana Keyhanmanesh
Tuberculosis and Lung Research Center, Tabriz University of Medical Sciences, Tabriz, Iran

Hassan Dariushnejad, Samaneh Ghasemali, Zohreh Sadeghi, Masoud Gandomkar Ghalhar and Zahra Davoodi
Department of Medical Biotechnology, Faculty of Advance Medical Sciences, Tabriz University of Medical Sciences, Tabriz, Iran

Nosratallah Zarghami and Mohammad Rahmati
Department of Clinical Biochemistry, Faculty of Medicine, Tabriz University of Medical Sciences, Tabriz, Iran
Department of Clinical Biochemistry, Faculty of Medicine, Tabriz University of Medical Sciences, Tabriz, Iran

Hossein Jafari Tekab
Department of Medical Genetics, Faculty of Medicine, Tabriz University of Medical Sciences, Tabriz, Iran

Hadi Valizadeh
Drug Applied Research Center and Faculty of Pharmacy, Tabriz University of Medical Sciences, Tabriz, Iran

Ramin Mohammadzadeh
Drug Applied Research Center and Faculty of Pharmacy, Tabriz University of Medical Sciences, Tabriz, Iran
Students Research Committee, Tabriz University of Medical Sciences, Tabriz, Iran

Behzad Baradaran and Bahman Yousefi
Immunology Research Center and School of Medicine, Tabriz University of Medical Sciences, Tabriz, Iran

Parvin Zakeri-Milani
Liver and Gastrointestinal Diseases Research Center and Faculty of Pharmacy, Tabriz University of Medical Sciences, Tabriz, Iran

Nasser Ahmadiasl
Drug Applied Research Center, Tabriz University of Medical Sciences, Tabriz, Iran

Shokofeh Banaei
Department of Physiology, Tabriz University of Medical Sciences, Tabriz, Iran

Alireza Alihemmati
Department of Histology & Embryology, Tabriz University of Medical Sciences, Tabriz, Iran

Behzad Baradaran
Immunology Research Center, Tabriz University of Medical Sciences, Tabriz, Iran

Ehsan Azimian
Department of Linguistics and Foreign Languages, Payame Noor University, Tehran, Iran

Narges Abdoli
Biotechnology Research Center, Tabriz University of Medical Sciences, Tabriz, Iran
Drug Applied Research Center, Tabriz University of Medical Sciences, Tabriz, Iran
Pharmacology and Toxicology Department, School of pharmacy, Tabriz University of Medical Sciences, Tabriz, Iran
Students' Research Committee, Tabriz University of Medical Sciences, Tabriz, Iran

Yadollah Azarmi and Mohammad Ali Eghbal
Drug Applied Research Center, Tabriz University of Medical Sciences, Tabriz, Iran
Pharmacology and Toxicology Department, School of pharmacy, Tabriz University of Medical Sciences, Tabriz, Iran

Venu Gopal Jonnalagadda
Shree Dhootapapeshwar Ayurvedic Research Foundation (SDARF), Panvel, Navi Mumbai-410206, Maharastra, India

Allam Venkata Sita Ram Raju
National Institute of Pharmaceutical Education and Research, Bala Nagar, Hyderabad, Andhra Pradhesh-500037, India

Srinivas Pittala
CSIR-Institute of Genomics and Integrative Biology, Near Jubilee Hall, Mall Road, Delhi-110 007, India

Afsar shaik
Gokula Krishna college of Pharmacy, Sullurpet - 524121, Nellore dist, A.P, India

Nilakash Annaji Selkar
National Institute for Research in Reproductive Health, Parel, Mumbai-400012, Maharastra, India

Abbas Delazar
Drug Applied Research Center, Tabriz University of Medical Sciences, Tabriz, Iran

Amirala Aghbali
Drug Applied Research Center, Tabriz University of Medical Sciences, Tabriz, Iran
Department of Oral and Maxillofacial Pathology, Faculty of Dentistry, Tabriz University of Medical Sciences, Tabriz, Iran

Behzad Baradaran
Drug Applied Research Center, Tabriz University of Medical Sciences, Tabriz, Iran
Immunology Research Center, Tabriz University of Medical Sciences, Tabriz, Iran

Faranak Moradi Abbasabadi
Department of Oral and Maxillofacial Pathology, Faculty of Dentistry, Qom University of Medical Sciences, Qom, Iran

Tahereh Mashhoody and Karim Rastegar
Physiology Department, School of Medicine, Shiraz University of Medical Sciences, Shiraz, Iran

Fatemeh Zal
Reproductive Biology Department, School of Advanced Medical Sciences and Technologies, Shiraz University of Medical Sciences, Shiraz, Iran
Infertility Research Center, Shiraz University of Medical Sciences, Shiraz, Iran

Ramlah Mohamad Ibrahim and Nurul Syima Hamdan
Department of Nutrition and Dietetics, Faculty of Medicine and Health Sciences, Universiti Putra Malaysia, 43400 Serdang, Selangor Darul Ehsan, Malaysia

Maznah Ismail
Department of Nutrition and Dietetics, Faculty of Medicine and Health Sciences, Universiti Putra Malaysia, 43400 Serdang, Selangor Darul Ehsan, Malaysia

Suraini Mohd Saini, Saiful Nizam Abd Rashid and Rozi Mahmud
Department of Imaging, Faculty of Medicine and Health Sciences, Universiti Putra Malaysia, 43400 Serdang, Selangor Darul Ehsan, Malaysia

Latiffah Abd Latiff
Department of Community Health, Faculty of Medicine and Health Sciences, Universiti Putra Malaysia, 43400 Serdang, Selangor Darul Ehsan, Malaysia

Naime Majidi Zolbanin and Parina Asgharian
Student Research Committee, Faculty of Pharmacy, Tabriz University of Medical Sciences, Tabriz, Iran

Elmira Zolali
Student Research Committee, Faculty of Pharmacy, Tabriz University of Medical Sciences, Tabriz, Iran
Biotechnology Research Center, Tabriz University of Medical Sciences, Tabriz, Iran

Hamed Ghavimi
Drug Applied Research Center, Tabriz University of Medical Sciences, Tabriz, Iran

Hadi Hamishehkar
Drug Applied Research Center, Tabriz University of Medical Sciences, Tabriz, Iran
Clinical Pharmacy (Pharmacotherapy) Department, Faculty of Pharmacy, Tabriz University of Medical Sciences, Tabriz, Iran

Nasrin Maleki-Dizaji
Department of Pharmacology and Toxicology, Tabriz University of Medical Sciences, Tabriz, Iran

Maryam Kouhsoltani
Department of Oral and Maxillofacial Pathology, Faculty of Dentistry, Tabriz University of Medical Sciences, Tabriz, Iran

Ali Poornajjari
Department of Medicinal Chemistry, School of Pharmacy, Ahvaz Jundishapur University of Medical Sciences, Ahvaz, Iran

Neda Adibpour
Department of Medicinal Chemistry, School of Pharmacy, Ahvaz Jundishapur University of Medical Sciences, Ahvaz, Iran
Department of Medicinal Chemistry, School of Pharmacy, Zanjan University of Medical Sciences, Zanjan, Iran

Mohammad Javad Khodayar
Department of Pharmacology and Toxicology, School of Pharmacy, Ahvaz Jundishapur University of Medical Sciences, Ahvaz, Iran
Toxicology Research Center, Ahvaz Jundishapur University of Medical Sciences, Ahvaz, Iran

Saeed Rezaee
Department of Pharmaceutics, School of Pharmacy, Ahvaz Jundishapur University of Medical Sciences, Ahvaz, Iran
Department of Pharmaceutics, School of Pharmacy, Zanjan University of Medical Sciences, Zanjan, Iran

Negin Seyed-Gogani and Mohammad Ali Hoseinpour-Feyzi
Department of Zoology, Faculty of Natural Science, University of Tabriz, Tabriz, Iran

Mohammad Amin Moosavi
Department of Zoology, Faculty of Natural Science, University of Tabriz, Tabriz, Iran
Hematology and Oncology Research Center, Tabriz University of Medical Science, Tabriz, Iran
National Institute of Genetic Engineering and Biotechnology, Tehran, Iran

Marveh Rahmati
Department of Biochemistry, Faculty of Medicine, Tabriz University of Medical Science, Tabriz, Iran

Nosratollah Zarghami
Department of Biochemistry, Faculty of Medicine, Tabriz University of Medical Science, Tabriz, Iran

Hematology and Oncology Research Center, Tabriz University of Medical Science, Tabriz, Iran

Iraj Asvadi-Kermani
Hematology and Oncology Research Center, Tabriz University of Medical Science, Tabriz, Iran

Elnaz Mehdizadeh Aghdam
Drug Applied Research Center and Department of Pharmaceutical Biotechnology, Faculty of Pharmacy, Tabriz University of Medical Sciences, Tabriz, Iran

Mohammad Saeid Hejazi
Drug Applied Research Center and Department of Pharmaceutical Biotechnology, Faculty of Pharmacy, Tabriz University of Medical Sciences, Tabriz, Iran
The School of Advanced Biomedical Sciences (SABS), Tabriz University of Medical Sciences, Tabriz, Iran

Abolfazl Barzegar
Research Institute for Fundamental Sciences (RIFS), University of Tabriz, Tabriz, Iran
The School of Advanced Biomedical Sciences (SABS), Tabriz University of Medical Sciences, Tabriz, Iran

Emmanuel Ike Ugwuja
Department of Chemical Pathology, Faculty of Clinical Medicine, Ebonyi State University, P.M.B. 053 Abakaliki, Nigeria

Behrooz Farhadi, Mahmoud Shekari khaniani and Sima Mansoori Derakhshan
Department of Biochemistry, Faculty of Medicine, Tabriz University of Medical Sciences Tabriz, Iran
Department of Medical Genetics, Faculty of Medicine, Tabriz University of Medical Sciences Tabriz, Iran

Index

www.ingramcontent.com/pod-product-compliance
Lightning Source LLC
Chambersburg PA
CBHW050446200326
41458CB00014B/5085